THE WORLD OF
THE AUTISTIC CHILD

THE WORLD OF THE AUTISTIC CHILD

◆ ◆ ◆

Understanding and Treating Autistic Spectrum Disorders

BRYNA SIEGEL, PH.D.

Langley Porter Psychiatric Institute
Department of Psychiatry
University of California, San Francisco
San Francisco, California

New York   Oxford
OXFORD UNIVERSITY PRESS
1996

Oxford University Press

Oxford   New York
Athens   Auckland   Bangkok   Bombay
Calcutta   Cape Town   Dar es Salaam   Delhi
Florence   Hong Kong   Istanbul   Karachi
Kuala Lumpur   Madras   Madrid   Melbourne
Mexico City   Nairobi   Paris   Singapore
Taipei   Tokyo   Toronto

and associated companies in
Berlin   Ibadan

Copyright © 1996 by Oxford University Press, Inc.

Published by Oxford University Press, Inc.,
198 Madison Avenue, New York, New York 10016

Oxford is a registered trademark of Oxford University Press

Library of Congress Cataloging-in-Publication Data
Siegel, Bryna.
The world of the autistic child : understanding and treating
autistic spectrum disorders / Bryna Siegel.
p.   cm.   Includes index.
ISBN 0-19-507667-2
1. Autism in children—Popular works.   2. Child
development deviations—Popular works.   3. Autistic
children—Education.   I. Title.
RJ506.A9S53   1995   618.92'8982—dc20   95-6888

2 4 6 8 9 7 5 3 1

Printed in the United States of America
on acid-free paper

To David

Foreword

Parents of children with autistic spectrum disorders [autism and pervasive developmental disorders] do not, in general, have a high opinion of professionals. Parents rapidly recognise whether a professional worker really knows anything about autism—and they tend to find that most do not.

There are only two ways of acquiring a depth of knowledge on the subject that earns the parents' respect. One is to be a parent oneself. The other is to work closely with the children over many years, observing and interacting with them and listening with great attention to the parents' descriptions of their children's development from infancy. This cannot be done sitting comfortably on the other side of a desk in a consulting room. You have to be part of the action to see it for yourself.

From reading this book, it is clear that Bryna Siegel is a professional who has learnt the hard way. She comprehends the emotions of the parents and the long painful process of coming to terms with their child's disabilities. She has empathy for the stress this causes the families. She has a wealth of practical advice on autistic behaviour and ways of encouraging the development of communication and other skills. The sections on evaluating educational programmes and how parents can relate to and work with teachers and other professionals are particularly helpful.

Bryna Siegel tackles incisively the subject of the unorthodox, untested "treatments," new varieties of which are currently appearing at an alarming rate. She is critical but fair in her judgements and gives parents guidelines to use when deciding whether to try one of these methods.

The book is full of sound common sense. I was therefore surprised to learn from one or two comments in the text that the author had worked with Bruno Bettleheim, the *Bête noir* of parents. It is a tribute to Bryna Siegel's ability to observe with clarity and to weigh up evidence that she has rejected Bettleheim's view of parental responsibility for autism and has no doubts about its origin in physical brain dysfunction.

The book is written for parents but should also be required reading for professional workers who see autistic children or adults, especially for its insights into parents' experiences of this strange, frustrating but fascinating condition.

Lorna Wing, M.D.
Centre for Social and Communication Disorders
British National Autistic Society

Acknowledgments

This book is actually a joint effort. It reflects what I have learned—and what I've been taught—by the autistic children and their families with whom I have interacted over the past twelve years. Without them, I would not have known what to write. What is written here is a reflection of all the impressions that have been made upon me by many, many children with autism and PDD, their caring and loving parents, wonderfully creative special education teachers, amazingly dedicated caseworkers, and other supportive therapists out to do their best, usually with limited resources.

I gratefully acknowledge the enthusiasm, commitment, and skill of the various colleagues, staff, and trainees (past and present) of the PDD Clinic here at the University of California, San Francisco, Langley Porter Psychiatric Institute, as well as those who worked with me at our first PDD Clinic at Stanford University's Division of Child Psychiatry and Child Development. I would particularly like to thank Dr. Sharadha Raghavan and Dr. Jelena Vukicevic for their dedication during our time together. Most central has been my collegiality with Dr. Glen Elliott, my close collaborator and friend for the past twelve years. At the time of this writing, our clinic has just completed assessing (and hopefully helping) just over 1,400 children with autism, PDD, and related problems. The efforts of all those involved in the PDD Clinic have been monumental. Of those who have been part of our clinic and research lab at Langley Porter, I would particularly like to thank Stephen Sheinkopf, Dr. Runa Lindblom, Dr. Anna-Marie Van Elberg, Karen Rabin, Leta Huang, Dr. Karen Biskup-Meyer, Dr. Eun Hee Park, Suzanne Pemberton, and Wendy Shapera. I have learned a great deal through collaborations and discussions with colleagues at other universities, beginning with the late Dr. Roland Ciaranello, Dr. Adrianna Schuler, Dr. Ivar Lovaas, Dr. Ed Ritvo, Dr. B. J. Freeman, Dr. Robert Spitzer, Dr. Fred Volkmar, Dr. Catherine Lord, Dr. Peter Szatmari, Dr. Sue Smalley, and Hillary Stubblefield.

Many thanks go to the families who have brought their children to our clinic. Some of you will see yourselves and your children in the vignettes in this book. I hope I've done justice to the stories you've shared with me, and that each of you feels that your confidentiality has not been compromised, but that there has been an opportunity created for other families who can learn from what you've experienced.

The opportunity to write this book has been an important watershed in my professional development. I'd like to thank my editor at Oxford University Press, Joan Bossert, for being the unseen reader in my head during 20 months of writing. I have greatly appreciated her supportive attitude throughout the development of this project. The book has been improved by the thoughtful comments of its OUP outside reviewers, Dr. Fred Volkmar at Yale University and Dr. Francesca Happe at University College, London.

I absolutely want to thank my family, especially since they put up with most of the writing for this project being done at home. My husband David Bradlow gave me the opportunity to discuss aloud much of what eventually got written down. It has been essential for me to have had David as a resource for working through the pain and grief I absorb from families of autistic children each clinic day at work. My daughter Alyssa put up with many hours where I'm sure she wished I'd been more accessible; and so do I. My stepson, Dan, contributed to this process by *trying* to make after-school snacks quietly so I could continue writing undisturbed. Catini faithfully stayed by my side throughout the writing process, although she largely slept through the whole thing. Last, I want to thank the Ghirardelli Chocolate Company for making semi-sweet morsels; even psychologists need positive reinforcers!

Contents

Introduction, 3

PART I. WHAT IT MEANS TO HAVE AUTISM

1. Defining Autism, PDD, and Other Autistic Spectrum Disorders, 9
   Diagnostic Signs of Autism, 9
   What Autism Is and Is Not, 13
   Autism versus Pervasive Developmental Disorder, 15
   Non-Autistic Pervasive Developmental Disorders, 20
   Chapter Summary, 24

2. Social Development in Autism and PDD, 25
   Early Signs of Social Isolation, 26
   Instrumental versus Expressive Relating, 27
   Disabilities of Social Understanding in Adults, 29
   Awareness of the Emotions and Feelings of Others, 30
   Seeking Physical Affection, 31
   Patterns of Comfort-Seeking, 32
   Difficulties in Developing Imitation, 37
   Lack of Social Play, 39
   Lack of Peer Friendships, 41
   Chapter Summary, 42

3. Communication Skills in Autism and PDD, 43
   Nonverbal Communication, 43
   Range of Emotional Expression, 48
   Atypical Features of Language Content and Use, 50
   Conversational Skill, 58
   Chapter Summary, 59

4. Autism, PDD, and the Child's Activities and Interests, 60
   Play and Imagination, 60
   Concrete and Functional Play, 64
   Intense Interest in Unusual Activities of Objects, 67
   Unusual Motor Movements and "Self-Stimulatory" Behaviors, 70
   Chapter Summary, 81

5. Getting a Diagnosis, 82
   "Labeling," 82
   Where Do You Get Autism or PDD Diagnosed? 84
   Components of a Developmental Evaluation, 85
   Assessment Methods in Developmental Evaluation of Autism and PDD, 91
   Early Diagnosis, 105
   Differential Diagnosis, 110
   Chapter Summary, 120

6. After the Diagnosis: Coping with a Sense of Loss, 121
   Natural Defenses and Grief, 121
   Initial Reactions to the Diagnosis of Autism, 123
   Concerns about Prognosis, 133
   Chapter Summary, 135

7. Family Issues, 136
   The Impact of Autism on Parents, 136
   The Impact of Autism on Brothers and Sisters, 148
   Acceptance of the Autistic Child Outside the Home, 154
   The Psychology of Choosing Residential Treatment, 159
   Chapter Summary, 162

PART II. TREATMENT RESOURCES

8. Finding Resources, 167
   Eligibility for Developmental Disabilities Services, 169
   Eligibility for Special Education Services, 176
   Legal Advocacy, 183
   Eligibility for Services through Medical Insurance, 186
   Books about Autism, 187
   The Autism Society of America and Other Parent Support Groups, 191
   Chapter Summary, 195

9. The Importance of Very Early Intervention, 196
   "The Sooner the Better" Philosophy, 196
   Support for Early Intervention from Theories of Neuropsychology, 197
   How Much Early Intervention Is Appropriate? 201
   Determining Frequency and Intensity of an Early Intervention Program, 204
   Chapter Summary, 208

10. Selecting a Classroom: Assessing Teachers, Aides,
    and Student Composition, 209
    Selecting a Classroom, 209
    Teachers and Teacher Training, 213

Making Classroom Observations, 215
Classroom Structure, 219
Mainstreaming and Full Inclusion, 225
Chapter Summary, 230

11. Behavior Management and Teaching Methods for
    Children with Autism and PDD, 231
    Primary and Social Rewards in the Classroom, 232
    Methods of Instruction, 242
    Chapter Summary, 252

12. Teaching Communication Skills to Children with Autism and PDD, 253
    Autistic versus Typical Language Development, 253
    Methods for Teaching Language to Nonverbal Children, 255
    Going with an "Oral Only" Language Approach, 262
    Early Oral Language in Children with Autism and PDD, 264
    Language Pragmatics Interventions, 267
    Multiword Language Development and Reading Skills, 272
    Chapter Summary, 273

13. Forks in the Road: The Elementary School Years and Beyond, 274
    Mental Retardation and Prognosis, 274
    Academic Skills for Higher Functioning Autistic and PDD Children, 277
    Vocational Choices for Higher Functioning Young People with
        Autism and PDD, 283
    Skills Training for More Cognitively Disabled Autistic Persons, 285
    Exemplary Adult Programs, 294
    School and Post-School Vocational Skills Training, 298
    Chapter Summary, 300

14. Psychoactive Medications, 301
    When Are Drugs Used to Treat Autism and PDD? 301
    Medications Most Often Used for Children with Autism or PDD, 308
    Monitoring a Child's Benefits from Medication, 317
    Chapter Summary, 320

15. Non-Mainstream Treatments for Autism, 321
    Evaluating Non-Mainstream Treatments, 321
    If It Sounds Too Good To Be True, It Probably Is, 322
    "Think Twice" Treatments, 324
    Chapter Summary, 332

Afterword, 333

Index, 335

THE WORLD OF
THE AUTISTIC CHILD

Introduction

This book is the result of twelve years of sitting with parents and explaining to them what it means for their child to be autistic. As many times as I have met and talked with parents confronting the diagnosis of autism for the first time, I know I cannot have the same feelings about the diagnosis of autism that parents do. I *do* know that many emotions present themselves. Both parental emotions and the child's treatment are very important issues that need to be thoroughly addressed. Over the years, I have become convinced that the parents' best defense against the potential emotional devastation of the diagnosis is to gain competence rapidly to get help for their child. I see treatment planning and implementation of treatment as positive coping that helps both child and parent function as well as possible.

This book, therefore, is about understanding the diagnosis of autism, the available treatments, and how—as a parent, teacher, or other child specialist—you can decide what is best for a particular child with autism or pervasive developmental disorder, depending on which areas of development are presenting the greatest challenges. This book is intended to be especially helpful to parents of younger autistic children who are trying to comprehend what autism is and what to do about it. Parents of older children, who already understand what autism is, may want to focus on the second part of this book, since it addresses educational treatment, medications, and longer term planning.

Autism and Pervasive Developmental Disorder (PDD)

One of the most difficult things in writing any book about children is that all children are different. With or without a developmental disability present, there are vast individual differences among children's personalities, temperaments, and abilities to learn. Books that tell the story of one particular autistic child can be especially misleading at first, because some of the things described may result from a particular form of autism, and other things may result from the individual's personality.

Various labels exist for a child with many or few symptoms of autism, or with severe or mild forms of autism. Sometimes phrases such as "autistic-like" or "autistic tendencies" or "pervasive developmental disability" (PDD) or "Asperger's syndrome" are used. In this book, I try to sort out what gets called "autism," what gets called "PDD," and so on, to help the reader who has heard one label or another applied to a particular child gain some idea of what material in this book pertains to that particular child.

How to Read This Book

Parents often tell me that the greatest difficulty with books they read on autism and PDD is that they feel jerked back and forth between realistic descriptions that they identify as being like their own child, and more frightening descriptions that are nothing like what their child does (and hopefully will never do). To avoid this difficulty, I have tried to be as clear as possible about how frequent different symptoms of autism are, which are more frequent in children with PDD, which correlate most strongly with mental retardation, and which symptoms are most often shared by children with severe language disorders, who may at times be mistaken for children with autism or PDD.

There are many section and subsection headings throughout the book. The reason for this is to guide the reader to the information that is relevant to the child he or she is concerned with. I encourage the reader to skip sections that refer to problems or behaviors that don't pertain to the child or children you have in mind.

The book is divided into two main parts: the first chapters explain what it means to have autism; in the second part, chapters concentrate on treatment resources and what to do to help. The first chapter is an introduction to the labyrinth of occasionally changing diagnostic terms used to characterize children with many or few symptoms of autism. The next set of chapters describe all the associated signs of autism in detail and try to give a sense of what it is like for a child who experiences a particular symptom. The final set of chapters in the first part of the book deals with steps to take in getting a diagnostic evaluation, the effects of the diagnosis on the child's family. The first chapter in the second part deals with a second labyrinth—the various services for children with autism and PDD, and how you can become your child's advocate to ensure that you get what you need. The next five chapters in the second part of the book deal with intervention through special education—beginning with a description of early intervention programs, how to select educational programs, and then moving on to how to implement behavioral training, as well as methods for teaching communication skills, academic skills, and everyday living skills. The next to last chapter deals with medical treatments for autism, and the final chapter deals with the constantly changing roster of new treatments that still have no proven track record but may present attractive alternatives to conventional therapies.

The mix of information on different topics in this book is based approximately on the balance of time I usually spend discussing each of these areas with parents of newly diagnosed autistic and PDD children. That is why this book will probably be of greatest interest to those gathering initial information about autism and PDD. Much of what is said focuses on young children. There *are* sections on adolescents and young adults, too. These sections are for the caregivers of such individuals, but also for parents of younger children to give them a sense of what life may be like down the road. The contents is a synthesis of clinical experience and years of following a wide array of literature on autism, PDD, and developmental disabilities. Whenever possible, I try to distinguish research-derived information from clinical experience, without going into the specifics of research studies. The information is presented in as nontechnical a format as possible so that training in developmental disabilities or special education is not needed to understand what is said.

There are many clinical examples in this book based on real cases of autism. In fact, there are *no* made-up hypothetical examples, as these could not possibly ring as true as the things that children have really done. The names of my patients are always changed, as well as details that would allow them to be identified by others. Some examples blend aspects of similar situations to illustrate a point succinctly, and to further protect the identity of the children and families I have had the privilege to learn from.

I hope my readers will find these contents useful. This book is an attempt to make the experiences of many families and the results of much research accessible to all who may benefit from it.

PART I

What It Means to
Have Autism

◆ ◆ ◆

Defining Autism, PDD, and other Autistic Spectrum Disorders

Diagnostic Signs of Autism

Autism is a developmental disorder that affects many aspects of how a child sees the world and learns from his or her experiences. Children with autism lack the usual desire for social contact. The attention and approval of others are not important to them in the usual way. Autism is not an absolute lack of desire for affiliation, but a relative one.

Terminology

Autism is the best recognized and most frequently occurring form of a group of disorders collectively known as the *pervasive developmental disorders* (PDD). This chapter will help develop a basic understanding of what makes up the diagnosis of autism and a closely related, but separately labeled diagnostic category called pervasive developmental disorder, not otherwise specified (PDD,NOS). Closely related diagnoses such as Asperger's syndrome, fragile X syndrome, Rett syndrome, and childhood disintegrative disorder will be described to show the ways each is similar to, but separate from, autism and PDD,NOS.

The use of slightly different ways of labeling autism and related conditions at different times in the past and in different countries can be confusing: The term pervasive developmental disorders (or PDDs) is most accurately used to describe autism (autistic disorder) plus an array of *non-autistic* PDDs (such as PDD,NOS, Asperger's syndrome, fragile X syndrome, Rett syndrome, and childhood disintegrative disorder). In this book, when we discuss autism and "PDD," I am really referring to "PDD,NOS," unless it is otherwise explicitly stated. This is because both parents and professionals tend to talk about children who have received a diagnosis of PDD,NOS as having "PDD." The full term PDD,NOS will be used only when PDD,NOS is being specifically compared with or contrasted to other non-autistic PDDs. The term PDD,NOS is an awful, awkward use of language that conveys virtually no specific information by the addition of the "NOS", but is meant to convey that the child is affected in the areas of both social and communication development in the manner of a child with a full syndrome of autism.

To further complicate the whole issue of terms used to refer to autism and related conditions is the fact that most people (outside of research articles) do not often use the term "autistic disorder," which is the technical term for autism in the official psychiatric diagnostic manual (called the *Diagnostic and Statistical Manual of Mental Disorders,* Fourth edition or DSM-IV for short). Just as most people refer to PDD,NOS simply as PDD, children with a diagnosis of "autistic disorder" are more simply referred to as autistic or as having autism.

It is most accurate to say that autistic disorder is a form of PDD, and that PDD,NOS is also a form of PDD. To make it a bit clearer, the term *autistic spectrum disorders* is used here to encompass autism plus the non-autistic PDDs and is meant to correspond exactly to what DSM-IV refers to collectively as PDD—that is, "pervasive developmental disorders."

Figures 1 and 2 illustrate where autism ("autistic disorder") stands among the various other PDD diagnoses, as well as its relationship to other developmental disorders with which it is sometimes confused. The diagrams cannot completely reflect the exact overlap, or the exact sizes of each of these diagnostic groups, but is instead intended to give a rough idea of how various diagnostic terms interrelate.

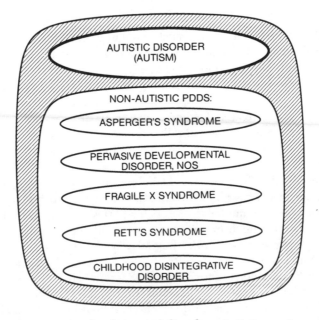

Figure 1   The pervasive developmental disorders: Autistic spectrum disorders.

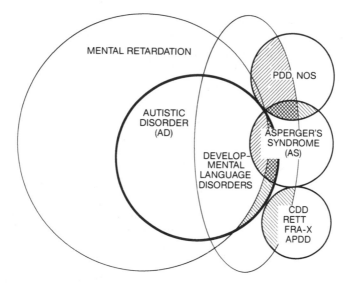

Figure 2 Autistic spectrum disorders and other developmental disorders. (PDD,NOS = pervasive developmental disorders, not otherwise specified; CDD = childhood disintegrative disorder; FRA-X = fragile X syndrome; APDD = atypical PDD)

The Concept of Developmental Disorders

The fact that autism and PDD,NOS are classified as developmental disorders means that they are conditions a child is believed to be born with, or born with a potential for developing. Autism is the result of an abnormality in the structure and function of the brain. Although technology still does not allow us to see much of how nerve cells grow or come together in the brain, or how information is passed from nerve to nerve, there is increasing evidence that the problems associated with autism and the other forms of PDD are the result of structural differences in the brain that arise during pregnancy—either due to something that injures the brain or due to a genetic factor that interferes with typical brain growth.

No series of studies to date have consistently found any specific structural brain difference or unique genetic abnormality that appears to be the physical cause of autism. About eighty percent of children with autism also have some degree of mental retardation. Most have mild to moderate mental retardation along with their autism, and a smaller percent have severe or profound mental retardation. Children who receive a diagnosis of PDD,NOS are less often mentally retarded than children who are diagnosed autistic; even so, close to half the PDD,NOS children have some degree of mental retardation, too. Of the twenty percent of children with autism who are not mentally retarded, about two-thirds have normal levels of nonverbal intelligence but do have more significant impairment in verbal intelligence (language). By the time they grow up, only about ten percent of children with autism have normal intellectual functioning in both verbal and nonverbal abilities. For many parents, the diagnosis of mental retardation along with the diagnosis of autism is a double whammy. In many cases, mental retardation can be detected at the same time that autism is diagnosed, and is important to take into account because it bears on the child's expected rate of learning, as we will discuss in Chapter 5.

Prevalence

Depending on the definition of autism that is used, slightly more or slightly fewer children will be considered autistic, or be considered to have another form of PDD. (In addition to the DSM-IV definition of autistic spectrum disorders used here, there is also a slightly different international set of diagnostic standards, as well as older sets of diagnostic standards like DSM-III-R and DSM-III.) In addition, the prevalence of non-autistic forms of PDD are less well studied than the prevalence of autism itself. Most experts generally agree, though, that if cases of both autism and non-autistic PDDs are considered together, and a fairly liberal definition of autism is applied, autistic spectrum disorders occur in approximately ten to fifteen out of every 10,000 children. Put another way, that's one out of 650 to 1,000 children. In a country the size of the United States, there are estimated to be about 450,000 children and adults with different forms of autistic spectrum disorders.

Usually, autism and PDD,NOS affect boys four to five times as often as they affect girls. Asperger's syndrome may affect boys as much as ten times more often than girls. In fragile X syndrome, some children are affected with autism or PDD,NOS as well as other behavioral difficulties not necessarily associated with the PDDs. Since fragile X is an X-linked genetic disorder (that is to say, a condition much more likely to affect boys most severely) fragile X and autistic spectrum disorders co-occur in boys much more often than girls. Clearly some families have an inherited form of autism, and in those families, girls seem more often affected (only about two autistic boys for each autistic girl instead of four or five). Children thought to have a genetic form of autism have either an autistic sibling or an autistic first cousin. It is not yet well understood how autism is inherited, and autistic children with more distant autistic relatives are now believed to have a genetic form of the disorder as well. The only time that symptoms of PDD occur more often in girls is when the girls are primarily affected by a disorder called Rett's syndrome. An autistic-like phase of development in early childhood (around ages two to five) characterizes many girls with Rett's syndrome; no boys are thought to be affected by Rett's syndrome.

Factors That Might Cause Autism

In addition to possible genetic causes of autism, cases of autism have been linked to a variety of risk factors associated with pregnancy and delivery. A "risk factor," however, is not the same things as a "cause," and it can be very difficult to say with confidence what "caused" any specific case of autism.

There are likely a combination of factors—genetic factors as well as factors related to the pregnancy and delivery that determine whether a specific child develops autism or another PDD. But it should be emphasized that "risks" associated with a pregnancy are not necessarily things that the expectant mother did wrong, but are often a variety of events over which she had no control. (This will be discussed in more detail in Chapter 5 in regard to the importance of giving a complete developmental history of a child at the time of diagnosis.) Relatively few cases of autism (perhaps three percent) are associated with another known genetic disorder like fragile X syndrome (which has already been mentioned), or tuberous sclerosis (a disorder involving the formation of abnormal brain and other tissue). In many cases, we do not yet know enough to say what may have caused the autism, except to guess that there might have been a spontaneous genetic mutation(s). There are many cases of autism or other forms of PDD where there is nothing that was apparently wrong in the mother's pregnancy or delivery, and where there are also no signs of a genetic cause—that is, no relatives with autism or another type of developmental disorder. Such cases are probably the ones due to currently unidentifiable genetic mutations, or to possible infections in the pregnancy that affected the fetus, but not the mother.

There is no evidence to support the idea that autism or any form of PDD is caused by the way a child is treated, although severely maltreated children and severely mentally retarded children sometimes do things that a casual observer might understandably confuse with autism. Years ago, some doctors suggested that autism might be caused by early rejection of the child by the parents, but such harmful theories have long since been definitively disproved.

Autism, or what was originally termed "early infantile autism," was first described by an American child psychiatrist, Leo Kanner. In 1943, he published a series of descriptions of eleven children who had a number of peculiar behaviors, but who all showed a marked lack of interest in the people around them. In the past fifty or so years, a great deal of scientific research and clinical study has resulted from Kanner's original observations. Kanner called the common thread he observed among these children "early infantile autism" because the disorder seemed to be present from the earliest part of infancy. In many ways, the autistic child's self-absorption and inability to take the perspective of others seemed similar socially to the limited way in which infants normally relate to the world during the early months of infancy when they are aware of nothing but their own satisfactions and dissatisfactions.

What Autism Is and Is Not

To determine whether a child is autistic or has another form of PDD, it is necessary to examine three things: First, one needs an understanding of what kinds of behaviors and behavior patterns are and are not part of the syndrome of autism. Second, one needs to understand the *function* as well as the *form* of the behavior—why the child does the things he does. Third, one needs to understand the formal diagnostic standards being used by the professional making the diagnosis. In this chapter, we'll explain the main diagnostic standards in use today, both in the United States and internationally, to diagnose autism and other forms of PDD and to distinguish it from other related disorders.

In Chapter 5, we'll discuss the distinctive features of other forms of non-autistic PDD such as Asperger's syndrome, which is believed to be genetically related to autism; the fragile X syndrome, a genetic disorder in which a number of affected children have some or all of the symptoms of autism or PDD,NOS; Rett's syndrome, a very rare, presumably genetic disorder affecting only girls, where many signs of autism are especially notable during early childhood; and childhood disintegrative disorder, an extremely rare form of later-occurring PDD. Much of what can be said about certain features of autism and PDD,NOS applies to other forms of non-autistic PDD. As various symptoms of autism and PDD,NOS are described, it will be noted when these are also symptoms of another non-autistic PDD such as fragile X syndrome or Rett's syndrome.

The Concept of a Syndrome

Autistic spectrum disorders constitute a syndrome—which means that affected individuals will not have *all* the associated signs and symptoms. Before their child is diagnosed with autism or PDD, parents often say that their child did not resemble the children they read about in books on autism. This is because no two autistic children are alike, any more than two normally developing children are alike. There may be certain striking similarities between two children in terms of very specific behaviors, but because they differ in other ways, it does not mean that both cannot be autistic. In a child with autism or PDD, a very careful evaluation needs to be undertaken in making the diagnosis in order to understand what behaviors are part of the child's autism or PDD, what may be a reflection of some degree of mental retardation, what is the child's personality, and what is a reflection of the way the child acts as a means of compensating for his or her disability. That is why it is important for a professional to consider *why* the child does what he does, and explain the meaning of unusual behaviors to parents in terms of what the child is trying to accomplish through his actions.

By the end of Chapter 4, you should have a fairly accurate picture of whether or not a particular child you have in mind has autism or PDD. However, making a diagnosis in a way that really helps sort out autism from mental retardation, and from personality and temperament, and from experience and learning is really a task for an autism specialist. This is because, as will be illustrated in later chapters, treatment planning is derived not just from a "label," but from a full understanding of how the particular signs of autism that are present in any one child fit together.

Autism versus Pervasive Developmental Disorder

For both parents and professionals who have had relatively little contact with autistic children, it can be difficult to distinguish autism from PDD,NOS. Many such people are of the opinion that it doesn't matter which way the child is "labeled." However, PDD,NOS implies the presence of fewer and, at times, less severe signs of autism. As such, children labeled PDD,NOS as a group tend to do better in a number of ways compared with autistic children as a group. Also, as a group, children receiving the PDD,NOS diagnosis tend to have less cognitive impairment than the group of children diagnosed autistic. There are, however, autistic children without mental retardation, and PDD children with severe mental retardation. The label of either autism or PDD is simply a shorthand for conveying information about likely developmental difficulties associated with autism, and their likely number and severity. Being labeled autistic rather than PDD doesn't fully convey how a particular child should be treated—that depends on which symptoms are present and how severely they are expressed.

From most of the research that has been conducted to date, the data support the idea that autism and PDD,NOS *are* variants of the same syndrome. A syndrome, however, is something that can have many different causes, but results in an overlapping set of symptoms. Depending on the cause of a particular case, there may be more or less overlap with other cases of autism where other causes were operative. As mentioned earlier, some cases of autism and of PDD are believed to be caused by multiple congenital or genetic factors, or combinations of the two. Even when the cause of autism or PDD is presumably the same in two children (such as with identical twins who both have autism), the symptoms of autism or PDD will be a little different in each child.

Generally, PDD,NOS can be thought of as essentially constituting a less severe, or less fully symptomatic form of autism. Research studies have shown that autism and PDD,NOS often have the same profile of symptoms but that the symptoms tend to be less numerous and less severe in the child diagnosed with PDD,NOS. Many people who conduct research on autism and treat autistic children have pointed out that the boundary between autism and PDD,NOS varies so much from doctor to doctor and clinic to clinic that the distinction is not reliable and is not worth spending too much time debating. Differences in treatment are based on the child's particular symptoms, and not on how he or she got that way or on which side of the autism/PDD,NOS "line" the child falls. What is important is recognition and analysis of specific symptoms and how they will be treated. By thinking of PDD,NOS as a generally less severe or less full-blown form of autism, one is accepting the idea that the symptoms of autism and PDD are on a continuum, even if the causes are not. The continuum of symptoms, however, is not just two-dimensional (that is, "more" or "less"), but multidimensional, since there are many different symptoms that each may be expressed "more" or "less."

In the material that follows, we'll distinguish between typical traits of children with autism and typical traits of children with PDD when possible, but the reader should bear in mind that everything said about autism can sometimes be true about PDD—but the degree of severity, or overall number of symptoms experienced, varies.

The DSM-IV Criteria for Autistic Disorder and PDD,NOS

At present, when autism is diagnosed in the United States, the clinician is probably using a diagnostic standard called the DSM-IV, which is an acronym for the *Diagnostic and Statistical Manual of Mental Disorders of the American Psychiatric Association, Fourth Edition*, which was published in 1994. Use of a standard diagnostic definition is designed to ensure that there will be agreement among doctors in different places as to what is being called autism, and where the line is supposed to be drawn between autism and PDD. But there are differences in how the DSM-IV criteria for autism are actually used. For example, doctors with different degrees of specialization in autism tend to use the label differently. This is because many adjectives used to describe symptoms of autism like "diminished" or "abnormal" or "impaired" or "atypical" may be interpreted to indicate different thresholds of severity by different professionals. It would be ideal if doctors had some sort of videotaped glossary of each symptom of autism that showed several examples of children doing things that were intended to be interpreted as meeting the criteria for various symptoms of autism, so that everyone could use the same yardstick to measure when "lack of awareness of others" really was "marked," or "ability to make peer friendships" was really "impaired." That isn't the case. It's one reason why the same symptoms can be differently interpreted at different diagnostic centers.

The twelve diagnostic criteria for DSM-IV Autistic Disorder are grouped into three areas—social development, communication, and activities and interests. Within each area are four specific criteria, each representing a different area of symptoms. Generally, the first criterion in each of the three areas is the one that can be detected at the earliest age, and the latter ones in each area are the ones that become apparent later on in development. In addition, each of the criteria should be evaluated according to the child's level of mental development so that developmental delay is not confused with autistic symptoms. The need to evaluate possible signs of autism according to the child's level of mental development is one reason why it is important to have IQ (intelligence) or adaptive behavior testing done as part of a diagnostic assessment. A child's developmental level can be estimated by an IQ test or a test of adaptive behavior, which is a way of measuring how/if the child uses his intelligence to adapt to the challenges of everyday life.

The Concept of Nonverbal Intelligence. Some of the most clinically useful research on diagnosing autism suggests that each diagnostic criterion be rated according to the child's *nonverbal* level of mental development. This is a very helpful way to think about the symptoms of autism because impaired *verbal* ability is, itself, a part of many signs of autism. By judging signs of autism in accordance with a child's nonverbal ability, there is a further check that other types of language delay are not confused with autistic symptoms. Nonverbal intellectual functioning includes nonlanguage abilities, which for young children can be assessed by how well they can put together puzzles, sort things, and copy actions they've seen. This can be contrasted with verbal intelligence that involves language use and understanding—which is always affected in certain ways in autistic children. Therefore, a measure of mental development for the purposes of assessing autistic symptoms is estimated through the child's functioning in areas not as directly affected by the presence of the symptoms of autism.

Using nonverbal intelligence as a way of estimating an autistic child's general level of mental development is not a perfect indicator, but it does provide a basis for separating many of the effects of mental retardation from the autism itself. Nevertheless, the majority of autistic children have some degree of mental retardation along with their autism, so it is important to find a way to measure it separately from the symptoms of autism. This is because delays in development due to autism or PDD and delays in development due to mental retardation are not always treated in the same way. By using the child's level of nonverbal IQ (nonverbal mental age) as a baseline, we are essentially asking "How does this child's behavior in each autistic symptom area compare to what a child should typically be able to do at this mental age?" Once there is a general fix on the child's nonverbal mental age (which a professional obtains through a combination of intelligence testing, observations of the child, and parent interviewing), it is possible to assess the child for the presence of autistic symptoms. (In Chapter 5 we will look at diagnostic procedures in more detail.)

Autistic Disorder. To be diagnosed as having autistic disorder, using the DSM-IV criteria, a person must have positive signs on six out of the twelve criteria. At least two of the criteria met must reflect difficulties in social development; two criteria must be met in the area of communication; and at least two criteria in the area of atypical activities and interests must also be met.

Pervasive Developmental Disorder, Not Otherwise Specified (NOS). If the child has a less severe form of the behavior described in a criterion, that may contribute to a diagnosis of PDD,NOS. If no criteria is met in the category of atypical activities and interest (part C in Table 1), but the child does show a variety of signs in the categories of social and communicative development, the diagnosis of PDD,NOS is also used. Sometimes, some doctors will use PDD,NOS provisionally when the child is so young that many of the criteria are felt to be too difficult to see. This is problematic, because other clinicians

Table 1 DSM-IV Criteria for Autistic Disorder and Pervasive Developmental
Disorder, Not Otherwise Specified (PDD,NOS)

To be diagnosed with autistic disorder at least one sign (each) from parts A, B, and C must be
present, plus at least six overall. Those meeting fewer criteria are diagnosable as PDD,NOS.

A. Qualitative impairments in reciprocal social interaction:
    1. Marked impairment in the use of multiple nonverbal behaviors such as eye-to-eye gaze,
       facial expression, body posture, and gestures to regulate social interaction.
    2. Failure to develop peer relationships appropriate to developmental level.
    3. Lack of spontaneous seeking to share enjoyment, interests, or achievements with others.
    4. Lack of socioemotional reciprocity.

B. Qualitative impairments in communication:
    1. A delay in, or total lack of, the development of spoken language (not accompanied by an
       attempt to compensate through alternative modes of communication such as gesture or
       mime).
    2. Marked impairment in the ability to initiate or sustain a conversation with others despite
       adequate speech.
    3. Stereotyped and repetitive use of language or idiosyncratic language.
    4. Lack of varied spontaneous make-believe play or social imitative play appropriate to devel-
       opmental level.

C. Restricted, repetitive, and sterotyped patterns of behavior, interests, or activity:
    1. Encompassing preoccupation with one or more stereotyped and restricted patterns of
       interest, abnormal either in intensity or focus.
    2. An apparently compulsive adherence to specific nonfunctional routines or rituals.
    3. Stereotyped and repetitive motor mannerisms (e.g., hand or finger flapping, or twisting, or
       complex whole body movements).
    4. Persistent preoccupation with parts of objects.

Abnormal or impaired development prior to age three manifested by delays or abnormal functioning in at least one of the following areas: (1) social interaction, (2) language as used in social
communication, or (3) symbolic or imaginative play.

Source: The Diagnostic and Statistical Manual, 4th Edition, American Psychiatric Association, 1994.

who are very experienced with young autistic children *can* tell fairly accurately
from the early profile of symptoms that *are* met whether the child has autism
or PDD,NOS. This is because they understand what the earliest forms of
autistic symptoms are. Using such early developmental guidelines, a clinician
who is experienced with young autistic children can often tell if a child is
autistic by a child's second birthday and sometimes sooner. As we'll discuss
later, it's important to get a diagnosis as early as possible. As specific symptoms
are discussed, we'll cover what the earliest forms look like.

One of the problems in using the diagnosis of PDD,NOS is that the lower
limit is not clearly specified. It is clear that to receive a diagnosis of PDD,NOS
a child should have difficulties in some of the areas listed in the social (part A)
and the communicative (part B) categories (see Table 1). However, some
clinicians might give a diagnosis of PDD,NOS to a child who meets as few as
two criteria for PDD,NOS (that is, one from part A and one from part B).
Although this is not strictly incorrect, clinically it matters a great deal *which*
criteria the child meets, as some of the problems that PDD children have are

also common in children with related problems like developmental language disorders. That's one reason why a diagnosis of PDD,NOS needs to be made by someone experienced with PDD children rather than by a clinician who is more experienced with other childhood difficulties and is relying strongly on the DSM manual for guidance.

ICD-10 versus DSM-IV Pervasive Developmental Disorders

While the American Psychiatric Association maintains its own standards, the rest of the world maintains theirs. ICD-10, *International Classification of Disease, Tenth Edition* is another diagnostic manual of medical terms. Its development and ongoing revision process is sponsored by the World Health Organization, which is based in Geneva, Switzerland. In 1994, ICD-10 became the newest international standard, and with it, new criteria for diagnosing autism appeared. There are close parallels between DSM-IV and ICD-10 criteria for autism, and a large international study of almost 1,000 children was carried out to ensure that the two sets of diagnostic criteria would essentially identify the same individuals. Therefore, it is fairly unusual to find a child who is diagnosed autistic by DSM-IV criteria and not by ICD-10 criteria, and vice versa. When a diagnosis of autism or PDD is made, the doctor making the diagnosis can tell you which standard is being used (See Table 2).

Table 2 ICD-10 Criteria for Autistic Disorder

A. Presence of abnormal or impaired development in at least one of the following areas from before the age of three years (usually there is no prior period of unequivocally normal development, but when present, the period of normality does not extend beyond three years):

1. Receptive or expressive language as used in communication.
2. The development of selective social attachments and/or of reciprocal interaction.
3. Functional and/or symbolic play.

B. Qualitative impairments in reciprocal social interaction:

1. Failure adequately to use eye-to-eye gaze, facial expression, body posture and gesture to regulate social interaction.
2. Failure to develop (in a manner appropriate to mental age and despite ample opportunity) peer relationships that involve mutual sharing of interests, activities, and emotions.
3. Rarely seeking or using other people for comfort and affection at times of stress or distress and/or offering comfort and affection to others when they are showing distress or unhappiness.
4. Lack of shared enjoyment in terms of vicarious pleasure in other people's happiness and/or a spontaneous seeking to share their own enjoyment through joint involvement with others.
5. A lack of social-emotional reciprocity as shown by an impaired or deviant response to other people's emotions; and/or lack of modulation of behavior according to social context, and/or a weak integration of social, emotional, and communicative behaviors.

C. Qualitative impairments in communication:

1. A delay in, or total lack of, spoken language that is not accompanied by an attempt to compensate through the use of gesture or mime as alternate modes of communication (often preceded by a lack of communicative babbling).

(Continued)

Table 2 ICD-10 Criteria for Autistic Disorder (*Continued*)

2. Relative failure to initiate or sustain conversational interchange (at whatever level of language skills are present) in which there is no reciprocal to and from responsiveness to the communications of the other person.
3. Stereotyped and repetitive use of language and/or idiosyncratic use of words or phrases.
4. Abnormalities in pitch, stress, rate, rhythm, and intonation of speech.
5. A lack of varied spontaneous make-believe play or (when young) in social imitative play.

D. Restricted, repetitive, and sterotyped patterns of behavior, interests, and activities:

1. An encompassing preoccupation with stereotyped and restricted patterns of interests.
2. Specific attachments to unusual objects.
3. Apparently compulsive adherence to specific, nonfunctional routines or rituals.
4. Stereotyped and repetitive motor mannerisms that involve either hand/finger flapping or twisting, or complex whole body movements.
5. Preoccupations with part-objects or nonfunctional elements of play material (such as their odor, the feel of their surface, or the noise/vibration they generate).
6. Distress over small, nonfunctional details of the environment.

E. The clinical picture is not attributable to other varieties of pervasive developmental disorder (Asperger's syndrome, Rett's syndrome, Childhood Disintegrative Disorder) nor to a specific developmental disorder of receptive language with specific socioemotional problems, reactive attachment disorder, mental retardation with some associated emotional/behavioral disorder, nor schizophrenia of unusually early onset.

Source: International Classification of Diseases, Tenth Edition, World Health Organization, 1994.

Non-Autistic Pervasive Developmental Disorders

So far, we have discussed how different diagnostic criteria are used for determining differences between what gets called autism and what gets called PDD,NOS. As has already been explained, PDD,NOS is one major form of non-autistic PDD. PDD,NOS can be understood as a milder form of autism in which only a few symptoms of the syndrome are present, though the causes of PDD,NOS and autism may be different. Since little is still understood about direct causes of autism or PDD,NOS in individual cases, different diagnoses within the spectrum of autistic disorders are based on whether distinct groups of individuals share a trait or group of traits not seen in other forms of PDD. That is how other terms for non-autistic PDDs like Asperger's syndrome, Rett's syndrome, and childhood disintegrative disorder have come into use. In addition, there are cases of PDD,NOS where the cause is known, such as in children who also have the genetic diagnosis of fragile X syndrome.

We now turn to the main features of the non-autistic PDDs. These non-autistic PDDs will be discussed in contrast to autism or PDD,NOS to illustrate—symptom by symptom—where the boundaries between these different groups fall. (In Chapter 5, those interested can find a more extensive description of Asperger's syndrome.) The best way to understand what needs to be done for a child with a non-autistic PDD is through an evaluation that looks, symptom by symptom, at the child to decide whether treatments used for a particular symptom of autism may also be appropriate for a particular PDD child—given his or her profile of symptoms.

Asperger's Syndrome

Asperger's syndrome (AS) was added as a new "official" diagnosis when DSM-IV and ICD-10 were published. In the past, children with AS were sometimes referred to as having schizoid personality, or schizotypal personality, and PDD,NOS. The possible causes, history, and changes in the use of "Asperger's syndrome" are described in Chapter 5. It is now recognized as distinct from autism. AS differs from autism in a number of key ways: First, children with AS may not be detected as early because they may have no delays in language, or only mild delays. In fact, it is usually not until parents notice that their child's use of language is unusual, or their child's play is also unusual, that concern sets in. Unlike autism, where the vast majority of children also experience some degree of mental retardation, children (and adults) with AS are rarely mentally retarded although many have low-average intelligence.

Children with AS are sometimes described as "active, but odd"—not avoiding others the way autistic children often do, but relating in a more narrow way, usually centering activity around their own needs and peculiar interests. In fact, having one or more areas of narrow, encompassing interest is highly characteristic of those with AS. (Again, this will be described in much more detail in Chapter 5.) Parents often ask whether AS is the same thing as "high-functioning autism." Research studies have addressed this question, and the answer is "no." One main difference is that children with AS tend to have fairly comparable verbal and nonverbal levels of intelligence, while higher functioning (that is, less cognitively impaired) autistic children tend to have nonverbal IQs that are markedly higher than their verbal IQs.

When younger, children with AS may stand out as socially "different" to adults (especially to nonparents), but adults usually can allow for these differences much the way they would when dealing with a younger or immature child's. Young children with AS usually don't give (nonparental) adults the impression that something is seriously "different," the way an autistic child does. On the other hand, the young child with AS typically has just as much difficulty really playing with others as autistic children do. This is because other young children, unlike adults, lack the skills to automatically adjust to the social "different-ness" of the child with AS. Sometimes a young child gets on relatively well with siblings who know and accept his quirks, but the child is rejected by peers—and quite often doesn't seem to care much that he is.

Rett's Syndrome

Rett's syndrome is believed to be genetic in origin because it affects only children of one sex—females—and is marked by a very characteristic hand-wringing movement that has to be frequent for the diagnosis to be made.

Rett's syndrome is an extremely rare disorder and may affect only one in 100,000 children. Girls with Rett's syndrome tend to begin life normally, and then lose acquired skills over time. Some develop a little language and then lose it. (Language loss, however, is very common in autism and PDD, so language loss alone in no way indicates the presence of Rett's syndrome.) The loss of abilities usually starts in the second year of life. Around that time, the hand-wringing movements begin to grow in prominence, often getting so severe that it is difficult for the child to feed herself or pick up objects without dropping them again, almost immediately. Careful observations of the hand-wringing movements show that there is actually one "master" hand that flails, and a "slave" hand that tries to catch it and hold it still. Nevertheless, girls with Rett's syndrome tend to persist in doing things with their dominant "master" hand, making most coordinated movements nearly impossible to complete. Eventually, most girls with Rett's syndrome lose the ability to walk and almost always develop severe to profound mental retardation. Between the second and fifth or sixth year of life, when Rett's syndrome is usually first diagnosed, the girl may also meet diagnostic criteria for autism or PDD because of a marked lack of social relatedness and the presence of other features of autism. Interestingly, however, the lack of social relatedness often fades after the preschool years, when the child becomes more social—which can be really gratifying for the child's caregivers. Rett's syndrome is included as a non-autistic PDD because its cause is not otherwise known, and because, for the period of time that the child with Rett's syndrome has autistic signs, she may benefit from teaching approaches used for autistic children (as we will discuss in Part II of this book).

Childhood Disintegrative Disorder

Childhood disintegrative disorder (CDD) is another fairly rare variant of PDD. Children with CDD have well-documented normal development early in life, but somewhere in the first five years they begin to "disintegrate" until their behavioral difficulties are basically the same as a child diagnosed with autism or PDD,NOS. The disintegration typically includes a loss of language, loss of a desire for significant amounts of social contact, and increasingly poor eye contact, and other forms of nonverbal communication such as pointing. Again, as is the case for Rett's syndrome, loss of language alone is usually not enough for a diagnosis of CDD. While about one-quarter to one-third of children with autism or PDD,NOS may lose an initial vocabulary of twenty or fewer words (or get stuck with a limited vocabulary for an extended period), children with CDD typically speak easily in phrases and often in sentences before they lose language.

The rationale for demarcating CDD as a separate diagnosis is that in the future it will allow us to study such children separately and determine whether they have a different cause for their autism or PDD compared with other children who have autistic spectrum disorders. So far, no clearly distinct differences in behavior have been attributed to children with CDD versus children with autism or PDD,NOS. Therefore, in terms of treatment, CDD is now treated in the same way that autism and other forms of PDD are treated.

Fragile X Syndrome

Fragile X syndrome is the most commonly inherited form of mental retardation. (Down syndrome, which is also a genetically caused form of mental retardation, is more common, but it is a one-time mutation rather than something passed from generation to generation.) Fragile X syndrome is identified by examining an individual's chromosomes (which are most often obtained from a blood sample), and looking at a particular location on the X chromosome to see if there appears to be a partial break or "fragile" site in the chain of materials that compose the chromosome. Males have one X chromosome and one Y chromosome, while females have two Xs. Males get their X from their mother and their Y from their father; females get an X from each parent, so if one X has a fragile site, the other X can substitute for it; this is why fewer females have problems associated with fragile X syndrome. Research indicates that as many as one-third of males with fragile X syndrome have signs of PDD, with a smaller proportion actually meeting the full criteria for autism. If the data are looked at the other way around, only a small percent (three to five percent) of autistic boys have fragile X syndrome. There is also a smaller number of females with a fragile X who have some form of PDD.

When Fragile X and autism occur together, the autism takes on a characteristic set of symptoms: Fragile X autistic children tend to have very poor eye contact; frequent stereotyped motor movements; very pressured, often high pitched, and rapid, burst-like speech; and significant amounts of echolalia (repetition of what is said by other people, as if by echo). (These symptoms and what they mean will be described in more detail in Chapters 2, 3, and 4, with further discussion of fragile X syndrome, symptom by symptom.) More children with fragile X syndrome have PDD,NOS than autism, and many of those with PDD,NOS and fragile X syndrome can be described as having an odd manner of relating to people, but are somewhat friendly and sociable in their own way. Fragile X children also have characteristic physical features like large, cupped low-set ears, longish faces, prominent chins, and very flexible joints (double-jointedness); the boys have large testicles. Sometimes the physical features are not that apparent until the child is older, or the child may not look so unusual because he may strongly rsemble the parent from whom he inherited his fragile X. An excellent reference book on fragile X syndrome is *The Fragile-X Syndrome* by Hodnap & Leckman (Sage, 1993).

Fragile X syndrome is not always considered strictly a "non-autistic PDD" because, unlike other PDDs, its cause is known. However, in terms of behavior, fragile X syndrome can be seen as a non-autistic PDD because of the numerous symptoms of autism or PDD in children with fragile X. When these symptoms do occur, and when the child with fragile X does meet criteria for autism or PDD,NOS, he will require the same treatment as any other autistic or PDD child with the same signs of autism.

Changes in Diagnoses Over Time

Diagnoses *can* change. But the great majority of children diagnosed as autistic when they are small will still be diagnosed as autistic when they are older. The numbers of symptoms of autism that are present and the severity of those symptoms virtually always change as children mature. In children who receive comprehensive treatment, there tend to be fewer and less severe symptoms with growth and development. For some autistic children, the number and severity of symptoms may diminish sufficiently so that the child becomes better described as having PDD,NOS rather than a full-blown case of autism. As mentioned earlier, some clinicians who see children at an earlier age choose to hedge their bets and diagnose a two- or three-year-old as having PDD rather than as having autism. If that child is then diagnosed as autistic at age four, it doesn't necessarily mean that his symptoms have become more severe, but rather that they are now more evident as language emerges and the opportunity to develop peer friendships leads to other noticeable problems. I always try to encourage parents not to think of a diagnosis in black and white. Each child's diagnosis needs to be given along with a band of certainty, and information of how likely it may be to change.

Chapter Summary

In this chapter, we have reviewed the labels for the different disorders in the autistic spectrum including autistic disorder, PDD,NOS, Asperger's syndrome, Rett's syndrome, childhood disintegrative disorder, and fragile X syndrome. In the next three chapters, we will focus primarily on autism and PDD to develop a more in-depth understanding of the specific signs of autism and PDD. The other non-autistic PDDs will be described insofar as they differ from autism and PDD,NOS. We'll explore not only *what* autistic children do, but our best understanding of *why* they behave the way they do. After reading Chapters 2, 3, and 4, which describe the social development, language, and play of children with autism and PDD, it should be possible to go back to the DSM-IV and ICD-10 diagnostic criteria given in the first part of this chapter and understand how a given child has been, or might be, diagnosed using a particular diagnostic standard.

◆ ◆ ◆

CHAPTER 2

Social Development
in Autism and PDD

This chapter will detail the signs and symptoms of autism that affect a child's social development. Atypical social relating takes many forms, as we'll discuss, and it is considered the core of the autistic syndrome. Often children with many signs of autism but relatively little impairment in relating to others are diagnosed as having PDD. As the information in this chapter is laid out, it will become clearer where boundaries between autism and PDD meet, and when it is useful to distinguish between the two. Figure 3 shows the various aspects of social development we'll be discussing in this chapter.

This most important criterion for diagnosing autism or PDD refers to whether or not the child relates to people as well, as often, and with the same degree of discrimination as other children his or her age. A child who is considered to show a marked lack of awareness of others does not necessarily avoid or resist all people at all times. In the autistic child, the level of interest in others and attachment to others are very different in *quality*. It's not that autistic or PDD children do not relate to others; it's that they do so differently.

Differences in how well or poorly, or how frequently, children relate to their important adults can make the difference between the diagnosis of autism or the diagnosis of PDD. Compared to other children their age, autistic children show a more pronounced and pervasive inability to relate to others. PDD children, on the other hand, do not relate normally, but under certain circumstances may seem to want or tolerate more contact with others. PDD children may approach others, but their interactions can have a self-serving quality; they do not consider, for example, the interests, feelings, or reactions of the other person. Autistic children are the same way, only more so. In most autistic children social interactions are less frequent and the quality of those interactions are different. Autistic children are often described as "aloof," "isolated," or "in their own world." PDD children are more often described as possibly wanting to relate, but not knowing how.

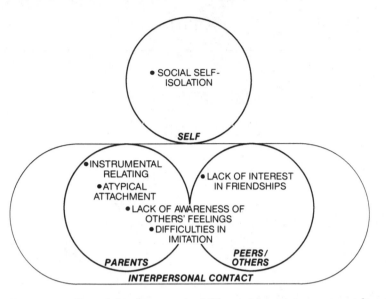

Figure 3   Aspects of social development in children with autistic spectrum disorders.

Early Signs of Social Isolation

Autistic children are very good at isolating themselves, even in a room full of family members. For example, in videotapes we've examined as part of a research project on autism in one- to two-year-olds, it is possible to see this isolation. The autistic toddler, although in a crowded room, doesn't seem to notice main events such as birthday presents being unwrapped, Grandpa arriving, or another child who is having a loud tantrum somewhere else in the room. Even by eighteen months of age, most toddlers naturally pay attention to such things as "main events" and somehow want to get into the act. A typical two-year-old will want to unwrap all the birthday presents whether or not it's *his* birthday; but an autistic two-year-old may be happy just to sit by himself and repeatedly wave a piece of ribbon.

Early Attachment Behavior

Left to themselves, many autistic children spend less time close by their parents and caregivers compared to other children. Those who do tend to stay close may look toward their caregiver to show off what they are doing far less often than other young children. Typically, a normally developing one-, two-, or three-year-old behaves almost as if he's attached to his mother by a rubber band: He can go a certain distance away, but if it's too far, the rubber band begins to stretch uncomfortably, stimulating the child's urge to return or visually check back. Autistic and PDD children seem to lack a "rubber band" (or have one that's very long, or with almost no elasticity). At the time his son was diagnosed with autism, a father described to me how he was concerned about his boy's lack of a "rubber band," deciding one day to test it at the beach. The father stood in one place and let his two-year-old toddle down the beach, to see how long it would be before he looked back. What this father reported was that the child went further and further, never looking back, until the child was so far away that the *father* felt uncomfortable about the distance, and ran off down the beach to retrieve his son. More often parents report concerns that their children readily wander off in parking lots, malls, and grocery stores, seemingly without a sense that they are going off alone. Other parents describe how their autistic toddlers and preschoolers will disappear into their bedrooms alone when company arrives. This is very different from other children the same age who either can't wait to be part of the goings-on, or who cling to their Mom or Dad until they get used to visitors.

Instrumental versus Expressive Relating

One of the main ways in which the quality of relating is different in children with autism and PDD is that relating tends to be *instrumental* rather than more purely *expressive*. Most normally developing children display a great deal of social expressiveness, meaning that they are constantly doing things to provoke an emotional reaction from someone or to show someone how they feel. This includes early behaviors like pointing and vocalizing at something interesting the child sees (but does not necessarily want), bringing toys to show parents, and looking toward the parent when the emotional state of someone in the room changes.

When a child mainly engages in an interaction *to get something he wants*, we define this as an *instrumental* style of relating. The "want" could be food, access to a place he can't get to on his own, or even physical-sensory stimulation like having his back scratched, being tossed in the air, or hugged. The parent is the "instrument" to get the child what he wants, when he wants it. An example of instrumental relating is when an autistic child hones in on one or two powerful words, like "bye-bye," and uses them whenever he doesn't like the situation—that is, too many people, unfamiliar people, a strange place, or too many demands that he behave a certain way. Sometimes this instrumental way of relating to people gives parents the feeling that the child is more interested in getting what he wants than he is in who gets it for him.

Many parents accurately perceive that their autistic or PDD child shows only an instrumental style of relating. What these parents often notice first is that the child mainly seeks them out to get food, or to get something else he can't get for himself, although the parents may also notice that the child usually does a great deal for himself. For example, parents will tell how their two-year-old opens the refrigerator by herself and will help herself to things she can reach. Usually this is seen as both very intelligent (to have figured out where to get things), as well as self-reliant, so at least at first the behavior seems quite desirable. However, what is also true is that other two-year-olds come get their parents when they're hungry—not so much because they can't do for themselves, but because getting someone else to do things for you seems so much more appealing.

Hand-Leading

Early on, many autistic and PDD children develop an instrumental way of relating described as *hand-leading*. This means that the child takes your hand and pulls it to something he wants. He may even use hand-leading to put a parent's hand on his back or arm if he likes being scratched or rubbed there. What makes hand-leading an autistic behavior is that it is not coordinated with looking at the parent, or looking back and forth from the parent to the desired object. It is a very physical way of bringing together two things that the child wants to see operate on one another (for example, a hand and an unopened bag of potato chips). When a child begins to be able to hand-lead, it means that visually, in his mind, he can now see the sequence of events he wants to happen, and that hand-leading is his best way of trying to make those things start to happen.

What is different about autistic hand-leading from what young children more typically do is that preverbal toddlers usually *point* rather than hand-lead. In autistic and PDD children, pointing often emerges very late, if at all. Normally, children do not have to be taught to point, but begin to do it spontaneously. Pointing implies that the child who is pointing understands that the other person will know that the point refers to something the pointer is thinking about. The capacity to understand that others think the same way you do is a capacity called *theory of mind*. Autistic and PDD children are very slow to develop even a partial theory of mind, and many never really develop it at all. Hand-leading is also used by other language-handicapped children, and by deaf children, but when they hand-lead, they combine gaze between the parent and the object with the hand-leading, making it a more social activity.

Social Referencing

Closely related to the observation that autistic children do not point or develop a theory of mind at the usual time is the observation that autistic children lack *social referencing*. Social referencing is an early form of social behavior that every parent recognizes: Usually social referencing first appears when the baby is about six to eight months old. For example, in a baby who is just beginning to crawl, a parent can observe social referencing when the baby sees an interesting toy a foot or so away that he'd like to put in his mouth. With great concentration, the baby will lean forward and squirm toward the object; next, grabbing it and shoving as much of it as he can into his mouth. The next thing the baby will do is look around to see who he can "share" this accomplishment with. If his eyes meet his father's, he'll smile (perhaps losing the object in the process). The baby might coo or otherwise communicate "Look at me! Look what I've done!" At this point the baby is very receptive to praise or some other "turn" the father will take to let the baby know his reaction to the new accomplishment.

The autistic or PDD baby does not or only rarely engages in social referencing. Although the same curiosity toward toys may apply, the need to share achievements is not intrinsically there. The autistic child is sufficiently pleased to please himself, and has little or no need to please others. Generally, parents observe that the autistic baby's approach to toys appears to be done with great seriousness. The autistic baby approaches something he wants, retrieves it, manipulates it, but shows little facial expression. Friends and relatives often comment that because of this the baby seems very focused, very intelligent, very serious and planful about his activities. Therefore, the early lack of social referencing is often not perceived as a warning sign that some essential component of social understanding is missing. The baby is so involved in his own experiments with the world that, like a tiny absent-minded professor, he is oblivious to others.

Disabilities of Social Understanding in Adults

Normally, social referencing is something that manifests itself throughout development as we mature into adults. All of us have a natural drive and desire to be acknowledged by others for our accomplishments. In autistic adults, we might see an individual who *can* do something (like bathe every morning), but sees no reason why he *should* just to please others or to conform to the rules of society. He sees no logical reason why his behavior should be referenced to someone else's social norms. Autistic people, however, are very different from individuals we label *sociopaths,* people who maliciously disregard and intentionally violate the values of society. The autistic person simply does not see why rules that other people feel are *important* to follow, like having a job to support oneself, if one can, should be seen as important for him. Therefore, in the mature autistic person there is little sense of shame or guilt over inappropriate behavior that typically would come from the awareness that others may be judging your behavior as bad, immature, or ignorant. For example, one young man I evaluated, who was found to be autistic but of normal intelligence, had written a bomb threat to his favorite radio station after it failed to broadcast an expected program one afternoon. Having been taught in school that envelopes need mailing addresses, return addresses, and stamps, he mailed his letter accordingly. When the police showed up at his house shortly after the letter had been received at the radio station, his older brother had to explain how his autistic brother simply didn't know how the police and the people at the radio station would interpret his actions, and that as an autistic person, his brother really would not be capable of planning and executing a bombing, but was simply expressing his frustration.

Autistic people learn to compensate for their lack of social understanding by learning many rules for social behavior—rules they tend to hold onto rigidly, even when the situation changes and the rule is no longer appropriate. There is a lack of flexibility in thinking and reasoning about social situations. An example of this is Dusty, a 25-year-old man with Asperger's syndrome who went through an intense period of riding public transit buses for up to ten hours a day. Dusty would greet anyone who sat down next to him on the bus. He had no way of judging which people would find this a passing friendly gesture and gladly reciprocate, and which people would feel this a clear violation of their own nonverbal signals declaring a desire to be left alone. Eventually, there were complaints made to the transit authority about Dusty. The only successful way of remediating his actions was to suggest the opposite behavior, urging him to be quite conservative and not greet other people at all.

Awareness of the Emotions and Feelings of Others

As might seem apparent to you at this point, something is wrong with how autistic and PDD children come to understand how others are the same or different from themselves. A fundamental part of this understanding is the perception of emotional states or feelings in other people. One thing that can be quite striking to a mother of an autistic child when a younger sibling comes along is that, by the time the younger one is fourteen to eighteen months old, the baby will know when her mother is feeling sad and will approach her, at least briefly, offering comfort of some sort (like patting her mother, or offering to share her bottle). This type of acknowledgement of the emotions of others, and the altruistic behavior that may follow, is much more unusual in the autistic or PDD child. Autistic children more often seem to perceive the intensity of emotion, but will fail to notice whether it is positive or negative. They tend to react to events in a "so-what-does-this-mean-for-me" fashion. The autistic child does tend to pick up on the arousal level of others around him (excited versus not excited), but is less able to discriminate among more subtle emotional states and how positive or negative they are. Therefore, it can be difficult for an autistic child to recognize when someone is acting mad or sad or angry or upset. This becomes very apparent when autistic children are older and attempts are made to "teach" them how to recognize emotional states (which will be discussed in Chapter 12). Parents who are accustomed to training their children by showing them how a particular action or activity has made Mommy happy or sad can be puzzled at the seeming indifference of the autistic child. An autistic or PDD child is not motivated to do something just because he will "make Mommy happy" or to be dubbed a "big boy" for doing it. Autistic children seldom adjust their own behavior in response to either the positive or negative emotions that others display towards their actions.

Autistic Aloofness and the Potential for Child Abuse

Particularly among parents who have more than the usual level of chaos in their lives aside from their autistic children, autistic emotional indifference or aloofness can be perceived as purposeful and hostile disobedience. In these cases, it can be very helpful for a parent to understand that the autistic child is not weighing his mother or father's appeals to behave well and then rejecting them. The autistic child is just doing what he wants to do, when he wants to do it, and sometimes it happens that the autistic child's activities are the opposite of what parents have asked the child to do.

If parents see the child's behavior as flying in the face of restrictions the parents have imposed, the risk that the child will be punished increases. Since a young autistic child is not understanding emotions (and often not understanding much language either), he often cannot link a punishment to his "crime." Punishments meted out to any children who do not have the capacity to understand what they are being punished for tend to be ineffective and also to make the child more anxious, and therefore likely to behave in an even more frenetic fashion, which may further increase the chance that he does something else that is bad. I sometimes see families where the autistic child is being hit rather severely for all sorts of behavioral infractions. Invariably, these parents assume their child *does* understand what he is being asked to do and not do. In these cases, parents need to remember that the child actually may *not* understand. The autistic child's lack of appropriate emotional response to being hit, along with inappropriate emotional responses in some autistic children (like giggling), is a dangerous combination that can send a stressed-out parent over the edge and result in unintentional (or, sadly, sometimes intentional) abuse of the child.

Seeking Physical Affection

Autistic children have characteristic ways of showing physical affection toward parents. It can be particularly difficult for first-time parents whose child is autistic to really appreciate the difference between the affectionate behavior of an autistic child, and that of someone else's child who is not autistic. Often, it is not until a baby sibling comes along that the contrast between "autistic" affection and normal one-, two-, or three-year-old affectionate behavior is really clear.

The first thing many parents say at the start of an autism evaluation is that they don't understand why a particular doctor or teacher could think their child was autistic, because the child *is* so affectionate. Yes, autistic and PDD children can be affectionate physically, but in ways that can be very different from other children their age. For most children, an interaction with a parent such as being hugged goes along with looking at, and talking to, or cooing to the person giving the hugs. A hug gives physical comfort and relaxation, but children normally want social comfort and reassurance along with a hug, too. Typically, children will eagerly hug whenever Mom or Dad offers one. One thing that parents of autistic and PDD children often mention is that their children like to be hugged—*but* only when the child wants it. The autistic or PDD child tends to be the one who decides when it's time for a hug or cuddle, and how long it will go on.

The affectionate contact between autistic children and their parents is different from that of other children of the same age. For example, the autistic child may drape himself across the parent's back or legs, or bury his head in his mother's shoulder, but without ever peeking out at her. Some autistic children back up into their parents rather than approach them frontally, and then plop themselves on their mother's or father's lap with their back to the parent. Sometimes parents even become concerned that the child has vision problems because of the perception that the child does not look at them while he is making himself so cozy. Watching these types of interactions, an observer gets the feeling that the parent is a giant teddy bear, favorite blanket, or a big bean bag chair. On one occasion in our clinic, a two-year-old autistic boy screamed and cried whenever his mother tried to leave the room. When she'd return, he'd run and grab her legs and be immediately comforted. Once, a staff member who was a large and ample woman, like the toddler's mother, entered the room while he was crying, he ran for her legs and calmed just as well. Since his comforting routine didn't actually involve looking at his mother's face, this type of substitution worked well for him.

What is also interesting to observe is how well parents adapt to their child's way of wanting physical affection. For example, many mothers of autistic children will hold out their arms and wait for their child to come, rather than approaching the autistic child and scooping him up. Unconsciously perhaps, the parent has recognized what the child prefers and what is more likely to produce more satisfaction on the part of the child.

Given this very different way of getting and giving physical affection, a doctor assessing a child for autism usually looks for when, how, and how frequently physically affectionate interactions take place. Important clues for this part of the diagnosis include how well the physical, visual, and verbal channels of interacting are tied to one another—that hugs should be accompanied by some prolonged face-to-face looking, and by happy sounds or words.

Patterns of Comfort-Seeking

Another facet of the diagnosis of autism is whether the child shows a developmentally appropriate level of comfort-seeking. Comfort-seeking is a natural need to be in reassuring contact with a familiar caregiver when distressed. Comfort-seeking is a key behavior in assessing the quality of a child's attachment to the parent. Key things that are assessed in a diagnostic history for atypical comfort-seeking include what it is that the child does when he is hurt or feeling ill, and how he reacts in relation to caregivers in situations of stress or fear.

Normal Development of Attachment Behavior

To understand how the attachment behavior of autistic children is different from other children, it's first necessary to understand what constitutes normal attachment. Normally, what is referred to as "attachment" is first in evidence around six to nine months when a baby begins to show a strong preference to being held or played with only by those he is quite familiar with—usually his parents. Even loving people the baby sees only occasionally and previously "liked," like grandparents or a favorite aunt, may get rejected during a certain period of development. Most adults are more or less aware that babies normally go through this "mommy-ish" stage and react by approaching the child more gradually or only when an attachment figure like the mother is holding the baby. Typically, this wariness of strangers peaks aroung thriteen months and is no longer as significant a factor by the time a child is beginning to talk (eighteen to twenty-four months). During this time period, babies will often cry when left in a room with even a very friendly stranger, and even with very interesting new toys. Even if a stranger is present and the parent is too, a normally developing child will tend to play quite close to the mother, and look or call back to her every time the strange person attempts to play with him. When the child becomes distressed by new people or other unfamiliar things, he seeks comfort by increasing his physical closeness, physical contact, eye contact, or calling out to his parent.

Non-autistic children can vary a great deal in how they attach themselves to their caregivers. Some of the variation in the quality of attachment *is* due to the quality of care they receive—but some normally developing children are naturally much more independent from caregivers than other, irrespective of whether their parents are warm and loving, or colder and more unavailable. The young autistic child's way of regulating her attachment to her caregiver tends to go beyond a desire for independence on the part of the child, and can often appear to be very actively avoident. A small number of autistic children show fairly normal patterns of attachment in terms of when they will go to their parents for comfort. However, these children still tend to show difficulties, but more subtle difficulties, in simultaneously using physical, verbal, and nonverbal communication to re-establish a sense of safety at being back with their parents.

Autistic Development of Attachment Behavior

In an autistic child, the normal stages of attachment are usually lacking. Either they are absent altogether, occur only partly, or are very delayed in emerging. Sometimes the normal "mommy-ish" stage that usually occurs around thirteen months of age does not begin until four or five years in an autistic or PDD child. Sometimes normal attachment behavior is present early on and then disappears early as well.

One of the basic ways attachment can be assessed in a clinical setting is by finding opportunities to observe naturally occuring separations and reunions between parent and child, or to stage such separations. In our clinic, for example, we routinely take the child into a room adjacent to the parent interview room to make behavioral observations of the child. Some autistic and PDD children protest this sort of separation a great deal. This is especially true for children with very little experience being separated from their parents. When you are a young autistic child who can't talk and ask questions about what's happening (nor understand explanations of why you're being taken into the next room), separation from what you know (your parents) can be very distressing, even if the way you typically behave toward your parents is more aloof (and seemingly less needy) than other children your age. Often little autistic children cry when separated, and if, once separated, the crying doesn't stop after various attempts to introduce interesting alternative activities, we take the child back to the parents. It is at this point that the autistic child's attachment system functions very differently as if the "volume knob" for seeking physical closeness is tuned way down. Instead of needing to approach the parent, get eye contact, get verbal reassurance, cling to Mom, sit on Mom's lap, and *then,* eventually, look out at the mean strange lady who took her out of the room, the autistic or PDD child will short-circuit this process. The crying may stop abruptly after coming into the room with only the barest glance in Mom's direction. If there is a physical approach, the child may stall part way, and veer off to a part of the room with no people in it. Sometimes the child continues to cry, but falls into a heap on the floor, making no attempt to approach his mother or look toward her. The need for contact or acknowledgment doesn't appear markedly in the child's actions. If there is physical contact, it tends to be without accompanying eye contact and without accompanying facial expressions that would indicate the child feels relieved. Although this type of natural experiment can be a good opportunity for clinicians to observe the autistic child's attachment, sometimes a mother, especially and experienced and responsive mother, "interferes" with our little experiment by running up to the crying child before he has a chance to decide to approach his mother or not, and picks him up. In such cases, we do not get a chance to really gauge the child's contribution to the attachment. Nevertheless, what is usually observed is a child who accepts being held for a relatively short period of time, compared to how long a similarly upset non-autistic child would want to be held. Typically, while the autistic child does remain in physical contact with this mother, there will be no eye contact or mutual talking or babbling as part of the interaction. All of this is to say that the autistic child *does* get comfort from the parent, but that the comfort-seeking pattern is very atypical because it is so "tuned down."

In PDD children in particular, the attachment pattern may look more normal, but it is often greatly delayed. For example, a six-year-old with a normal

IQ might only be entering the stage of being completely miserable when separated from his mother. On being reunited with his mother, this child might crawl into her lap, look into her face, pat her cheeks, smile, and then triumphantly begin to suck his thumb while looking out at the examiner who had taken him away from his mother earlier. While this pattern of behavior would have been wholly normal at age two or three, at age six it is very delayed compared to other six-year-olds. Interestingly, it often seems that children with these delayed-but-normal patterns of attachment do ultimately develop better social skills; however, this is something that has not yet been thoroughly studied.

Some young autistic children may appear to be attached in some situations but not in others. For example, a mother might report, and a father will independently confirm, that their child runs to his father to be picked up as soon as the father returns home from work each night. Next, father and son might have a routine of bouncing on the sofa, or reading a favorite book together. Strangely however, the same boy may fail to greet or approach his father when reunited with him in our clinic playroom after the boy has been crying. Why? Parents and the activities they provide become part of a secure routine that autistic children like to count on. To some extent, this is true of any child who counts on a bedtime story or going to the playground after school. The difference with the autistic child is that the reunion with his father each evening is part of a larger routine, a larger "whole" or gestalt, and not something that is a satisfying experience on its own or in another context.

In assessing attachment in autistic children, the clinician must always take into account that there will be individual differences, and differences as a function of experience, just as there are in non-autistic children. Some normally developing children have had more experience with separation from parents, such as children who've been in day care a great deal since they were infants. It may take more stress to activate attachment responses in such children, but when activated, the comfort-seeking of non-autistic children will look more typical than in an autistic child. For example, a normally developing toddler who has been around many different adults may be quite pleased to have any friendly stranger help him put a puzzle together. But, if the friendly stranger suddenly tries to pick him up, the toddler may be expected to fuss and run back to his mother. When he does, he'll likely look at her face, want frontal contact and want to talk about what happened—all normal attachment responses, albeit ones that took a while to trigger. Because of inconsistent parenting, some normally developing children have very avoidant or resistant attachments to parents. Especially with abused or neglected children, a pathological attachment is formed to caregivers which may look a lot like an autistic child's attachment. Only careful history-taking and following the child once he's out of the abusive situation may reveal what the main problem truly is. However, because the difficulties experienced by autistic children go well beyond attachment, it is actually seldom that there is a real question of whether a child is autistic, or whether a child has been maltreated. In my own experience, this has only been at issue when the maltreated child has a dis-ability related to autism, such as a severe developmental language disorder, so that the maltreated child, like the autistic child, appears impaired in both her ability to communicate *and* to relate socially.

Coming for Comfort or Help When Hurt

Assessing the parent-child attachment relationship is the most direct and important way to evaluate a potentially autisitic child's social development when he is a baby, toddler, or preschooler. Another way to look at comfort-seeking is to examine what the child does when hurt or ill. With children at later developmental stages and older chronological ages, the attachment ob-servations that are so helpful with younger children don't tell you much since no one expects an eight-year-old confronted with a stranger to run to his mother's lap. What is expected is that the child will depend on the caretaking adult for help when in distress. A normally developing five-year-old child who cuts himself, or even falls down and gets a little bump, will run to his mother to show the hurt, get it kissed, and have it made all better. It's quite normal for even near-imaginary bumps to be presented in this way when the child is feeling tired or stressed. This is something the autistic child seems to need to be "taught" to do. If the procedure of coming for a kiss is there at all, it may be ritualized, and not accompanied by a need for verbal explanations or reas-surance. Sometimes a child may be "taught" to come for comfort when he gets cuts and bruises, but then does not come when really distressed. Once when interviewing a mother of a PDD boy about this, she gave several convincing examples of how her ten-year-old son Nathan would show his hurts to receive Band Aids and other nurturing. Later though, when talking about some of Nathan's fears, she described how the thing he was afraid of most was thunder-storms. At these times, Nathan would retreat into the bathroom (the only room of the house with no windows), take blankets and pillows, and hole up alone until well after the storm was over. Thinking about this later, I realized this was a striking example of abnormal comfort-seeking—that when most fearful and distressed, what Nathan wanted most was to isolate himself from others.

Many parents of autistic children are struck by the lack of comfort-seeking, or like Nathan who was afraid of thunderstorms, the need to be alone when distressed. Some parents even recall that as infants, their crying or fussy autistic babies calmed down better when put down in their cribs than when Mom or Dad tried to bounce, cuddle, or soothe them verbally. In infancy, these children typically were not suspected of being autistic, and this pattern of calming down more readily when put down than when held generally was not regarded with much concern since most parents were quite satisfied at finding anything they could do to quiet a crying baby, especially something that didn't require their prolonged attention at three in the morning.

As toddlers and preschoolers, many autistic children can be observed crying in response to pain, frustration, tiredness, or hunger, but they do not direct their outpouring of emotion to an individual. This is quite different from the normally developing toddler: Typically, a toddler who has been punished or frustrated in her attempts to do something she shouldn't do will cry. But even though angry at the parent who is thwarting her willfulness, she will cast sidelong glances at the parent to see what effect her tears and screaming are having on her audience. The autistic child will just stand and cry and scream at no one in particular. Watching this happen, one sometimes has the sense that the child is not really connecting the cause and effect of what has happened to him. Eventually, the crying, screaming autistic toddler usually calms down spontaneously. No one has gone up to him at that particular moment (although earlier interventions may have been tried); the crying just stops. And without a glance around, the little boy or girl continues on his or her way. In fact, parents of children who act this way soon learn that trying to comfort the screaming child just adds insult to injury and leave their children to "cry it out."

Difficulties in Developing Imitation

Early in development, babies discover imitation as a means of taking in information about the world. Through imitation the baby uses and practices what he sees. It is one of the most basic forms of human communication. Through imitation, a baby can acknowledge the existence of someone else by copying him. If you can catch a newborn in just the right stage of quiet alertness, and pace things so the newborn can follow your actions, you can even get a newborn to stick out her tongue in response to your sticking out your tongue. Early imitation is a nonverbal means of information-processing in which a template of something seen is used to shape one's own behavior in a similar fashion. The desire to imitate appears to be innate. In normal development, a baby is not taught the *idea* of imitating. Only in the second half of the first year do parents usually begin to *teach* through soliciting imitation. Learning to wave bye-bye is one of the earliest social imitation tasks that parents often try to teach to their babies. How parents teach a baby to wave bye-bye shows the many social ways in which an infant of that age is typically already predisposed to learn: Typical teaching strategies include waving bye-bye to the baby at every chance it pertains, using a loud, exaggerated, high-pitched tone of voice the baby is likely to pay attention to, and taking the baby's hand and waving bye-bye with it while saying bye-bye. The learning of this task on the baby's part consists of copying a particular action upon receiving a verbal cue, satisfying his desire to be praised when he accomplishes the right thing, and eventually, learning that bye-bye marks a certain class of events that happen to him.

By the end of the first year of life, the autistic of PDD child usually fails to show basic development imitation, like waving bye-bye. Partly, the autistic or PDD baby is not motivated to do anything (including waving bye-bye) simply to receive social praise. But there seems to be more to it than that. The innate drive to imitate seems to be missing too. And the more "social" the imitation, the harder it is for the autistic child to master.

The development of imitation skills in autistic and PDD children can be divided into three levels of increasing difficulty. The first, and easiest, level can be called "spontaneous object use," meaning that the task provides its own model of what to do. For example, a pegboard with square holes and square pegs is a spontaneous object-use task. To know what to do, the autistic child does not need to rely on what anybody says or imitating what anybody does to know how to proceed. Autistic children tend to do very well in these types of activities. Next in complexity is the type of imitation that involves "motor object imitation," meaning the child has to watch how an object is manipulated and then do it too. A simple example would be folding a piece of paper in half to make a "book"—something that most toddlers at eighteen to twenty-four months can do. Interestingly, many four-year-old autistic children can do "spontaneous object-use" tasks that normal four-year-olds can do but still can't do "motor object imitations" as well as most two-year-olds. To take this one step further, the next most complex type of imitation for an autistic child is "body imitations," which involve copying an action with your body (rather than using an object like a piece of paper). Waving bye-bye is a form of body imitation. Again, most young autistic children who can do pegboards or puzzles, and even those who can fold paper in imitation, usually still don't wave bye-bye, something one-year-olds often have mastered. So it seems, the more the form of imitation involves a human model and has meaning as part of social interaction, the relatively more difficult it is for the autistic child to master.

Why is it that autistic children should have so much difficulty spontaneously imitating and learning through imitation? One possible explanation is that it is difficult for an autistic child to pay attention to a human model. When we discussed attachment difficulties in autistic toddlers, it was explained how the "volume" on the "attachment knob" seems tuned up too high. Therefore, autistic toddlers may need very little parental contact to restore emotional equilibrium after becoming distressed. The same "volume" problem seems to be the case with "tuning in" to another person's actions in order to develop templates needed to copy or imitate. (In Chapter 9, the development of imitation skills will be discussed in terms of strategies for overcoming this sort of difficulty.)

The desire to copy another's actiona seems to be missing in autistic children. Instead of imiating, the autistic child tends to come up with his own novel ways of doing things. For example, Joseph, one of the first autistic children I ever worked with, taught himself to swim not by imitating people but by imitating an object—by, as he said, "being a washing machine" and pumping his whole body up and down like the agitator in the middle of the washer drum. He was uninterested in learning how to swim by copying the swim instructor or the other children at camp. In fact, it could even be said that Joseph was *unaware* that he could learn to swim better by copying others.

Developmental Aspects of Imitation

At each stage of development, age-appropriate forms of imitation are largely lacking in children with autism and PDD. Obvious forms of imitation in young children include copying the activities they see their parents doing around the house: Ten-month-olds will pat babies. Eighteen-month-olds will hold toy telephone receivers to their ears. Two-year-olds will grab spare screwdrivers and pretend they are screwing screws. In the preschool and early latency years (five to eight years old), imitation consists of even more socially complex behaviors such as dressing up and prancing around in dramatic hats, gaudy dresses, and high-heeled shoes, or adopting the macho style of walking used by TV tough guys. As children mature, imitation becomes tied closely to imagination which is another area of development where children with autism or PDD often have difficulty. Imagination often consists of imitating something real and then adding to it, or confabulating various real events in new combinations. (Difficulties autistic and PDD children have in the development of imagination will be discussed in more detail in Chapter 4.)

When autistic children do use some imiation, it tends to be very concrete or one-to-one rather than like the more "as if" play of their agemates. For example, an autistic three-year-old may try to screw things with a real screwdriver, but is less likely to be applying his "screwdriver" skills to a pencil which he *pretends* to use as a screwdriver. Actions tend to be concrete rather than representational.

Normally, teenagers imitate one another a great deal, conforming in dress, actions, and values. But even rather bright teenagers with PDD will display behavior that appears to be "off" for their age. They button the top button of their Izod tee-shirt and then tuck the stylized tails of the tee-shirt into their pants. They wear black nylon socks with sneakers instead of cotton crew socks, and insist on having their hair cut in a way that embarrasses their teenage siblings. By the time a young person with autism or PDD is an adult, the lack of imitation of subtle (and more obvious) social conventions signals to others that he is different, and constitutes an unintentional form of nonverbal communication by the autistic young person that he is not like others. This can present painful and awkward social situations for the teenager or young adult with PDD or autism who tries to interact socially but is grossly inept in his idioms of speech and physical mannerisms, and in addition has an odd appearance and unconventional habits. Social skills training programs for higher functioning autistic and PDD young people, though, do offer specific interventions for ameliorating these awkward characteristics. (Such interventions will be discussed in detail in Chapter 13.)

Lack of Social Play

When an autistic child has a family where there are older siblings or many cousins around, or lives in a neighborhood with lots of other toddlers, parents sometimes begin to notice when their child is around age two-and-a-half that something is very different about how he or she plays with others. Usually by this time there is also some concern about language development, so the first thing parents think is that other children don't want to play with their child because he can't talk, and he doesn't want to play with them because they can't understand him. But on closer observation, it is possible to tell that there is more to it than that. For example, I remember that as a graduate student, I'd sometimes visit the playground in a large graduate student housing complex at Stanford, where I was studying. There would be babies, toddlers, and preschoolers from many different countries on the playground. These children typically only spoke their native language, but you couldn't tell that these children couldn't verbally communicate with one another by watching the two- and three-year-olds play with one another. They would watch one another, pause, smile, and copy. They could somehow organize themselves to push one another on a Hot Wheels, or play together in a sandbox. All this communication basically came from reading each others' faces and nonverbal communication like pointing. The autistic child is unable to understand this type of communication, and so attempts by other children to engage him in play are aborted even when peers use nonverbal cues to compensate for the difficulties. Another three-year-old may try once or even three times to engage an autistic three-year-old, but if the autistic child doesn't answer back, either verbally or nonverbally, the other child will likely walk away. This is what parents of autistic children being to notice. Sometimes parents notice differences at an even earlier age because the usual amount of unabashed staring at one another that eighteen-month-olds do is not there in autistic toddlers.

Autistic Children's Play with Siblings

As autistic and PDD children get older, social play either remains absent or occurs only in limited ways. Usually, an autistic child with a sibling plays a little with him or her—often more than with anyone else. This is because the sibling, through extensive trial and error, has the opportunity to learn what forms of play his sibling will or will not accept. For example, because many autistic children really like movement stimulation, favorite activities with a brother or sister may consist of being chased, tickled, jumping on the bed, or other roughhouse play. However, as in other forms of social interaction the roughhousing for autistic children is usually not accompanied by looking into the face of the person doing the chasing, or verbalizing to the other child who is doing the tickling.

Autistic children often do play *near* their siblings, especially after their siblings have learned to mostly leave them alone. Sometimes this "nearby play" is taken to be "parallel play." The two types of play are actually different: Parents will report their children "played" together meaning their children do play near one another, and may have read that "parallel play" is normal for two-year-olds and so they judge the play of their two-year-old autistic child to be normal. Parallel play, however, is actually an early form of social play that implies that one child watches and then imitates the play of another child—doing the same thing, maybe not at the same time, but in the same physical vicinity—producing "parallel" activity. When asked to think about reciprocal play between the autistic child and her siblings, most parents realize that their children play near each other but that there are few if any instances where their autistic child copied something her brother or sister had just done.

In older autistic children, there may be limited, concrete, or fairly immature play with much younger children. A ten-year-old autistic boy, for example, may develop a friendship with a five-year-old non-autistic boy that is based on his Ninja Turtle or Power Ranger action figures. The relationship may be fairly well circumscribed to include doing things with the action figures, and the five-year-old is likely to be the one who suggests what they'll do next. Similarly, playing board games, where rules and turns are structured, can be a limited form of social play that an autistic child engages in. Double joystick Nintendo is another example we hear more and more about in our clinic. Turn-taking at video games allows the autistic child to play alone while still playing with another child.

When a child is described diagnostically as having an absence of social play, it means that the full range of play activities that would be expected at that age are absent—although some more limited play, like some of the activities just described, may occur. Like other symptoms of autism, the autistic or PDD child seldom displays a complete absence of age-appropriate behavior. More often the frequency or quality of behavior is different from other children the same age.

Lack of Peer Friendships

Children who do not engage in social play do not have peer friendships. Sometimes the absence of friendships is a more prominent signal to parents that something is wrong than the absence of truly sociable play, which can be more difficult to judge. Since most children these days are in day care by age three, or at least attend some sort of play group, there is usually some opportunity for parents to observe their child in relation to other children. By age three, children usually begin to ask for another child from day care, preschool, or a play group by name, and express a desire to have that child come over, or to be able to play more with that child. Autistic children, however, don't seem to notice other children as the most interesting other thing in the room besides themselves, as children of almost any age typically do. On one occasion in our clinic, at a time when we had a very small waiting room, two fathers whose autistic boys had been in the same class for the previous four years encountered one another. As the fathers greeted one another and chatted, the two boys (both about eight years old) made no acknowledgment of one another, even though they were typically together five days a week, six hours a day. I had thought there might at least be some sort of reaction to seeing a familiar "object" in an unfamiliar place, but, no, neither recognized the other.

Even older, high-functioning autistic people who are quite verbal have a hard time giving you a definition of friendship, or naming someone they might consider to be a friend. When they do name a "friend," it might be the person who drives their bus each morning and greets them, or their caseworker who takes them shopping on Thursday afternoons. In such cases, the autistic person has learned to define friendships according to rules that fit the particular situation: A bus driver may be a friend because you see him regularly, and you always greet one another. A caseworker may be a friend because you go out together, and she talks with you about things you are interested in. The more intrinsic desire to form bonds with someone who is in some way like oneself, to share similar interests, and to give as much as you get from a relationship, is basically absent. To those around the autistic person, this can seem like self-centeredness or egocentrism taken to the most extreme degree. In some ways it is. However, an autistic person's self-centeredness comes from his lack of awareness that others have thoughts and feelings, too. This is different from a severely emotionally disturbed person who knows that everyone has feelings, but just doesn't care. As we discussed in the last chapter in the section on Asperger's syndrome, it can be hard for an older autistic person to even know what to do to develop or maintain a friendship when they *do* express a desire for friends.

Chapter Summary

In this chapter, we've covered several areas of the social development of autistic and PDD children that are different from normally developing children. At each developmental stage, there are different benchmarks for social development, and it is through an assessment of the degree to which the child has reached these benchmarks or not that the social symptoms of autism or PDD are judged. The social impairments of autism and PDD are considered the most central features of the disorder. The use of language for the purpose of communicaton is a social phenomenon as well. In the next chapter, we'll examine how language development is characteristically different in children with autism and PDD.

♦ ♦ ♦

CHAPTER 3

Communication Skills
in Autism and PDD

It is when autistic and PDD children begin (or fail to begin) to use language, parents begin to detect how different their children are. Most obvious is when a child does not begin to speak at all. Because all children vary in their developmental patterns and use first words at somewhat different ages, the presence of a language delay alone is not the easiest way to detect a problem like autism or PDD. First words are just one indication of how communication skills are taking shape. A careful history can reveal whether other related milestones in development, such as pointing and certain forms of imitating, are developing on time. These related milestones give the clinician a way of predicting what types of language problems can be anticipated, and how they can be helped. In the first part of this chapter, we look at spoken language as well as forms of nonverbal communication that toddlers learn to use. Both verbal and nonverbal ways of communicating are assessed when a clinician considers whether a child may have autism or PDD. Figure 4 shows the various aspects of communication skills that will be discussed in relation to autism in this chapter.

Nonverbal Communication

Even though the absence of spoken language is the first thing most parents worry about, before the appearance of speech there may likely be other signs of a difficulty. Long before meaningful words are first spoken, infants and toddlers are communicating through the use of gaze, facial expressions, sounds, and gestures. These means of communication are not as precise as spoken language in terms of the content they convey. Nevertheless, nonverbal communication is a rich method for getting across reactions to things that happen to the child, and feelings that the child wants others to know he is experiencing. In children with autism and PDD, this early nonverbal commu-

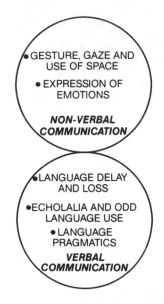

Figure 4   Development of communication skills in children with autistic spectrum disorders.

nication is usually quite limited or absent. Babies quickly develop an innate ability to communicate with nonverbal signs such as facial expressions of emotion, looking between an object of interest and another person, and anticipatory reaching to gain physical contact with a caregiver. Autistic children, however, need to learn nonverbal communication, just as an adult would need to learn a foreign language. In fact, it is usually harder for an autistic child to learn to use nonverbal communication than it is for an adult to learn a foreign language, because the autistic child tends to find the task unpleasant, overly stimulating, and without much meaning at first. Early difficulties in using nonverbal communication are virtually universal among children with autism, PDD, and Asperger's syndrome.

Theory of Mind

In thinking about the nonverbal communication of an autistic child, it is important to distinguish between nonverbal cues that the responsive parent just knows how to read (like a little boy who keeps playing, but holds the front of his pants when he has to go potty) versus *intentional* messages that the child is sending to the adult (like a little boy who looks at his mom with a pained expression and wiggles up and down while holding the front of his pants). True nonverbal communication involves a type of "mind-reading"—knowing that what you're thinking is somehow going to be conveyed to someone else through you facial expressions or gestures, and without the use of words. In recent years, a whole body of research, much of it from England, has focused on autism and "theory of mind." Simply put, a theory of mind is the belief or "theory" you hold that others have a "mind" capable of understanding things the same way your mind does. In the last chapter, we discussed how a lack of theory of mind results in unawareness of others' thoughts and feelings, and so contributes to the lack of interest on the part of autistic children in sharing their triumphs and failures with significant adults (that is, what was described as a lack of social referencing). Similarly, when it comes to communication, a lack of theory of mind makes it difficult for the autistic child to know where to start in sharing his experience—nonverbally or verbally. For example, if an autistic child does point at, or reach for something she wants, she may do so without first ascertaining whether anyone is there to get her "message."

Use of Gesture

The Anticipatory Reach. In recent research we've been doing, we've learned that one of the first things that may strike parents of an autistic child as different is the absence of an *anticipatory reach.* An anticipatory reach is when a baby who is old enough to sit up (or stand) puts his hands up signaling that he'd like to be picked up. Many autistic children never raise their hands this way. Of the children who do, they may not look at the parent while being picked up, or may look only fleetingly (instead of gazing steadily at the parent's face until they are really "up"). Some only want "up" when they want something they can't get for themselves—like to get out of their crib so they can crawl to an interesting looking object. The anticipatory reach of an autistic or PDD child is seldom social—that is, wanting just to be held, or to be talked to, or to be admired by the adult doing the holding. More often, the reach, if it is there at all, is intended to recruit the adult as an aide in getting something the child wants.

Pointing and Hand-Leading. At about eight to ten months of age, babies usually begin to point. (In Chapter 2, pointing was discussed as a social behavior that babies use for sharing interesting experiences with significant adults.) Nobody teaches babies to stick out their index fingers in the direction of something they want; they just do it. As a forerunner to spoken language, pointing can be described as a *referential* form of communication. The finger, as we all know, "refers" to an object to be found in the direction the finger is pointing. Being able to point is the first indication we have that the child knows that *you* can deduce what is at the end of the limaginary line, just as he can. Autistic children either do not have this ability, are very slow to acquire it, or have to be taught it, because, as we've discussed, they lack a theory of mind.

Instead, autistic children typically develop hand-leading instead. This means that the child takes the hand of the adult and puts it directly on the thing she wants the hand to manipulate—for cxample, the front door, the TV "on" button, or the spigots for the bath tub, whatever is her pleasure. The adult's hand is being used as an instrument. The autistic child seems to be operating from a visual understanding that this adult hand can operate the object in the desired way, and thus meet the child's need to go outside, watch a Disney video, or take a bath. Hand-leading is a very functional means of communication, but it *is* atypical of most children. Although it is a nonverbal mode of communication, it is something normally developing children seldom do. Normally, children point before they can walk. Hand-leading develops after the autistic child can walk, and before the autistic child can point (if he ever does). The normally developing child never really needs hand-leading, because pointing (and verbalizing along with it) is generally more expeditious. So the absence of pointing and the presence of hand-leading are things a doctor looks for in assessing a toddler for autism or PDD, well before the child is two to two-and-a-half-years old, which is when pediatricians typically begin to be concerned about the lack of language.

Facial Cues

Smiling. Another major form of nonverbal communication is eye-to-eye gaze and smiling. Around two to three months, a baby usually recognized the face of her mother and father and looks back with a fixed gaze, brightens, and smiles to show recognition and pleasure. Interestingly, most, though not all, parents of autistic and PDD children remember their baby's first smile. There is some evidence that the very earliest smiles are not controlled from the same area of the brain as later gazing and smiling. (We know that some early smiling *is* reflexive, such as when babies smile in their sleep.) Perhaps some of the early smiles that we think of as "social" smiles are somewhere in between reflexive smiles and true social smiles, and that's why we see them in babies who become autistic. Or, it may be that the brain dysfunction that causes autism does not start until later in the first or second year of life. It may also be that early smiling is a response to all sorts of interesting sights—including faces. As the child matures and the subtle variations of smiling emerge, the processing of a smile may be too stimulating for an autistic child and create a sort of social "overload" which the child responds to by turning away and avoiding facial gaze. This "overload" phenomenon is the same difficulty we discussed in the context of difficulties autistic children have in "overloading" on parent responses to their distress, and "overloading" socially in a context where they might otherwise be able to learn by imitating something they see.

Eye Contact. By the end of second year of life, virtually all autistic and PDD children show some degree of abnormality in eye contact. This can take the form of eye gaze being absent, or fleeting, only looking at others when they don't look back at you, or being wooden and fixed. Usually, autistic children make better eye contact with familiar people than with unfamiliar people. Most children with autism and PDD make some eye contact, and it's important to take note when eye contact does occur. Many children with PDD, and some with autism, will make eye contact fairly regularly but usually only briefly, and usually only when they want something. Such children tend to make much less eye contact just to see if you are noticing the same interesting thing that they are noticing, or to see if you will praise or encourage their activities. Autistic children with punitive parents tend to look before beginning to do something they are sometimes punished for, but the tendency to please themselves rather than to please the caregiver is usually stronger, and they'll tend to proceed even if the caregiver responds with a nonverbal warning.

For autistic children, making eye contact with most people seems to be as difficult as staring down someone very threatening. One way I sometimes explain this to parents is to say that for an autistic child, giving eye contact is like it might be for you, if you suddenly found yourself at a crowded party, in a strange country where everyone felt it was quite normal to talk to you from within four inches of your face, and ignored signals you might make to indicate you wished to move further away. In that case, *you* would probably try to avoid eye contact and turn away, too. One of the things that may contribute to a diagnosis of PDD rather than autism is that the child may make fairly frequent eye contact, albeit only in "instrumental" contexts when he wants something specific from someone, or to quickly note a reaction when anxious. This indicates a greater innate awareness of the social function of eye contact, but the child with PDD has the same difficulties an autistic child has in finding eye contact overstimulating if engaged in for more than the usual durations.

Use of Interpersonal Space

Autistic children regulate the space between themselves and others differently from other people. As with eye contact, getting too close to other people seems to be difficult and even threatening for autistic children. Like eye contact, physical closeness with familiar people usually is easier than closeness to unfamiliar people or unfamiliar peers. Ethologists (behavioral biologists who study social behavior in animals) have made some interesting observations that may help us understand how autistic children regulate the space between themselves and others. In fact, during his retirement, one Nobel laureate ethologist, the late Niko Tinbergen, wrote a book on ethology and autism with his wife, who was a teacher of autistic children, called *Autism: New Hope for a Cure* (see Chapter 15). Although autistic children are certainly different from the herring gulls on whom Tinbergen built his fame, he made a number of good observations about how autistic children can be told apart from other children as a function of how they use interpersonal space. Autistic children often tend to keep farther distances between themselves and others. For example, on a crowded playground, autistic and PDD children drift to the periphery. When concentrating on an activity, an autistic child is more likely to keep his back turned to others than to face them. Even approaches to parents and other well-liked adults may be unusual in that the child may approach and then back into the adult's lap rather than facing forward. I remember one four-year-old boy with PDD coming back for a follow-up at a clinic I was visiting. He had worked for some time with a wonderful language therapist there who had really made a lot of progress with him. As he caught sight of her at the end of the hall, she knelt down, held out her arms, and called his name. He came running. Then, when he was two feet away, he stopped dead, turned himself around, and backed into her lap! It was clear he was glad to see her, but he really needed to regulate the closeness of their contact in his own way.

Autistic children often prefer to sit side by side with parents rather than facing them while they play together. When wary or apprehensive about a new situation, autistic children will sometimes circle, or pace, as if staying prepared for the type of "fight or flight" response that an animal on the alert might have. This wary circling may lead us into thinking an autistic or PDD child is hyperactive if he is just observed in a group setting like a classroom, although the same child may not be that way at all when left alone.

All of these differences in nonverbal aspects of social interaction can be observed in the preverbal autistic or PDD child. For the experienced clinician, they can be some of the best early indicators of autism, before the absence of speech or atypical development of spoken language can be fully assessed.

Range of Emotional Expression

Very early in development, babies begin to use tone of voice to convey different emotional states. Happy babies coo. Excited babies giggle and burble. Irritable babies make fussy noises and pout. Angry, frustrated babies scream and cry. These expressions on the part of the baby usually provoke characteristic reactions on the part of caregivers, who lend words to their babies' emotional expressions. A caregiver may mirror back the baby's expression to acknowledge that the baby's communicative attempt is being received by the adult. The sending and responding to such signals does not usually work quite the same way with autistic babies. One study showed how sounds made by young preverbal autistic children were more difficult for people not familiar with the child to interpret in terms of emotional content, and that the sounds these children made were more unusual and repetitive.

Autistic and PDD toddlers tend to operate with a diminished range of emotional expressions. Autistic children seem to have fewer moments when spontaneous emotional reactions cross their face. One qualitative way that autistic and PDD children may differ is that in some PDD children, emotions seem governed by an "open window" versus "closed window" phenomenon: PDD children show many fewer moments of emotional expression overall, but every now and then the "window" opens for some reason (often direct and familiar play with a caregiver), and for a few brief moments, emotional reactions appear much more normal. However, it seems that the child with PDD just can't sustain such contact. Nevertheless, these "open window" moments provide a different starting point for treatment than in the autistic child, who seems to lack comprehension of emotional expression altogether.

Quite often, parents note that it is the finer shades of emotional response that are missing—that the child's reaction goes to one extreme or the other. Often, it appears that autistic children express only two emotional poles: positive excitement and displeasure. Shades of positive emotions—anticipation versus satisfaction or a response to humor—seem lacking. Similarly, negative emotions such as anger versus frustration versus disgust also seem poorly differentiated. Emotional responses to pleasure often occur as a reaction to nonsocial rather than social stimulation. Usually delighting stimulation such as seeing a spinning top, or kinesthetic stimulation such as being tickled or bounced, may produce laughter more easily than a game of peek-a-boo.

Sometimes emotion (what clinicians call *affect*) is present, but not linked to any apparent situation. Some parents express concern because of a child who suddenly begins laughing or crying for no particular reason. This can even go on during sleep. Much of the time, autistic and PDD children express little emotion, even at times when other children would. For example, after working long and hard to complete a puzzle, an autistic child may not even crack a smile or look up at anyone. Sometimes, if the child does smile, he does it to himself rather than looking up and sharing his smile and his accomplishment with an adult who has been watching. This type of response detracts from the expected social meaning of a smile. The seeming lack of much positive emotional response to one's own successes adds to the impression often given by autistic or PDD toddlers that they are very intelligent because they look solemn and serious as they pursue their various activities.

I am often asked whether autistic children are more beautiful or handsome than other children. Autism certainly has no obvious identifying physical traits (dysmorphology) the way Down's syndrome does. Perhaps part of this impression of beauty comes from the lack of emotional expression on their faces. Autistic children constantly convey the same sort of feeling we get from non-autistic young children when they are sleeping and their faces are so beatific and calm.

Prosody or Tone of Voice

When an autistic child does talk, we often can detect another difference in the quality of the language—the tone of voice is unusual. Almost all autistic children with spoken language have an atypical tone of voice. Many PDD children do too, but a significant number of PDD children can have fairly normal-sounding speech. Sometimes the tone of voice used by autistic children has a flat, atonal sound that makes parents concerned that the child may have a hearing problem, because his voice sounds somewhat like a deaf child's. Sometimes, instead of the voice being flat, it is high-pitched and unmodulated. Sometimes speech is sing-songy, rising and falling rhythmically, rather than rising and falling according to the words that most need to be accentuated. This is probably because autistic children can't comprehend the additional (emotional) meaning that tone of voice imbues to what they are saying. It's also almost as if the autistic child is having to deal with two languages at once—a "language" of intonation and cadence, and a second language of content. The language of intonation and cadence expresses the emotionally laden part of the language, and this is precisely the type of information an autistic person has trouble understanding.

The best way I can relate personally to what it must be like for autistic children to try to comprehend prosody and word content at the same time comes from an experience I had in Beijing, China, while watching the English BBC news (picture and voice) broadcast in my foreign guests' hotel while there was a simultaneous Mandarin overdub. Even though I don't understand Mandarin, and can't even distinguish among its units of sound very well, it was very, very difficult for me to follow the English because of the simultaneous "noise" the Mandarin soundtrack introduced. Like an autistic child, I was having great difficulty understanding anything because I was being forced to listen to two languages at once. Many parents describe how their autistic children are drawn to the robotic synthesized voices on computers, or dialogue from children's movie videos that they watch over and over again. This may be because the tone of voice remains fixed with each piece of dialogue, no matter how many times you replay the videotape (and this probably helps comprehension). In everyday speech, we say the same word a little different each time, depending on the context. This very likely contributes to making language very difficult for the autistic child to decode. (In Chapter 12, we will talk about some treatment strategies to get past problems in prosody decoding and into better language comprehension.)

In most autistic children, tone of voice is consistently "off" in some way. In PDD children, there tends to be some interesting compensations that make prosody sound more normal, at least some of the time. For one thing, some speech may consist of "delayed echolalia," things the child has heard in the past. Delayed echolalia often reflects both the contact and prosody of what the child has heard in the past. The fact that in producing delayed echolalia, autistic and PDD children tend to memorize prosody and content together provides a major clue to the fact that these two channels of communication are received together as one unit of meaning. Since autistic children do not preceive prosody as a separate "channel" of information, they have difficulty extracting meaning from tone of voice alone.

Atypical Features of Language Content and Use

Onset of Language

There are a number of ways in which the language of autistic children is used differently from that of other children of the same age. In autistic children, the rate of early language development is almost always slow. In children with PDD, language may start out with little or no delay, but it doesn't take long until the use and content of the child's language begin to strike parents as unusual. In fact, it is the unusual quality of the language that is often a first indicator that something is atypical about development. When autistic or PDD children first begin to speak, parents often don't realize that something is wrong with the language because it seems more "creative" than the first words that older siblings used. For example, Simon, a little boy with PDD who did not speak at all until three and a half, used as his first words "sausage" and "bacon"—said perfectly clearly the first time he ever spoke. It almost goes without saying that these were his two favorite foods, and he spoke these words while watching them being prepared.

Some parents get the feeling that it is almost painful for the child to speak, because the child won't speak unless the situation gets very distressing. These children usually have a small speaking vocabulary, and when a word does come out, it is usually something like "More!" or "Stop it!"

Mutism

There is also a small number of autistic children who, although they are almost always mute, very occasionally (maybe once or twice a year) *do* say something. When you first hear parents report "talking" in a child that is obviously mute, you tend to be skeptical. But after you've heard about this phenomenon from many parents who are otherwise very reliable, you have to begin to wonder why it is that this small number of children have the capacity to speak but do so only very rarely. Much like the "window" described earlier which allows the child to express emotion for a brief and fleeting moment, it also seems there is a random window of opportunity (perhaps some type of neurological event) that happens (or doesn't happen) that allows otherwise mute autistic children to speak. One mother reported driving in her car with her sixteen-year-old daughter in the front seat and her mute nine-year-old autistic son, Sean, in the back. They heard: "It's a stop sign." Mother and daughter looked at each other and simultaneously realized that Sean was the only other person in the car! Another mother recalled taking her mute eighteen-year-old autistic daughter to a friend's house and being mortified when her daughter said "I don't like the damn furniture."

Depending on what studies are surveyed, about twenty-five to forty percent of autistic children are described as remaining mute throughout life, and never speak, or may speak only a few words or sounds that have communicative meaning that is mainly understood by them and familiar caregivers. These are usually the autistic children who also have moderate to severe mental retardation. Some autistic children who remain mute understand language fairly well, but some mute autistic children who are also very retarded can have persistent and significant problems with language understanding as well. While many autistic children are mute, not all mute children are autistic. Mute children who have severe expressive language disorders, or who are mentally retarded but not autistic, tend to compensate for lack of language with more than the usual amount of gesture in order to get their messages across. As we discussed earlier in this chapter, autistic and PDD children rarely use gestures or understand them.

If a child uses gestures to compensate for communication problems, it can be an important clue in differentiating among mute children who are autistic and mute children who have severe language problems. For example, we recently evaluated Deena, a six-year-old, for PDD but found instead that she had a severe expressive language disorder. While I was speaking with her mother, Deena approached me enthusiastically, babbling incoherently but with great emphasis in her voice, repeating several unintelligible "words" (or perhaps "phrases"). Her narration aparently had to do with an imaginary tea party, as she brought her mother, her grandmother, and myself tin teacups of Play-doh, indicating with her own cup that we should drink up.

Many fewer children with PDD remain mute. Children with PDD tend to have less cognitive impairment along with their autistic symptoms, and mutism is fairly well correlated with degree of mental retardation, meaning the more mental retardation that accompanies a particular case of autism, the more likely it is that the child will remain mute. With other non-autistic PDD (discussed in Chapter 1), such as childhood disintegrative disorder, children become mute after using language for a few years. Children with CDD tend to have fairly normal language for their level of development, but then lose some or all of it. (This is different however, from the 'developmental set back' of language in the twenty-five to thirty percent of autistic children who initially have single words and/or a few phrases which they lose before they are two to two-and-a-half years old.) Generally, autistic children who do not begin talking by age six remain mute. This may be especially true of autistic children who have already received significant amounts of appropriate language training by age six, and may be somewhat less true for those who received little or no language help before age six. (This is discussed further in Chapter 12 where we cover the development of language skills in autistic children.)

Language Loss

About one quarter of parents with autistic children report that their child initally seemed to develop language normally, only to stall, or lose it entirely, a few months later. There are the typical patterns of early language loss. In one, the child develops a small vocabulary, usually of ten to twenty words or short phrases, which then disappear entirely. The second pattern is one in which the child develops the same small number of words, but then vocabulary size seems to "plateau" rather than grow; and when new words are learned, old ones seem lost. Words a child might be expected to use daily, like "bottle," are heard perhaps only once a week or once a month. Typically, language loss begins around ages fifteen to twenty-two months and lasts several months or until speech therapy begins—or, in some cases, is permanent. Careful examination of the histories of some children with language loss suggests that other "developmental setbacks" may be occurring at the same time. These may include less eye contact, a decrease in sociability (such as the child suddenly not minding being left alone in his playpen when others leave the room), and a loss of interest in toys. This phenomenon is often described in the developmental histories of autistic children, but it is very poorly understood. Some parents link the change they see in their child to an illness (such as a high fever), some to an injury (for example, falling off a swing onto the head), some to an emotional trauma (for instance, the father leaving the home); some suspect physical or emotional abuse (they wonder whether the child was maltreated in day care); and some voice a concern that the child was pushed too hard developmentally (for example, by moving him from a crib to a bed too soon). Because parents offer such a range of explanations, it makes a clinician skeptical of any one of them—and turn to explanations that might be superordinate, such as a developmental failure of a neurological process, or activation of some sort of dormant virus. The pattern of early language loss and other developmental setbacks that may accompany it remains unexplained, but we do know that when it is experienced by children with autism or PDD, the language that re-emerges after the loss (or plateau) tends to be characteristically autistic in the ways that will now be explained.

Instrumental Language

There are two prominent features of autistic language that cut across all levels of language development. The first is the fact that autistic language is primarily "instrumental" rather than "expressive." The second is that most of the language is "elicited" rather than "spontaneous."

Autistic and PDD children use language primarily to get their needs met. Of course, we all use language to get our needs met, and little children probably spend more time trying to get others to meet their needs than older people do. What is meant by *instrumental* language is that the language is focused on provoking an action or obtaining an object that does something for the autistic child and that he wants right now. This includes declarative statements like "Go now!" or "Want sandwich!" or requests for particular toys.

Instrumental requests generally do not take into account whether it is appropriate or expeditious or polite to fulfill the request at a particular moment. For example, at a recent Autism Society meeting, I encountered Paul, a twenty-year-old man of normal intelligence with Asperger's syndrome who was there along with his mother, a long-time Autism Society stalwart. "Say hello to Dr. Siegel," his mother prompted. Paul shot me a fleeting glance, held out a limp hand, and intoned "Hello, Dr. Siegel . . . Go, now, Mom?" (Paul is sometimes more conversational than this, especially when the topic is the solar system, but a darkened auditorium, amid a crush of people, did not seem to Paul like a great place to hang out and chat.) For autistic people, chitchat in a casual setting like a group meeting is about as unpleasant and overstimulating to them as it might be for one of us if someone was talking while we were trying to pay attention to an absorbing movie in a theater. With conversation being this difficult to attend to, no wonder autistic children generally limit themselves to instrumental requests.

Immediate Echolalia

One of the hallmarks of autistic language is "echolalia." As the name implies, this is speech that consists of echoing back what the child has just heard. Although echolalia is very common in autistic children when they first begin to speak, it is also seen in children with severe receptive or expressive language disorders (sometimes also referred to as *aphasia* or *dysphasia*).

The reason that echolalia is used is because the child has poor comprehension of what is being said to him. In a way, it is as if you were in Spain with only some rusty high school Spanish at your command. You might muster your resources and formulate a sentence asking for directions to the train station. When given the response in Spanish, you might then find yourself repeating aloud what had just been said to you. This would do several things for you. It would give you a chance to let the words sink in. It would demonstrate to the person you are speaking with that you have received his "signal" and are actively trying to decode it. And it would give that person an opportunity to repeat or modify all or part of what he said to you in case you introduced any errors into his statement. So the echoing provides the speaker who has poor comprehension of the language a chance to digest meaning. If you were at a loss for other Spanish words, but thought you did comprehend enough to figure out in which direction to travel to find the train station, you might repeat part of what you were told a couple of times, and then just nod, smile, and point in what you thought was the direction of the train to see if you got further assent. You would in effect be using echolalia in the same way as the person with a severe receptive language disorder.

This process works a little less well for autistic children since a very social part of the communication—the ability to send or receive communicative gestures—is almost always significantly disabled. However, the echolalia still serves several compensatory uses: (1) it lets the listener know he has been heard, (2) it may indicate that the information is actively being decoded, (3) it may indicate agreement with what has been said, or (4) it may even indicate disagreement with what has been said if repeated in an agitated or upset voice. Parents usually come to understand the particular way their child uses echolalia, and try to respond accordingly. So, for example, a mother might say "Do you want more raviolis, Michael?" Then, Michael might excitedly reply ". . . want raviolis, Michael!" to indicate that he, indeed, very much wants more raviolis. Another child might use echolalia to indicate negation, for example, Martin, who would say, "Don't want no sandwiches!" whenever offered a disliked food. As long as he was with a caregiver who knew he disliked sandwiches, Martin's statement served to accurately convey his desire to refuse the offered food.

Pronoun Reversal. Years ago, when psychoanalysts still had some interest in studying autism, they made much of the way in which echolalia produced "pronomial reversal," meaning that autistic children seemingly confused pronouns for "I" and "you" and seemed always to refer to themselves in the third person rather than as "I." For example, a mother might say: "Do you want me to pick you up?" And the child might respond: ". . . me pick you up?" This was interpreted as an ego deficit, an inability to have a completely formed sense of self, an estrangement from one's own self. It was also seen as a failure to have complete boundaries between the child and (usually) the mother, since much of this strange echolalic speech was elicited by her as the primary caregiver.

Given what we know now, it is abundantly clear that echolalic speech is just that—echoing, which means that the child attempts to comprehend, but ends up with language coming out pretty much as it has gone in. As language comprehension grows and improves in the autistic or PDD child, personal pronouns remain a problem, not because of ego boundaries, but because they don't have a fixed, concrete meaning like nouns, which are more easily learned by autistic children.

Auditory Processing. The reason that autistic children usually go through a significant stage of echolalic language is that there are disproportionate rates of growth in certain cognitive abilities. The growth of auditory memory (memory of sounds that are heard) proceeds at a fairly normal rate, but the ability to comprehend lags behind. (Pure auditory memory matures earlier than memory of "digested" information.) It is pure auditory memory that allows us to memorize the words to little songs like "Frère Jacques" in French without being able to translate a single word. To compenste for lack of comprehension, autistic children at times naturally use their strengths—their auditory memories—to try and make up for their weaknesses and their inability to understand. This is what produces echolalia.

In normal language development, there is a certain amount of echoing that goes on too. Usually, it is limited to a few words at a time and is not the predominant mode of expressive speech. It also occurs at the same stage at which the child begins to initiate many things of his own to say. Normally, children can echo when they want to be part of the conversation but don't know what's going on. For example, a 22-month-old Lizzy who is definitely not autistic, was recently at my house while a football game was on. She was asked: "How about them '9ers?" She nodded and smiled ". . . the '9ers." Then, she was asked, "What do you think of the Eagles?" Again, she looked up from the TV, nodded and smiled ". . . the Eagles." This same type of "parrot" dialogue continued for another six or seven NFL football teams even though, as her mother pointed out, Lizzy didn't even know what a football was. Conversational use of echolalia is kind of like Peter Sellers' character of Chauncey Gardener in the movie, *Being There.* In the movie Peter Sellers' language is interpreted metaphorically rather than as a reflection of his lack of language understanding. Most parents figure out that echolalia is the child's attempt to communicate and understand by trial and error and learn to respond accordingly.

Delayed Echolalia

Delayed echolalia occurs when language that was heard sometime in the past is "played back." Delayed echolalia usually emerges later than immediate echolalia because it requires even more developed auditory memory. Some children who are classified as having PDD or Asperger's syndrome never go through a stage of immediate echolalia, but may go through a prolonged and quite elaborate period of delayed echolalia. There are two kinds of delayed echolalia—functional and nonfunctional.

Functional Delayed Echolalia. The presence of delayed echolalic language also highlights another kind of cognitive problem that autistic children have— breaking wholes into parts. Once a language segment is accquired whole in a particular context, where its meaning may be understood for that context, it can get overgeneralized. There is classic example of this in the writing of Leo Kanner, who first described autism: A boy's mother had shouted at him "Don't throw the dog off the balcony!" After that, the boy would say "don't throw the dog off the balcony" to indicate the word "No." Aaron, a four-year-old patient of mine, protested going to another playroom with the phrase "'No, no, I won't go,' said Thomas the Tank Engine." This was a passage from a favorite video of his.

Just as immediate echolalia has an anlogue in normal development, delayed echolalia has an analogue as well. Overgeneralized use of phrases usually happens with single words in the normal language development of one-and-a-half to two-year-olds, and is called *overextenstion*. For example, a baby may have a kitty at home, and at first refer to a kitty as "kitty," but then also refer to dogs and even cows as "kitty." Next, the baby may get the idea that there are little animals *and* big animals, all of which are either "kitties" or "cows," and finally, that among household animals, there are separate words for "kitties" and "doggies." PDD and autistic children who use delayed echolalia in lieu of more spontaneous words are also overextending the meaning of words.

Nonfunctional Echolalia. Sometimes PDD and autistic children produce delayed echolalia that has no apparent bearing on anything. Sometimes a favorite phrase can be repeated so many times that everyone around the child is driven to distraction. Probably the closest cognitive experience most of us have that is like nonfunctional delayed echolalia is when we hear a song on the radio in the morning, and then it sticks in our heads all day, silently playing itself back. It is hard for a person to predict what song might get stuck in his head, and when it will happen. The same seems to be true of what autistic children select. Like the parroting speech of immediate echolalia, the child usually does not comprehend all of what he is saying. The language *expression* becomes more advanced than the language *comprehension*. We know this because researchers have compared the segments of spontaneous (nonechoed) language spoken by autistic children to segments that are part of delayed echolalia routines, and they found that the spontaneous segments of language are much less sophisticated.

Interestingly, over the last few years, I've been seeing more cases of delayed echolalia developing at an early age. Why? With the advent of home VCRs and the relatively inexpensive cost of classic Disney and other children's movies, autistic children are watching the same movies over and over again. Typically, parents report that their child has one or two favorites that he has watched more times than anyone at home cares to count. Usually by the third showing of a video an autistic child will begin to memorize, recognize, or even anticipate certain segments. Over time, certain segments may become favorites, to be rewound and played, over and over. Woe be it to anyone who tries to interrupt this process! In Chapter 12 on language interventions, we'll discuss the relative benefits and drawbacks of letting young autistic children watch lots of videos repeatedly.

Idiosyncratic Word Use and Jargon

A topic that is closely related to the emergence of delayed echolalia is the presence of idiosyncratic word use or jargon. This is when a child acquires his own personal meaning for a word based on his own experience. The word or phrase is subsequently used irrespective of whether there seems to be a likelihood that the listener will know what the child is referring to. In young autistic children, sometimes meaningful communication is idiosyncratic use of delayed echolalia, as in the "No, no, I won't go . . ." example. Sometimes, however, an autistic child repeats a phrase he's heard just because it appeals to him. To know whether delayed echolalia is meaningful or not, you have to know the child's experience and where the phrase or word he is using originally came from. For example, Samuel, five-year-old boy with PDD, was disturbing his parents by constantly saying "Soon I will die and go to heaven." They even feared that Samuel might be suicidal. As they reported this to me, Samuel's second-grader sister, who was along for the appointment, interrupted: "I know why Sammy says that . . . they say that in the movie *All Good Dogs Go to Heaven.*" Indeed, it turned out that the family owned this video and that Samuel (and his sister) watched it frequently. In actuality, Sammy understood neither the concept of dying nor heaven, but picked up on the phrase, probably because of particular dramatic music when it was said, or because it was said in a tone of voice that interested him.

In adults with autistic spectrum disorders, some idiosyncratic word use can be quite clever, and the meaning apparent though not obvious to others with a different frame of reference. For example, Julie, a rather large woman with Asperger's syndrome, who was *very* interested in the biology of plants, came into one of our playrooms which was furnished with preschool-sized tables and chairs. Not being that eager to talk to me in the first place, Julie looked at the furniture and declared "I won't sit in those *zygote* chairs! I won't sit at that *fetus* table!" Because it is difficult for the autistic individual to take the perspective of another person, the use of such idiosyncratic language may not even strike them as unusual (and certainly not humorous) in any way.

Conversational Skill

In autistic teens and adults, the conversational use of language becomes theo-retically possible as enough vocabulary and syntax are acquired. However, the nature of the conversations tend to be characteristically unidimensional. After someone had helped Julie and me replace the zygote chairs with adult-size chairs, we began to talk. I found myself asking many, many questions about the growth of hanging houseplants to keep the conversation moving. (Julie was also interested in large tropical fish, but in the lobby, I had mistaken her pocketbook, which was shaped and painted exactly like a rainbow grouper, to be a parrotfish, and she wasn't eager to discuss fish with me anymore.) Some higher functioning autistic people and most people with Asperger's syndrome will talk about topics that interest them with just a little encouragement. This demeanor has sometimes been characterized as "active, but odd," and is different from that of higher functioning autistic people who simply won't converse at all. On topics that are not their 'special' topic, they are much more cursory (but usually accurate) in their responses. Interestingly, higher func-tioning people with autism, PDD, or Asperger's syndrome seldom lie, though they may not be open in disclosing information. Being able to lie convincingly also requires the "mind-reading" ability associated with a theory of mind—an ability that such individuals lack or have only to a very limited extent.

Language Pragmatics

The *language pragmatics* of autistic and PDD children are rather abnormal, even when the vocabulary and information about the world that is needed to converse is present. Abnormal language pragmatics means that, even though the content needed for conversation is there, there is little understanding of how to express what one may have to say. The first element of this is turn-taking—knowing if the listener is listening (and interested), knowing how much time to leave (or not leave) after the person talking with you has finished her turn, and knowing how and when to look at someone to signal that you know you are in a conversation together. Deficits in language pragmatics, taken out of the context of the rest of the symptoms of autism are sometimes referred to as a semantic-pragmatic deficit. Children who have just a semantic-pragmatic deficit tend to make up for their lack of words, or lack of understand-ing in how to use them, by using more nonverbal forms of communication.

By examining language pragmatics in nonverbal interactions, or even in one-word interactions, it is possible to detect emerging difficulties in the area of conversational ability even in toddlers. For example, at two years, when a child is still primarily communicating in single words and short phrases, there already is "conversation." Although the child's response may be mainly single words, the child can convey what is wanted, what the child sees, and how the child feels. Gestures and tone of voice are used to convey meaning as well as actual words. But few autistic and PDD children have such "conversations" even when their vocabularies are developed at this stage, and so this absence of conversational ability can be judged diagnostically, even in very young children.

Another aspect of language pragmatics is topic maintenance. In fully verbal, older autistic children and adults, it is almost impossible for them to realize when the listener has heard enough talk on one topic or when enough has *not* been said: Rules of topic maintenance also require that you say enough on a topic. For example, in asking an autistic person the question "Do you like coming to visit San Francisco?" the autistic person might reply "Yes." (Silence.) Of course, in response to that sort of question, the person being questioned would usually say something about *why* she likes San Francisco (if she did), all the while looking at the questioner to determine from nonverbal cues how much more information might be enough. So, even when adequate language for conversation is present, individuals with autistic spectrum disorders tend to choose not to elaborate unless the topic itself stimulates them in some idiosyncratic way.

Chapter Summary

Thus far we have examined the social and behavioral difficulties autistic and PDD children have, as well as how disabilities in social perception make it difficult to learn and implement language for the purposes of communication. In the next chapter, we focus on a third aspect of social impairments that are associated with diagnostic signs of autism and PDD—characteristic differences in the way the child plays and generally shows interest in his environment.

◆ ◆ ◆

CHAPTER 4

Autism, PDD, and the Child's Activities and Interests

Several aspects of how a child may observe and react to the world around him can give us a clue to whether that child has autism or PDD. The activities, interests, and responses of children to their environment comprise a third area that clinicians study to determine whether there are any difficulties associated with autism. We first looked at social development, and then language. Play is the third dimension of a triad of social impairments associated with autism. In this chapter, we discuss differences in how autistic children play with toys; how differently they react when excited, bored, or frustrated; and how they are different in the way that they develop particular narrow interests, routines, and rituals. Figure 5 shows the areas of interest and activities of autistic children that will be discussed in this chapter.

Play and Imagination

Parents who have had other children before their autistic child comes along almost always notice that their child does not play with toys in the usual way. They do not show interest in the same toys at the same stages of development. Some parents notice that the child simply doesn't seem interested in toys at all. When this happens to new parents, the parents sometimes feel that they have not bought developmentally appropriate toys, and go out and buy more; or they may think that the child is particularly bright, because he seems to become easily bored with new things. But as experienced parents realize, most infants and toddlers without developmental problems will find a way to play with almost anything.

Often the young autistic child plays relatively infrequently with either toys or other objects. He may wander around touching various things, but never really become engaged in anything for very long. Things that *are* picked up are often dropped soon after, seemingly without notice. Very young autistic children and autistic children with severe retardation seem to show this pattern

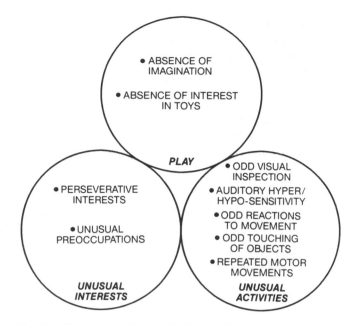

Figure 5   Development of play in children with autistic spectrum disorders.

most markedly. By contrast, young PDD children often show greater intensity of interest in objects, but tend to have a rather limited range of what catches their fancy, and the play itself quite often has certain hallmark characteristics.

Attachment Objects

Some young children with autism or PDD do develop a preference for a particular object, and occasionally that object *is* a toy. Usually, the object is not the typical cuddly toy, like a teddy bear or doll, that a normal child might choose. More often it is an object with some sensory characteristic that the child finds particularly appealing. Parents will report that their children carried around all sorts of things for weeks, sometimes months on end. One boy carried a Downy fabric softener bottle (presumably because of the smell); another a smooth wooden Russian Matrushka doll (perhaps because of its smooth surface); one boy favored a rubber corn-on-the-cob (again touch); one girl, a plastic Strawberry-Shortcake doll (perhaps because of its smell); and the most unusual object I can remember, a little boy carried around a butter knife which had a carrot on top of its blade (perhaps because it was visually stimulating). Even when an autistic child does select a fairly common attachment object like a teddy bear, parents can tell that the autistic or PDD child regards their "luvy" differently. For example, the little girl with the Strawberry-Shortcake doll would frequently smell it, but seldom look at its face. Another little girl, Cassie, carried a "My Little Pony" lunchbox everywhere full of "My

Little Ponies"—small hard-plastic iridescent horses. She would line them up, but never have them play with her, or with one another, or act out a story.

There are times when an object serves as a secure base for an autistic child. Sometimes so much so that it is preferred to the comfort offered by caregivers. Some autistic children have favorite blankets, usually one with something particularly nice to touch on it, like a silky edge. Like other young children, many young autistic children will want their blanket when distressed. Unlike most other young children, some young autistic children seem to want their blanket *more* than parents, and calm down more easily once they have their blanket and are left on their own to pull it over their heads and block out the world.

Why do autistic and PDD children tend to reject the most usual type of attachment objects like stuffed animals and dolls? For one thing, they seldom seem to recognize that stuffed animals or dolls resemble real animals or people. This may be an early indication that the child has not developed a "theory of mind," as discussed in the last two chapters. When "theory of mind" does not begin to develop at the expected time, we may see it as a failure to "read the mind" of a teddy bear and decide he might be hungry, too. Normally, nine- to ten-month-olds, and sometimes even younger babies, have this type of recognition of a teddy bear's "needs," and will cuddle a doll or teddy bear, or try to feed it some of what they themselves are eating. The absence of this development in autistic children is the forerunner of some of the difficulties they have later on in taking someone else's perspective or realizing that someone else's thoughts or feelings are like their own.

Sensory Play

The earliest form of play that infants and toddlers typically pursue is sensory (also called sensorimotor). It involves physical action on things in the environment. At an early stage, everything goes into the mouth. Autistic children often persist in this stage far longer than other children. One reason is that their development is often slower, and so they are slower to leave this stage. Second, autistic children tend to remain oriented by their senses, even after they develop more sophisticated means of exploring objects. Some researchers have suggested that whatever is neurologically wrong with autistic children causes them to pay too much attention to "proximal," or near, sensory information, such as taste and touch, and too little attention to "distal" senses, such as seeing and hearing things that are not right next to their eyes or mouth.

Perseveration

One thing that is often different about the sensory play of autistic children is its repetitiveness. This is often referred to as *perseveration.* Instead of pulling the string or handle on a talking, spinning "Speak 'N Say" toy five or six times, the autistic or PDD child may engage in such an activity for twenty minutes without stopping. At first, a parent may be impressed by the child's attention span, but after a while, a parent may also be frightened by the almost maniacal singlemindedness that characterizes how intensely the activity can be carried out. Sadly, I remember a videotape of a severely retarded autistic boy that was made two days before his death from an unrelated illness: Dwayne had always been quite perseveratively preoccupied with spinning tops and "Speak 'N Say" toys. Propped up in his hospital bed, the nurse handed him a "Speak 'N Say." Weakly, Dwayne grabbed for it, managed to pull the string a few times, watched the dial in the center of the toy spin, and then fell back exhausted.

Perseverative behaviors are not unique to autism and are found in other children with a variety of syndromes associated with mental retardation. The likelihood that an autistic child will develop some highly perseverative behavior is correlated with the degree of mental retardation—meaning the more mental retardation an autistic child has, the more likely perseverative behavior is. What is unique in autism is that the perseverative behavior is often sensory activity, especially when the child is young or still nonverbal. Once the child gets the urge to perseverate an activity, it can be very difficult to interrupt him or her. For the autistic child, being interrupted while engaged in a favorite perseverative activity can be like having someone switch off the TV at the most suspenseful part of a movie. The child tends to react with annoyance and anger and may not easily accept the finality of the interruption. In later chapters we'll discuss how to introduce limits on perseverative behaviors.

Preoccupation with Parts of Objects

Another aspect of the sensory play of autistic children is their tendency to become preoccupied with selective parts of objects and not to see the object as a whole, or more specifically, as something designed to have a particular purpose. For example, in our clinic, we have had generation after generation of "Speak 'N Say" toys, a perennial favorite among autistic children (as illustrated by the earlier example of Dwayne). These toys have a pull string that activates a spinning dial in the center of a round toy. The dial has an arrow that can be pointed at a particular animal, letter of the alphabet, etc. (depending on which model), and then the toy announces the name of the animal, letter, etc., in a mechanical voice. Many young autistic children only watch the pulled-out string retract into the "Speak 'N Say." Others only watch the dial spin. I'm not sure I ever saw anyone, other than a parent or staff member, set the dial to a particular animal or letter, which is how the child is supposed to use the toy. Instead the autistic child attends to just one feature of such a toy. Another example is a toy vacuum cleaner we have in our clinic. It lights up, makes a whirring noise, and colored styrofoam balls (representing dirt) jump around inside. Some autistic children put their ear to the toy vacuum and listen to the sound. Others flick the on-off switch and watch the light flicker. Others stare at the jumping balls. Almost no one pretends to vacuum with it (although normal preschoolers pretend to vacuum, and surprisingly, find it an attractive activity).

Concrete and Functional Play

The play of autistic and PDD children lacks the imagination other children display at the same level of mental development. Play allows children, even without language, to work through their attempts to understand things they see and hear about. That is why children whose parents have new babies at home often have a resurgent interest in baby dolls, why a child being potty-trained takes Pooh-Bear to the potty and remonstrates with him, and why Ninja Turtle action figures have sword fights. Very young autistic children seldom represent (reenact or play back) play they have seen in a way that would demonstrate that they understand the toy's function. PDD children sometimes display representation (for example, rolling a car along the floor), but little or no play that is not based on something they've already seen. The key difference between children with autism or PDD and other children is that when children with autism or PDD do play with toys, they do not add their own thoughts, feelings, or interpretations to what they have seen. As a generalization, we might say that autistic children usually lack both "reenacting" play as well as "spontaneously composed" play, whereas PDD children sometimes do reenact but, like autistic children, seldom add spontaneously composed themes to their play. Often, this reenacting type of play is essentially a form of *echopraxia*, meaning gestures are played back just as language is played back in delayed echolalia. Some researchers who study autistic play call this *playlalia*.

Playlalia. On the surface, playlalia can look the same as the play of other children the same age. For example, many two-year-old autistic children will "play telephone." They pick up the receiver and punch the buttons on a toy phone. Then they put the receiver down. Less often will you see the autistic two-year-old yammering, as if talking to someone. What is really never seen is successive "calls"—say to grandma, Big Bird, Barney, or the family dog. That type of elaboration on a play theme is beyond the scope of imagination of most autistic children. Instead, the physical actions, copied strictly from what has been observed in the past, is the "playlalia."

Sometimes playlalia is more subtle. The components of the play *are* initially made up by the child but don't get elaborated; instead, the play tends to get played out, over and over in an identical way, and ideas do not get linked and relinked in new ways as the play time progresses. A good example is Matthew, a rather bright autistic boy of five. He would gather all sorts of objects from around his house and configure a "dashboard" on the sofa. If he did this only once, we could call it imaginative. However, Matthew would become irate if anyone moved a single piece of his "dashboard," *and* if overnight, his parents put the pieces away, he would rebuild it exactly the same way, the next time he had a chance.

The Relationship Between Imagination and Language

There is a rather direct relationship between imagination and language. Imagination helps language to grow. Toddlers use what is sometimes referred to as "private speech." Basically, this means that they talk to themselves as they play. Typically, not all of this speech is clearly audible and not all is well articulated. When dedicated child linguists follow two- and three-year-olds around to get private speech samples, they find a jumble of phrases the child has heard, as well as the immature grammatical structures characteristic of the child's age. It is a child's opportunity for language rehearsal. It is not clear what drives private speech, but without private speech, the autistic or PDD child misses out on this opportunity to advance his development. Play and language do not drive one another: First, the inability to engage in varied play makes for a dry landscape of activities to attach the private speech to in the first place. Second, the absence of language ability means that language is not there to illustrate the play and to serve as a self-guidance system to creative further play. There are different theories regarding whether the primary deficit in autism is language of whether it has a social basis. Either way, we can see why there are joint difficulties in both language and play for autistic and PDD children. Normally, language and play grow off of one another. When both are impaired, they are likely to mutually inhibit the development of the other. In later chapters we'll discuss strategies for promoting language through play, and promoting play through language—depending on the one the child is naturally most advanced in.

The Need for Sameness: Insistence on Routines and Resistance to Change

One of the most striking features of autism, when it is present, is that the child can insist on peculiar routines and resist small, seemingly insignificant changes in his surroundings. While this behavior can seem puzzling and inexplicable, and is the stuff that TV specials on autisum abound in, it can be understood fairly easily if we consider the context of how the child with autism or PDD sees the world. The need for sameness is not present in all autistic individuals. It seems present more often in higher functioning autistic children and older autistic individuals compared to younger and more mentally retarded autistic individuals. At young ages, this cluster of signs can take very basic forms. Joseph, at 27 months, would tip over all the dining room chairs on their backs, and look at them for long periods of time. He'd become inordinately upset if his mother tried to right them. (Like Matthew-the-dashboard-builder's mom, she would wait until he went to sleep at night to reorganize the dining room.) Joseph's interest in positioning objects could be seen in other settings as well. He came to our clinic, found our toy vacuum, carefully positioned it upright in the middle of the room, and watched it in a prolonged manner, jumping and flapping his hands at it while he circled it. While he was doing this, and we were watching him through a one-way window, his occupational therapist arrived with a videotape of some puzzling behavior he said that Joseph showed at school. We discovered that the occupational therapist's room had the same kind of toy vacuum, and that Joseph engaged in an identical activity there. Most often, this insistence on having things arranged in an unusual way has an inexplicable origin. One autism researcher suggests that it may go back to when the object was first noticed, and that at that time, a fixed template emerged for how the object should fit with the rest of the world. The template, however, often seems to be one that is formed without being subjected to analysis of whether the "fit" is functional. For example, a parent may note that their autistic toddler always used to drink apple juice out of a blue plastic bottle, but now won't drink apple juice any more at all. Sometimes this sort of thing can be traced to an occasion where, for some reason, the usual blue bottle wasn't available and an attempt had been made to substitute a bottle of another color, for example, resulting in both the bottle and future apple juice being completely rejected. To most of us, what makes a baby bottle a baby bottle is that it is a container, and it has a nipple on top. For autistic children, however, it is more difficult to discern what may be seen as the main perceptual characteristics of things—for example, what makes a bottle a bottle. It may have been the "blueness" or the "plasticness" that caught the attention of the autistic child—features we know to be irrelevant. It may also have been that the blue plastic bottle was viewed as inseparable from the apple juice in some subtle way, in terms of its taste or color, and that when altered by a clear bottle or a glass bottle it became as repulsive as if you or I were made to drink apple juice mixed with milk. In this context, insisting on a blue plastic bottle makes a little more sense.

At an older or cognitively more sophisticated level of functioning, the autistic child's insistence on sameness can seem almost like an obsessive-compulsive disorder where an otherwise fairly normal person feels an uncontrollable urge to repeatedly check things and redo things because of an insecurity that something may go very wrong if that "something" is not done exactly right. One frequently mentioned example of this phenomenon in autistic children is the insistance on specific routes. Often, these can be walking or driving routes. One parent described how his four-year-old autistic son would go for a walk around the neighborhood with him each evening—always bending down to touch the ground in the same place, sitting briefly on the same benches encountered along the way, and always touching each streetlight pole he passed in the identical fashion. This little boy's routine was benign since taking a walk allows for stops and starts along the way, but other children have routines that, when not followed, can greatly disturb them or others. Bridget, an eight-year-old girl with PDD would insist on a certain route home each day. Her mother was well aware that attempts to stop or deviate from the route with Bridget in the car was asking for trouble. Nevertheless, one day, the choice was to stop at a gas station or run out of gas. Bridget screamed hysterically the entire duration of the stop—much to the embarrassment of her mother, who felt (probably correctly) that people were looking at her like she was some sort of childnapper. Another boy, Alan, who had been interested in maps since an early age, had been dubbed his family's "Roads" scholar by age nine, because he would take maps in the car and announce which way to turn next whenever they went on familiar trips from home.

While this type of insistence on routines or resistance to change in the familiar environment can have its intriguing (or annoying) aspects, it has some analogues to early normal development. Among normally developing children, very young children can become temporarily fearful if a familiar person changes drastically—if Daddy shaves off his beard or gets new glasses, or if Mom gets a radical haircut. Also, developmentally delayed children, who are *not* autistic, also tend to do better with a high degree of routine and structure in their lives. For children with moderate to severe mental retardation, as well as for most autistic and PDD children, the presence of day-to-day structure and routines usually is accompanied by a reduction in tantrums and an increase in compliance. This is because if you have limited ways of understanding what is going on around you and you don't have language that is proficient enough to ask questions, routine is reassuring and lends a predictability that minimizes the need to be on-the-alert and anxious about what may happen next. But while many children with developmental disabilities generally prefer routine, the thing that is particularly symptomatic of the insistence on routines in autism is that the preferred routines are characteristically ones with little or no functional value. Sometimes, the need for a routine is noticed because the child has great difficulty switching between equally functional ways of going about an activity. For example, an autistic child may protest severely if he is moved to a new place at the dinner table, or if he is bathed one night before dinner instead of after dinner.

Intense Interest in Unusual Activities of Objects

Of all the signs of autism, the one that has received the most attention in the media is the special interests and abilities that autistic people may show. Sometimes, the special abilities of autistic individuals are referred to as *splinter skills*, or as *islets of ability*. Sometimes, autistic individuals with marked talent in an area like drawing or music are referred to as *autistic savants*. These terms refer to the idea that it is possible for certain aspects of intelligence to develop unimpeded by the sources of brain dysfunction that have caused the autism. Like other signs of autism, having peculiar interests or abilities is a sign that not all children or adults with autism or PDD have. Some of the more elaborate interests or special abilities are found in the relatively small proportion of autistic people with little or no mental retardation accompanying their autism. Some of these special interests are discussed further in the section on Asperger's syndrome in Chapter 5. Like other symptoms of autism, having a tendency to focus on narrow, peculiar interests seems to follow some sort of developmental trajectory, becoming more complex in older children. For example, Brian, a ten-year-old autistic boy writes out pages and pages of calendar dates each day (for example, "Monday, December 5, 1994"). Jonathan, an eighteen-year-old autistic boy, likes to calculate in his head the day of the week on which December 5, 1994, would have fallen. In both cases, the attraction to the finite, concrete, absolute, and mathematical qualities of the calendar is the same.

In the young autistic child, the predilection for this sort of behavior is first seen in the tendency of the child to make his own sense out of an object rather than to naturally apprehend how others might think of using that object. For example, very commonly, many young autistic children start by lining things up to make long neat lines, or particular precise patterns with a variety of objects. Jonah, age twenty-six months, for example, loved to play with crayons according to his mother—but he never colored. When he came to see me, Jonah did indeed play with crayons for quite a long time. But instead of coloring with them, he lined them end to end, or arranged them in sunburst patterns. On a home videotape of eighteen-month-old Matthew's Christmas morning, his Mom and Dad urged him to unwrap presents. He was totally uninterested. Finally, from behind the camera, Dad said "Just leave him alone and let's see what he does." Little Matthew shoved and leaned against the big boxes, pushing them all into single line. From off camera, Matthew's mother can be heard saying "That's amazing! Look what he's doing! He's lining them up perfectly!" In these very tiny kids, the lining up of objects seems closely related to the search for certain kinds of sensory stimuli which we discussed earlier. Sometimes, when the line is complete, the child stares at it, gets excited, and flaps his arms or hands. There seems to be something very visually satisfying for them in seeing these precise fixed patterns. At other times, the tendency to show a perseverative interest in a particular class of objects leads to later adaptive behavior: Many two- and three-year-old autistic and PDD children love to line up the letters of the alphabet or numbers, and through this routine teach themselves to read and count at quite an early age.

As cognitive development progresses, the drive to obtain satisfaction from things that are precisely ordered or form a precise set seems to be satisfied more through mental activity than through something physically present, as is manifest in the lining up and arranging behaviors. The drive for mental orderliness and repetition is expressed as a tendency for rituals and routines in everyday activity. Some children develop an interest in a particular kind of object. The object, or class of objects, may initially be satisfying because it has certain perceptual characteristics, such as a shape or color that is attractive. For example, Alan (the "Roads" scholar, mentioned earlier), at age three and a half was fascinated with the round orange logo for Union 76 gas stations. He would point out Union 76 stations while in the car, insist on driving past them, and at home draw the Union 76 logo repeatedly. As he got older, he became more generally interested in street signs. I recently saw him (he's now nine), and we played with blocks and built street signs (at his initiation), and he asked me my favorite intersection. In further discussion about road signs, I was almost able to accurately recall the name of the main road in his town—El Cerrito Boulevard, but called it El Cerrito Road instead, and this was very unsatisfactory to him. Whatever it is that drives these interests, there is an absolute concreteness to it in which being close gets you no cigar. As Alan gets older, we might expect he'll become interested in world maps and perhaps geography. Often with higher functioning autistic and PDD adults, it is possible to trace a special interest back for years, through earlier stages of cognitive development. The earliest interest I have been told about was David's, age seven, who was fascinated by fireplace accessories. His parents trace his interest in fireplaces back to when he was six months old, when he would creep and roll himself toward the fireplace when he was placed on the livingroom floor. As proof of this early fascination, David's parents have photos of him as a baby, next to the hearth which was blockaded with pillows so the baby wouldn't roll into the bricks and hurt himself.

In autistic people with high levels of cognitive development, we often see a special interest that involves quantification. Naturally, numbers and mathematics are a big attraction. However, there is typically a rote and repetitive quality to the pastime that is intrinsic to the satisfaction it provides. This is the case with Brian who was described earlier, who is currently writing out all the days of the week and dates for every day since January 1, 1900. His father said Brian's in the 1930s now and works on his project a little most days after school. On IQ testing, Brian comes out about average. He is capable of doing more with numbers than this, but this is the type of activity he is drawn to and selects.

Sometimes it can be difficult to assess how narrow or exclusive a child's interests are, and whether the interests do in fact have the intense and unusual quality that would be supportive of a diagnosis of autism. For example, many higher functioning autistic boys that I now see are rather exclusively interested in Nintendo. Despite the fact that they show no interest in learning to read, for example, or any other organized instructional activity in school, such children may be able to play Super Mario Brothers II until the end of the game, when the little Egyptians come out and dance. Jefferson, a six-year-old boy with PDD, began to play Nintendo so obsessively that he would refuse to stop for meals, wet his pants (although toilet trained), and developed a blister on his thumbs from operating the joystick. Severe screaming tantrums lasting up to two hours would result when his mother would finally unplug the Nintendo and lock it in a closet. Of course, many otherwise quite normal seven- to twelve-year-old boys can be quite insistent about Super Mario Brothers II, too. The point is that these autistic special interests have a more obsessive and insistent quality than they do for normally developing children. As parents and professionals working with such autistic and PDD children, our challenge is to transform the "special interest" into a functional, useful activity or learning strategy.

Unusual Motor Movements and
"Self-Stimulatory" Behaviors

Many, though not all, autistic children display repetitive motor movements of some kind or other; these frequent, almost mechanical repetitions of the same posture or movement are called *stereotypies*. Presence or absence of these stereotypies (also referred to as stereotyped motor movements) does not mean the child does or does not have autism. In some children, stereotyped repetitive motor movements are transitory and minor, lasting only a few years during early development; in other children, they develop into lifelong patterns that are in evidence for hours each day. Stereotyped motor movement includes waving the hands or arms repetitively (called flapping), toe walking, tensing, rocking, head-banging, and other patterns of repetitive movements. This section will explain what motor movements are most specifically characteristic of autism and what our understanding is of why autistic and PDD children sometimes do these things.

Sometimes parents notice stereotyped motor movements without, at first, realizing the behavior is atypical. At first, it may seem like the child is just doing something to show his or her babyish form of excitement such as waving arms up and down, or dancing from foot to foot on tip-toes. The parents of two-year-old Laurel called the tip-toe dancing their daughter did her "happy feet." After a while, some parents get the sense that the child is showing these same exact physical expressions of excitation a little too frequently, or in precisely the same (and unusual) context each time. Laurel, for example, would show "happy feet" each time she saw a cascade of water falling from the roof gutter onto the backyard deck. It was at this point that Laurel's parents became concerned that the "happy feet" might be part of some neurological problem. Sometimes before parents are consciously aware that there is something unusual in their child's movements, a doctor, teacher, or more experienced parent may notice the stereotypy as a problem, because they don't see it as having an "explanation" the way the parents do.

There is no fixed time by which an autistic child will absolutely develop motor stereotypies or not. There are, however, some general developmental patterns to the emergence of different motor stereotypies, and they'll be described in the order that they are most often first in evidence. First, though, we'll examine why autistic and PDD children sometimes develop these motor stereotypies.

What Function Do Stereotyped Motor Movements Serve?

Like many of the other signs of autism that have been described thus far, stereotyped motor movements often seem to serve as a response or reaction to difficulties that the child has in properly regulating the perceived intensity of different types of sensory stimulation. When sensory or social stimulation is too intense, some sort of overflow tends to occur. In normal development it's easy to think of this in terms of some newborn babies who quickly overflow and cry out as soon as they feel a little hungry or uncomfortable in some other way. However, we also know that some babies are born mellower than others, and that from the first day of birth, it takes more to get some babies to cry. Most babies, though, develop more tolerance with time, and by the end of the first year, you see a lot less crying than at the beginning of the first year. Like crying, stereotyped motor movements *also* are a way of indicating overflow. The critical difference here may be that the innate mechanisms that allow the baby or child to tolerate certain levels and kinds of stimulation without feeling overwhelmed are not functioning properly in the child with autism or PDD.

This type of overflow problem is not unique to autism, but is in fact present in many infants and toddlers who are still neurologically not well organized. Mentally retarded children with motor stereotypies constitute one of the largest categories of inaccurate referrals to our clinic because they too are neurologically not well organized. However, as autistic children get to be about three or four years old their motor stereotypies (as well as other difficulties) become more specifically associated with autism and include complex repeated patterns of arm movements or pacing as well as flapping and tensing associated with close visual inspection of certain objects.

Repetitive Movements as Self-Regulation of Arousal. In addition to stereotyped motor movements serving as a possible overflow response, there is some evidence that they also can function as a way of self-regulating the level of auditory, visual, or motor stimulation the child perceives as most pleasurable. In the 1960s when transcendental meditation was popular, people were encouraged to chant "O-o-o-o-m-m-m" to reach a state of consciousness where one could become relaxed through a significant reduction in the amount of stimulation entering conscious awareness. It seems that, at times, autistic children engage in repetitive behaviors for the same purposes. Some autistic children will carry out stereotyped movements even when there are no apparent demands being made on them, and even when there is no increasing level of sensory input. At these times, the stereotyped movements are the main focus of activity and appear to be quite pleasurable to the autistic child. While engaged in prolonged periods of stereotyped motor movements, like rocking or hand-flapping, the rhythmicity seems to serve the purpose of shutting down access to other forms of stimulation. Thus it is usually more difficult to get the attention of an autistic child who is rocking or flapping in this manner, than one who is not. While this type of activity may be pleasurable to the child at the time, it is cutting him off from possible participation in other activities that could potentially be more meaningful. For this reason, such behaviors are often called "self-stimulation"—or in some of the treatment literature, "self-stims" for short.

It should be emphasized that not all autistic children and even fewer PDD children have stereotyped motor movements. Despite the TV documentary prototype of the furiously rocking autistic child, there are relatively few who rock furiously. Many children develop only a mild form of such movements or display them as a transitory activity in toddlerhood.

Earliest Emerging Movement Disturbances. Often, rocking is one of the earliest forms of stereotyped motor movement parents recall when they look back at the early development of their child. Sometimes the baby will have rocked a great deal on all fours from the point when crawling was about to begin. Other babies rock back and forth in their cribs as a prelude to falling asleep. For other autistic babies, rocking begins with walking, when the child begins to do stiff-legged rocking from foot to foot, either on his own, or when the general level of environmental stimulation begins to rise (for example, when noise increases to an uncomfortable level, when in a new place, or when among strangers). Interestingly, many parents will note that their autistic child's sibling did a lot of rocking too as a toddler, or that they themselves rocked, or *their* siblings did as children. It does seem that many individuals who rocked as children grow up normally. Whether this is something that may be genetically related to autism, or is just a very common trait in the population, has not, as far as I know, been specifically studied—although parents understandably ask about this.

Another early movement disturbance that usually starts early is toe-walking. As the label implies, the child walks up on the balls of his or her feet as if wearing invisible high-heeled shoes. Usually toe-walking begins around the time the baby first starts to walk, and can be fairly persistent through the first three or four years. Many autistic and PDD children only toe-walk when excited, but some do it almost constantly. Like rocking or head-banging, toe-walking is not unique to autism, and in one recent study, we found that only about twenty-five percent of autistic babies had toe-walked, but over fifty percent of non-autistic children who had been preemies did as well. Many of the young autistic toe-walkers we see also have an extreme aversion to wearing shoes, because it makes the toe-walking more difficult, and they can be very clever and very fast at getting their shoes and socks off. Often autistic and PDD children who toe-walk subsequently develop other motor stereotypies as well.

In addition to rocking and toe-walking, some autistic babies and toddlers bang their head, although this is not nearly as common a symptom as rocking. Only a tiny proportion of autistic children ever head-bang, and if they aren't head-banging by the time they start to talk or hand-lead (and thus able to relieve frustration by some form of communication), it is highly unlikely they will ever develop head-banging.

There seem to be two types of head-banging. When head-banging starts very early, it often takes the form of fairly gentle, almost exploratory, banging of the top of the head or forehead against various surfaces. And some babies do bang the backs of their head, especially when upright. In these instances, the head-banging seems to be almost a form of sensory exploration, as if the baby is checking out how hard the object is, wondering what sound the banging will make, or taking note of how it makes his head feel. Some gentle head-banging is probably a form of desirable movement stimulation, akin to swinging on a swing, or riding a rocking horse—which such a child may also enjoy. The second type of head-banging gets reported more often—either because it's more frequent or more of a problem, or both. Autistic toddlers sometimes get into the pattern of head-banging when frustrated or overwhelmed. This can be a reaction to the child's desire for something to be done a certain way, or at a particular time, and the child is frustrated because his desire remains un-fulfilled. Sometimes the parent is carefully trying to avoid the head-banging tantrum by agreeing to the child's wishes, and sometimes the parent is just a helpless onlooker with no idea of what is bothering the child. Head-banging definitely *has* a powerful effect on parents, who try hard to stop it and worry that the child will hurt himself. Angry autistic toddlers will bang their heads on wood floors and even concrete and *do* have to be stopped. Usually the tod-dler's head-banging ceases once the child is able to establish some form of communication.

A number of years ago, as a graduate student in a class given by Dr. Bruno Bettleheim, I tried to discuss head-banging with him as my way of highlighting the neurological aspects of autism. He told me, after two months of Socratic torture, that the real reason autistic children bang their heads is that "it feels so good when they stop." There really is little support for that hypothesis. Instead, as we will discuss later, some autistic and PDD children, especially when younger, have a diminished perception of pain, and that, coupled with head-banging, can make for a dangerous combination because there is no natural feedback of a pain sensation telling them to stop. One theory about head-banging in autistic children suggests that they have a sort of anesthesia for pain perception, and that therefore the negative (emotional) aspects of pain are not perceived. Instead, the autistic child may have the same sort of percep-tion that an adult would have from pinching his lip after having Novocaine for some dental work. Just as playing with a numb lip can result in a sore lip when the anesthetic wears off, autistic children may have a similar morbid fascina-tion with finding their pain threshold. As with other kinds of information processing we have discussed, an autistic child's ability to perceive pain seems yet another sensory area where the perceptual "volume" is poorly adjusted.

Head-Banging as a Self-Injurious Behavior. There is a *very* small number of older autistic children, particularly some of the adolescents in the moderately to severely retarded range, who begin self-injurious head-banging around ten to fifteen years of age. The origin of self-injurious head-banging is not well understood, although the hormonal changes associated with puberty are prob-ably contributory. When adolescent autistic children head-bang, it may be when they are frustrated, for the same reason it occurs in the two-year-old autistic child; or it may be more spontaneous with no real noticeable "cause." Some have suggested the possibility that head-banging is an attempt to self-treat a migraine or other serious headache. On a number of occasions, older, higher functioning autistic people have been able to describe things like "lightning in my head" or "exploding bombs." Sometimes caregivers notice an increased photosensitivity or other signs that might support the presence of migraine. When head-banging becomes self-injurious in older autistic children, *which is very rare,* it needs to be taken seriously and often treated with special medications designed to reduce self-injurious behaviors; a very few autistic children will bang hard enough to cause bleeding foreheads, nosebleeds, and bleeding inside their skulls.

Other Self-Injurious Behaviors. There are a few other self-injurious behaviors (sometimes called SIBs) that appear very occasionally in autistic children, particularly in autistic children with low IQs. Of these the most common is hand-biting. Characteristically, autistic children who hand-bite do it about one third of the way up from the wrist on the inside of the lower arm, or below the index finger near the intersection with the thumb. (I have often wanted to check out these specific points with an acupuncturist or acupressurist, to see if there may be some underlying neurological basis of the biting, but haven't pursued this conjecture yet.) Hand-biting seldom draws blood, but sometimes results in a callous on the arm or hand if biting is unremitting for a substantial period of time. Hand-biting generally responds well to behavioral treatments, and it's my clinical impression that there is a lot less hand-biting now than twenty years ago, when behavioral methods and training in early communication skills were not frequently implemented or well understood. This supports our understanding that SIBs are often the result of frustration and lack of communication skills. Other SIBs seen in autistic children can include hitting the side of the head or repetitive scratching of certain parts of the body. Brady, a seven-year-old autistic boy, developed a pattern of hitting the side of his head and pulling his ear. He eventually ripped off some of his outer ear tissue and caused a partial hearing loss through his actions. This degree of self-injury is very unusual and occurred, I believe, because those involved in his treatment persisted in using behavioral treatments exclusively for the SIBs, resisting our suggestions that a medication specific for self-assaultive behavior be tried. (There will be further discussion of SIBs and psychopharmacological treatments of them in Chapter 14.)

SIBs are frightening behaviors. Because of this, some parents naturally fear their children will develop them once they've seen some other signs of autism. Unfortunately, this fear is played upon by the media, and many television programs on autism (which form the basis of what most people know about autism until they have an autistic child) tend to overemphasize SIBs *because* they are so dramatic and frightening. Therefore, it's important to state here, again, that these behaviors are rare—only a very small number of autistic children (probably less than five percent) ever develop any of them—and they are largely quite treatable. It is even more rare to see SIBs in autistic or PDD children who are not also moderately to profoundly mentally retarded.

Hand Regard and Flapping. In the autistic child's second year of life, his or her parents sometimes begin to report that their child stares fixedly at things. All babies can be somewhat mesmerized by a spinning top, but autistic babies can become fixated to an extent that their parents may find disturbing. The autistic baby's attention span for seeing the top spun and re-spun may seem endless. A similar fascination with light or movement, such as watching telephone poles go by while in the car or staring out the window at tree branches moving in the wind, may be noted. (We have some ornamental hazelnut trees with peculiarly fine and twisted branches outside the windows of our clinic. Often we have to close the window shades to reduce the significant degree of distraction this causes to some of the autistic children we see.) Sometimes the autistic or PDD toddler will be seen holding out his hand and staring at it fixedly, or moving it side to side, or front to back. After a short period, this *hand regard* tends to develop into what is called *flapping.* Some children hand or finger flap; others arm flap; many do both. Finger-flapping consists of rapdily waving the fingers, usually in response to something very exciting. Some children just flick one or two fingers so that it looks like a nervous twitch. Hand-flapping is when the whole hand is flapped at the wrist, usually with the fingers loose. When finger-flapping or hand-flapping occur alone, the arms are usually held rigid, elbows bent tightly upward, or elbows locked and fully extended. Arm-flapping (some call it arm-waving) refers to flapping of the whole arm—either the lower part, or the lower and upper parts together. Once you've seen autistic or PDD children do this a couple of times, you recognize it when you see it again. In fact, many parents think flapping is a peculiar habit their child has developed and are surprised that when the child starts a special school there are two or three other children in the class doing the very same thing. Conversely, when flapping first appears in a two- or three-year-old already attending school, parents often ask me if he has learned this "bad habit" from imitating another child in the class whom the parent previously observed flapping. The answer is basically "No." Flapping is a neurological sign of the brain dysfunction that underlies autism and PDD. Either you have this propensity from birth or not. While certain types of environmental stimulation tend to make flapping more pronounced, there are also effective ways to correct this dysfunctional behavior (see Chapter 11).

Later Complex Motor Rituals and Mannerisms

Sometimes as autistic children get older, they develop more complex, unique patterns of motor movements. These can be behaviors of short duration, like the uttering of a particular sound, extending the neck in a peculiar way, or waving the arms around as if signaling an unseen person with a particular message. Some grow complex, such as one fifteen-year-old boy who would reach his hand down the front of his pants for a second and then proceed to reach down the neck of his shirt. Even though this young man had a well above average IQ, and knew other students saw his behavior as "weird," he could not/would not stop doing it. There are as many different forms of these motor stereotypies as children who have them. Like some of the other motor stereo-typies that have already been described, these behaviors often seem to fulfill a self-stimulatory function. Because they can sometimes occur seemingly without cause, however, they are often first suspected to be evidence of seizures or motor tics. Careful observation and evaluation, and sometimes neurological testing, may be needed to rule out a neurological and uncontrollable event. A tic or seizure won't respond to behavioral interventions, but self-stimulatory behavior will. In a child who clearly meets all of the diagnostic criteria for autism or PDD, these brief oft-repeated motor stereotypies are more likely to be self-stimulatory than they are to be tics or seizures, although it is usually worthwhile to get an experienced professional's opinion on the matter. When seizures or another movement disorder is suspected, a neurologist or movement disorder specialist should be consulted. Odd patterns of movement can also be the result of side effects of certain psychoactive medications used in the treatment of autistic children (see Chapter 14).

Autistic teenagers, and adults particularly, sometimes develop very complex motor rituals. Most often, these complex patterns are seen among the more mentally retarded in the autistic population. Some of these rituals, like the brief motor stereotypies seem to be self-stimulatory. When autistic individuals are left alone for a free play period in our clinic observation room, we have seen a number of amazingly complex examples of these motor rituals. For example, one young man, Jim, paced in an exact square, executing a complex hand gesture each time he arrived at the fourth corner. Other children with complex motor rituals look like they are dancing some new dance, only you can't hear the music. Often complex motor rituals feed off themselves, and their pace picks up as the person engaged in the ritual becomes more involved in it.

Other complex motor rituals are more akin to what might, on the surface, be described as an *obsessive-compulsive disorder* (OCD) in a person without any of the symptoms of autism. Complex motor rituals that border on the features of OCD are often seen in higher functioning individuals with PDD, perhaps even more often than in individuals with the full syndrome of autism. The difference between a complex motor ritual in a person with PDD or autism and an obsessive-compulsive ritual in a non-autistic person is that the PDD or autistic person usually appears quite content when engaged in his ritual, while a person with obsessive-compulsive disorder most often feels oppressed by the need to engage in the repetitive behavior. For example, Phyllis, a twenty-eight-year-old autistic woman, had rituals that involved her purse. Each time she sat down, she would move its long strap over her shoulder diagonally in a certain fashion, and then line up the purse on her lap very evenly. If the strap or purse placement wasn't right, or became misaligned during attempts at conversing with her, all else would cease while purse placement resumed. It bothered the examiner, but not Phyllis, that purse placement frequently had to be attended to. Occasionally, higher functioning autistic people will develop symptoms of OCD that really are OCD and not just complex motor rituals: Tom, a twenty-two-year-old autistic man with an IQ in the 120s, had many very time-consuming motor rituals. Before sitting on a chair, Tom would have to touch its sides, back, and the seat in a certain way. If, for some reason, he felt he had not done this just so, he would immediately do it again, however many times it took until he got it "right." When arriving home, he had to walk up the front path a certain way—stepping certain places and not others, again, until he got it "right." Unlike a classic example of someone with OCD, Tom was not able to articulate *why* he couldn't stop doing these things, but the longer he would try to get something "right," the more agitated he would become.

Most motor rituals and the OCD traits that autistic children display are remediable using behavior therapy methods (which will be discussed in Chapter 11). Like other, related symptoms of autism, motor rituals are not present in all autistic children. Motor stereotypies of some sort are found in the majority of autistic and PDD children at some time in their lives, but a very small number develop complex motor rituals or OCD traits.

Maladaptations to Input from the Senses

One of the most basic problems that many autistic children have, and a problem that parents may notice the earliest, is overreactivity or underreactivity of the senses. Some researchers have suggested that problems in dealing with sensory information may even be the primary abnormality that results in the rest of the symptoms of autism. (However, until we have a better idea of the exact location and type(s) of structural brain abnormalities associated with autism, we won't really know if sensory processing abnormalities *are* the primary problem.) Many autistic and PDD children show difficulties in reacting either too much, or too little, to things that are seen, heard, touched, and that move. Various sorts of sensory stimuli seem either overmodulated or undermodulated, and these sensory maladaptations take a few characteristic forms.

Auditory Hypersensitivity and Hyposensitivity. One of the first things parents may notice about their autistic child is that she doesn't respond to sound in the usual way. The cumulative observations about the child's hearing may appear puzzling: There appears to be selective hearing. On one hand, there may be some concern that the child has a hearing loss, because she doesn't respond to her name being called, to people talking to her in "baby talk," or sometimes even to loud sounds staged just in back of her to informally test hearing. On the other hand, a specific jingle on TV, the sound of the back door being opened, or the sound of water running into the bathtub may get a clear response from the child. Since many young autistic children (and many young children in general) have chronic and recurring ear infections, this "selective hearing" may be blamed on blockages due to fluid in the ears. If ear infections *are* a concern, then a hearing test is usually given, which can verify the fact that the child does hear. (More about diagnostic testsing, especially tests for hearing loss, in Chapter 5.) Although the child really *is* hearing, he seems to be blocking out much of what is said, as effectively as most people can block out the sound of an air conditioner in a room in which they are sitting and talking to someone. When autistic and PDD children seem to block out sounds that other children readily attend to, the phenomenon is referred to as *auditory hyposensitivity.*

On the other hand, a number of the very young autistic children who attend poorly to speech sounds appear more interested in nonspeech sounds. Sometimes the earliest sounds attended to and imitated are vacuum cleaners, fire trucks, and garbage disposals. However, in other autistic children, these same sounds may be perceived as unusually offensive. The observation that certain sounds *are* offensive can be surmised by the fact that some children will scream or cover their ears every time the sound occurs. These reactions seem to be idiosyncratic to a given child. Some autistic children are hypersensitive to low sounds (like the vacuum or garbage disposal), while others are set off by higher pitched sounds such as the cry of a particular baby. (On more than one occasion, I have had mothers tell me that they have been asked to take their child out of a day-care arrangement because their child screamed and threw terrible tantrums whenever a particular baby cried. It is an even more difficult situation when the offending baby is the autistic child's own baby sibling.) As autistic children grow up, some discover that covering their ears works not only as a portable soundproof barrier to offensive sounds, but can also help create a buffer between themselves and new unfamiliar things they don't want to pay attention to. Later we'll discuss methods for structuring the environment around the child in a way that minimizes his need to cover his ears or use other avoidance behaviors.

Visual Regard. Another form of sensory regulation gone awry is visual regard that is intent and persistent. This takes the form of the child picking out a specific object, or more often a class of similar objects, to stare at and visually inspect repeatedly in an intent manner. As with the presence of auditory hyposensitivity, parents who first notice their child holding an object close to his eyes and scrutinizing it carefully may have the impression that the child has poor vision. However, as with the observations about selective hearing, the parents remain unconvinced that the child *really* can't see well because they've also noted that their child can spot and grab an errant M&M on the coffee table while running by it. Usually a vision test by the pediatrician rules out low vision definitively.

There are a few very characteristic forms that visual regard (or visual detail scrutiny, as it is sometimes called) can take. Many children are attracted to objects with a strong horizontal axis such as twigs, pens, chopsticks, or bits of toys with horizontal characteristics such as Lincoln Logs. Another type of preferred object for visual regard is something that can be wiggled, such as a long loose and flexible string, belt, rubber band, or blade of grass. Typically the object is held at a fixed distance from the face. Some children hold objects quite close, others at arm's length. A number prefer to hold the object on the periphery of their visual fields (generating the hypothesis of partial blindness). During a period of fixed staring, the child may shake the object or keep it still; in either case, she becomes quite transfixed. After a period of staring, the child may appear clearly excited by the activity, which is demonstrated by some motor behavior such as flapping the hand that is not holding the object, toe-walking, or tensing the whole body. Sometimes parents worry if this might be a kind of seizure. There is no evidence that it is, and this type of behavior, when it is present, does not go away with the administration of antiseizure medications.

The Proximal (Near) Senses: Touch, Taste, and Smell. Just as a child may become fixated visually, a child may become fixated by the tactile qualities of an object, (sometimes referred to as *tactile detail scrutiny*). Smooth objects are often preferred, including satin blanket edges, nylon stockings, or smooth wooden surfaces. A preference for something like a satiny-edged blanket may seem pretty normal for a child under four, but this behavior begins to bother parents as the child grows older and the blanket becomes a decrepit shred that must nevertheless go everywhere with the child. Most objects of tactile scrutiny are not carried about as attachment objects the way a teddy bear is, but are appreciated as a part of an object that has one particularly attractive dimension—a heating grate with a repetitive pattern to the grill, a textured carpet, a chain-link fence, and so on.

For other children, the important channel for repeated sensory stimulation can be taste. Justin, age four, carries around a barely recognizable stuffed kitty whose limbs and nose have been chewed on for quite a long time. Other autistic children repeatedly put gravel, twigs, or leaves in their mouths. Sometimes there is a question of whether such children should be diagnosed as having *pica,* a condition where various nonfood items are indiscriminately eaten. While, on the surface, the autistic child's behavior looks like pica, the autistic child's objects are usually tasted but not eaten. Other autistic children will develop a mannerism of checking out new objects by tapping them against their teeth or lips.

Still other autistic and PDD children become fixated by smell. They can be observed smelling almost anything much the way another child who is not autistic might touch a new object to explore it. Most often, abnormalities of proximal sensory processing are seen in young children with autism and PDD as well as those children with moderate to severe mental retardation, and less often as the children grow older, and less often in those with initially higher IQs.

Overreactivity to Movement. Just as some parents notice that their autistic child is overreactive or underreactive to certain sounds and sights, there is a similar phenomenon with respect to movement. (Sometimes, responses to movement are referred to as "vestibular" responses.) Some autistic or PDD children seem to love certain forms of stimulation they receive from movement, while others have a similarly strong reaction that takes the form of hating and fearing it. Some autistic children may love one type of vestibular stimulation like swinging, but fear another form, like escalators. Young autistic and PDD children will often participate most willingly in activities that include a lot of movement, like jumping on a bed with a sibling, chasing, or wrestling and being tickled. They are drawn to swings, merry-go-rounds, rocking horses and trampolines, elevators and escalators. Parents often ask if it's bad to let their autistic child receive "too much" vestibular stimulation. There are two answers to that question. One, it *is* too much if it attenuates the child's opportunities to be learning through doing other things as well. Two, highly desirable movement stimulation (like going on a little exercise trampoline) can be saved as a "reward" to be used after the child does some other activities he needs to be learning; or movement stimulation can be incorporated into teaching to make learning a more positive experience, as we will discuss in Chapter 11.

Elijah, age ten, once clearly illustrated how obtaining movement stimulation can be its own reward: On one occasion, Elijah, a consummate autistic escape artist, ran away from our inpatient unit at Children's Hospital at Stanford. Needless to say this caused extreme panic among the staff. Where did he go? He walked across the street to the shopping center he knew well. He was observed by a plainclothes security guard, acting odd and wearing a hospital ID bracelet, and repeatedly riding the three-story escalator in a Nordstrom department store. After the incident, I tried to explain to some of the unit's staff that he was not so much running *away* from the hospital, as running *to* the escalator.

Another type of physical sensation that some autistic children crave is deep pressure stimulation. This is the type of sensation one experiences with a massage. The difference with autistic children is that they are often not comfortable if the deep pressure is delivered by someone other than themselves; or unless they can control when the contact (say, from the mother) starts and stops. Some autistic children like to be squeezed between sofa cushions or gym mats. Temple Grandin, a high-functioning individual with PDD, who has co-authored a book entitled *Emergence* about her experiences growing up, developed a "squeeze machine" that allows autistic people to give themselves deep pressure stimulation through a mechanical device they can control themselves. She developed this idea after watching cattle go through cattle chutes in a stockyard.

Some autistic people react to movement stimulation with great apprehension—refusing to enter elevators or screaming fearfully at attempts to take them on a carousel at the zoo or park. As with children who cover their ears in response to particular sounds, certain forms of movement we consider within the normal range seem to them to be like going for a ride on the scariest roller-coaster at Disney Land—involuntarily. Such children need to be gradually introduced to normal levels of movement stimulation in order to develop a tolerance.

Chapter Summary

The preceding three chapters have presented our current understanding of the various symptoms of autism. From the case examples, it should be clear that each child with autism or PDD is different. Each has different symptoms that are most characteristic of his or her particular case of autism or PDD. It cannot be emphasized too strongly that no child, of course, will have all, or perhaps even most, of the specific symptoms described in the last three chapters. Some descriptions will ring true. Some will not. Much depends on the mental and chronological age of the particular child, the severity of his autistic impairments, and probably, the yet-to-be understood causative factors that underlie each case. In the next chapter, with this definition of autism and PDD in hand, we will discuss how these disorders are usually first detected by parents, primary-care providers, and teachers, and what steps are needed to get a definitive diagnosis. Chapter 5 will also cover what you may learn from a diagnostic evaluation, such as information about possible etiology or cause, and the prognosis in a particular case.

CHAPTER 5

♦ ♦ ♦

Getting a Diagnosis

Getting a diagnosis really has two important purposes. First, a diagnosis is a label. It means that what is wrong is a recognizable problem that has happened before. The "label" is important insofar as it is a shorthand for a treatment plan. The second very important purpose of a "label" or a diagnosis it that it is a ticket to services. If your child is very young and you are just starting to think about going to doctors to find out what is wrong, and what you need to do, this is an important chapter for you to read. For professionals involved at the time of diagnosis, this chapter is intended to illustrate questions parents often focus on, and the support and guidance that are helpful in assuring parents that helpful treatments are available.

"Labeling"

Labels frighten many parents. A label alone, especially of a fairly uncommon disorder like autism of PDD and especially when applied to a very young child, can seem like a death sentence or imprisonment with no hope of parole. No one intends parents to come away with that message. But, unfortunately, there are many doctors and evaluation teams who use labels without realizing the effects they have on patients and their families, and ultimately on parents' willingness to seek the needed treatments associated with the label. When a diagnosis is given without an explanation of what it tells about the treatments the child will need, parents can feel that the diagnosis is much like a prison sentence. Like a criminal trial, for several days, "evidence" in the form of all the various assessments the child is subjected to, is collected and weighed. Then a "verdict" is handed down. The parents gather along with all the experts ("judges") who have been involved in the case. The only hope of appeal for the child's "sentence" is if the parents decide to seek out another team of experts (a new "court") to see if a new diagnosis ("verdict") will be rendered. If the parents have put their trust in the system at the beginning of this process, they may feel any "appeal" would be futile. The "prison term" ahead can seem dark and forbidding, empty, and with no hope for parole. Many parents talk about how helpless they have felt when first hearing a professional say, "Yes, your child *is* definitely autistic."

As bad as getting a diagnosis can feel, it is the mandatory first step of developing a plan for treating a child's autism or PDD. No two cases of autism or PDD are identical. Each case presents a somewhat different configuration of symptoms, and this mixes with the individual personality and learning characteristics of each child. A diagnosis should tell you not only whether or not your child has autism, but something about what kind of autism he or she has. By "kind" of autism I mean getting a good description of which symptoms of autism are present in your child, which symptoms seem most prominent and which more mild, and what relative strengths and weaknesses are present in your child overall. Only then can treatment plans begin. The logical thing to do, once you know a child's strengths and weaknesses, is to come up with ideas about how to use the strengths to help compensate for the weaknesses. There will be many specific examples of this in Part II as we talk about treatment plans for specific areas of development.

I must admit that I sometimes feel irritated with some colleagues who see autistic children for diagnostic assessments and mainly produce five to twenty-five page long reports describing back to the parents everything the parents told them—and not much more. Along with recasting what the parents have said in professional jargon, they enumerate various statistical scores from tests the child was given. It's not that such reports are bad; they can be marvelously detailed. When I read such reports, I can picture just what the child is like. But, what I don't like is when these reports conclude with only these two lines

Diagnosis: Autistic Disorder (299.0-DSM-IV/ ICD 10)
Recommendations: 1. Referral to school district.
2. Return for reassessment in 6 months.

What have parents who receive such reports learned about what to do for their child? Probably not much. Parents need to be told what they personally can do for their child, day-to-day, to help him improve. Just turning the child over to the schools, and coming back for more evaluation in the future, gives the parents no control in a very stressful situation where having control can be very therapeutic. Often, parents I meet who have just been through evaluations that have not explained enough and told them what to do, are the ones who are most gun-shy about further evaluations. They feel further assessment will just "label" (read "life-sentence") their child, again, and deepen feelings of hopelessness. For parents, a diagnostic evaluation should tell *what to do,* not just *what is wrong.* Most parents after all basically know what is wrong before they ever see a doctor, or wouldn't have gone in the first place. It is not the label, per se, that is important, but what that label implies for treatment.

Because a diagnosis is a label or shorthand for treatment, it needs to correspond to the services the child needs in the immediate future. As a child improves, obviously, he may need different kinds of services. Sometimes a re-diagnosis is helpful for that reason. Diagnoses can change as a child improves, as was pointed out in Chapter 1. In many children, the severity of the symptoms diminishes, but the diagnosis stays the same; still, new treatments may be needed. In some children, however, it is warranted to shift from a diagnosis of autism to a diagnosis of PDD or Asperger's syndrome. In others, the shift maybe from a diagnosis of PDD to perhaps a diagnosis of a developmental language disorder—or to perhaps no diagnosis at all. While the vast majority of autistic children improve, the vast majority also remain autistic. Unfortunately, changing a diagnosis does not make a child better (as some parents who argue for a diagnosis of PDD over a diagnosis of autism might dearly wish), but a changed diagnosis may mean that the child *is* better.

Getting a Diagnosis: Why Sooner Is Better

After your pediatrician has gone through some developmental screening of your child's milestones, he or she may suggest that you go to a specialized autism center or developmental disabilities center for further assessment. Often a pediatrician will also give the option to "Wait and see." From what is known about intervention for children with developmental disorders, "Wait and see" is not the best approach. The earlier intervention starts, the better. (The rationale for early intervention will be discussed in detail in Chapter 9.) If it turns out that a child is misdiagnosed as PDD or autistic but really is just a little slow, it will not have hurt him to have been in an infant stimulation program or to have gotten (unnecessary) speech and language therapy. What we do know is that most brain growth, and most fundamental aspects of learning, takes place in the first six years of life. This is really the prime time for intervention. You can think of it as a period of time when you can get in there and re-wire the circuits or re-write the software—and that the efforts will be more effective early rather than later.

Where Do You Get Autism or PDD Diagnosed?

Since autism or PDD occurs only about once in every 1,000 births, it is a disorder that many general pediatricians, and even many child psychologists or child psychiatrists, have rarely seen. A good standard of practice is for such professionals to pass along cases of possible autism to specialists who focus on developmental disabilities, or preferably, autism. It *is* possible for a good pediatrician to make a diagnosis of autism in some cases. Also, some cases *are* more easily diagnosable than others. However, as we've already discussed, a diagnosis should also be tied to treatment plans, and for that, you will need the diagnostic opinion of a professional who has experience with many autistic children who have difficulties similar to your own child's.

There are various ways to obtain an evaluation from an expert on autism. Often your pediatrician can recommend the best person for your child's evaluation. Even if your pediatrician doesn't have much contact with developmentally delayed children, he or she probably knows another physician who does. If your pediatrician con't provide you with a referral, or just doesn't share your concerns, you can certainly proceed on your own. Many parents are under the impression that to have a child evaluated for a possible developmental problem there has to be a referral made by another professional first. Usually, this isn't true. Most centers serving children with special developmental needs are very sensitive to the importance of early intervention and will evaluate any child potentially in need of services. In the United States, if you do need some kind of referral, many states have departments of developmental services or regional centers for individuals with developmental disabilities. Your pediatrician may refer you to such an agency, or you may be referred there by your school district. The state or county agency for developmental disabilities usually provides case management, meaning that they help you find services (and perhaps pay for services) rather than providing them directly themselves. In other countries, there is often a similar setup, either with a municipal council holding responsibility for children with learning handicaps, or a central hospital that provides services.

A parent can also directly explore community resources, such as a local university or children's hospital which may have a department of developmental disabilities, child psychology, or child psychiatry. You can call and ask whether there is a clinic where children can be evaluated for autism or pervasive developmental disorder. Another alternative is to call (or write) to the national office of the Autism Society of America, or to call your state chapter of the Autism Society (see Chapter 8 for addresses and telephone numbers). They should be able to recommend a center or a particular doctor in your area.

If you live in a more rural part of the country, you may want to combine a trip for a diagnostic evaluation with a vacation or visit to family in an area where there are specific resources for autistic children. In some ways, it's more important to go out of your way to get a detailed expert diagnosis if you *do* live in a rural area, because you will probably end up with more of the responsibility for your child's needs than if you lived in a region with more diverse social and educational services. We will talk more about being an advocate for your child in Chapter 8.

Of course, many parents who are seeking a developmental evaluation of their child have no idea that autism may be the problem. In such cases, a center specializing in a range of developmental disorders can be the best place to go. If a child has other developmental problems as well, such as concerns about motor development or seizures, this is all the more reason to go to a center that treats a broad range of developmental disabilities.

Components of a Developmental Evaluation

An evaluation to check for autism or for PDD is one and the same. As described earlier, both autism and the various forms of non-autistic PDDs form a spectrum of autistic disorders. When an evaluation is done to examine a child for autism the examination will include consideration of whether any other autistic spectrum disorders might be present instead. When making an appointment for an evaluation, a parent should not hesitate to ask what procedures may be done, why they will be done, and how much they will cost. It is not always possible for the professional who is gathering "intake" information from you to give you the full picture in advance since initial findings may influence what procedures get included as you go along. But you should be able to get some idea in advance or what you may hope to learn from the steps taken by the clinician. There are a number of basic components to an evaluation for autism or PDD.

Behavioral Testing as Part of a Developmental Evaluation

Behavioral versus Physical Markers of Autism and PDD. The most important aspect of a developmental evaluation (that is, an evaluation of the child's strengths and weaknesses in developing) the assessment made of a child's behavior. Autism is a disorder that can be classified as a *behavioral* diagnosis as opposed to a *physical* diagnosis. This is not to say that autism does not have a physical cause; only that, at present, we have no specific physical markers. Therefore, a diagnosis of autism of PDD is based on how the child behaves. Unlike Down syndrome, a common form of mental retardation in which there is an extra chromosome in the twenty-first pair of chromosomes, there is no such chromosomal, blood, brain, or other physical marker for autism that we know of right now.

A number of investigators are looking for abnormal genes and abnormal antibody responses, and studying pregnancy and birth trauma, but none has yet found a marker that is unique for autism. For example, a few studies have reported abnormalities in brain structure or in immune system function. When other researchers then try to replicate such findings with other groups of autistic children, they typically find that either the newly reported finding doesn't hold up, or that the finding isn't unique to autism—perhaps encompassing other children with mental retardation or language disorders.

Similarly, we know that certain pregnancy and delivery risk factors occur more often in the case histories of autistic and PDD children. However, we also know that (1) most children whose mothers experienced these same risk factors turn out to be completely okay, and (2) that among those who may have been compromised by exposure to a pregnancy or delivery risk factor, only a small proportion are autistic or have PDD, and the rest have other kinds of developmental disorders. Thus, it is important for a doctor to ask whether certain risk factors may have been present during pregnancy, and whether other family members have any of the autistic spectrum disorders. But, an affirmative response to either type of question does not confirm or rule out a diagnosis of autism or PDD.

Since there are no specific biological markers for autism or PDD (and therefore no markers to differentiate among autistic spectrum disorders), the diagnosis is dependent on demonstrating the presence of specific behaviors. What this means is that the diagnosis of autism is made on an assessment of the child's behavior, including testing his social relatedness, intelligence, expressive and receptive language, adaptive behavior, and the presence or absence of specific signs of autism. Each of these will be taken up one at a time in this chapter.

Medical Testing as Part of a Developmental Evaluation

Medical tests that are carried out as part of an evaluation for autism are done not to actually confirm the diagnosis of autism, but to rule out other possible causes of the child's difficulties—conditions that have a known physical basis. There are no known physical disorders that can produce autism, except the fragile X syndrome which is sometimes considered an autistic spectrum disorder, as discussed in Chapter 1. When conducting a diagnostic evaluation for autism, some centers routinely prefer to do extensive "rule-out" testing first—even if the child appears to be autistic—and despite the knowledge that no physical markers exist for autism. Rule-out testing can include various blood tests to look for inborn errors of metabolism, cytogenetic testing to look for chromosomal abnormalities, brain-imaging studies such as CT (computed tomography) scans or MRI (magnetic resonance imaging) studies. When brain-imaging studies are conducted, the doctors are looking for *any* sign of neurological abnormality, not for signs that are specific to autism. As mentioned earlier, a few research studies have begun to suggest specific abnormal results on the MRIs of some autistic children, but these findings are not yet well replicated (or functionally understood) so as to constitute any kind of diagnostic test for autism.

One question that parents often ask is how important is it to do genetic, blood, and brain studies as soon as a developmental disorder is suspected. My own opinion is that if autism or PDD is suspected and there are no obvious signs of brain damage, it is important to establish the diagnosis of autism first, and get treatment underway, and then do further tests (at a more leisurely pace) to accumulate further reassurances that any number of other unlikely "rule-out" conditions aren't *also* a concern. Of course, if there are specific reasons to suspect another disorder, tests for that disorder should be promptly carried out. For example, if a child is having "blanking out spells," neurological studies should be made of the brain and nervous system to rule out a seizure disorder. If a child has an unusual physical appearance, it may suggest a specific genetic abnormality, and this should be checked out through cytogenetic testing. As was mentioned, the only genetic disorder known to occur with any regularity in autistic children is the fragile X syndrome. Therefore, it is probably the most commonly given test for children suspected to have autism. In the last section of this chapter, a more detailed description is provided of exactly what fragile X syndrome is, and how it may overlap with autism.

Roles of Different Professionals in the Developmental Evaluation

Developmental evaluations for autism may include child psychologists, child psychiatrists, developmental-behavioral pediatricians, child neurologists, speech and language pathologists, educational specialists, occupational therapists, or social workers. Some clinics make sharp disciplinary distinctions among professionals and the activities they carry out; other clinics do not.

It is important that the clinicians evaluating your child be experienced with autism. An excellent clinician who has not also seen a number of autistic children is not going to be able to put your child into a realistic context—that is, be able to tell you what the child can learn next, how he can learn it, and how far he is likely to go. In contrast, an experienced clinician who has seen many autistic children *can* give you specific information about treatment and tell you something about the future. No doctor has a crystal ball, in spite of what many parents may wish. Through accumulated experience, both of seeing certain autistic children as they grow up and seeing children at different ages, and by studying the research literature on the prognosis for autistic children, an experienced doctor has some sense of the trajectory of any autistic child's development.

Parents often have strong feelings that ricochet between wanting to know what they are in for and *not* wanting to know all the details, but wanting instead to take it one day at a time. It can be true that a parent may not yet be "ready" to hear certain kinds of information about prognosis. A good clinician is trained to meter information about a child: to prepare parents to understand new and often difficult-to-accept information and help parents to ask questions when they are ready to handle the information. In university-based centers where a great deal of training of new doctors takes place, parts of a developmental evaluation may be carried out by a trainee, such as a psychology intern, a child psychiatry fellow, or a developmental pediatrics resident. Such trainees are always reporting directly to supervisors, and in highly specialized clinics, the supervisor usually becomes directly involved in discussing results of an evaluation with the child's family. As a parent, if you ever have a concern about the accuracy of something a trainee has said, or don't feel your questions are being fully answered, you should ask for a chance to discuss matters with a supervisor. This really is your right and should not be taken as an insult by the trainee.

Roles of Members of a Developmental Evaluation Team. Usually the main clinician involved in a diagnostic evaluation for PDD or autism is a child psychologist or child psychiatrist. This person will usually work in conjunction with other doctors, therapists, and educators who together provide all the pieces of data needed to make a diagnosis and to develop a treatment plan. The components of the evaluation that need to be coordinated include taking a developmental history of the rate and pattern of the child's acquisition of new skills, some type of systematic observation of the child's behavior, and intelligence testing. At the completion of all of that data-gathering, the clinician in charge, and perhaps other members of his or her team, meet with parents to discuss findings and recommendations. It can often be helpful for parents attending such evaluations to come with a speech and language therapist or infant educator who is currently working with the child (if there is one). A professional who already knows a child may be able to provide shorthand information to the diagnostic team that is trying to get to know the child, and afterward can be available to help parents weigh the information and recommendations given.

The Role of the Psychologist. One aspect of developmental evaluation that is typically the exclusive domain of psychologists is intelligence (IQ) testing. This is because using IQ tests requires a specific background and training, just as the medical tests that physicians use require medical training. Some psychologists focus on IQ testing, but for school-age autistic and PDD children, it may be more important to focus on educational testing that assesses the child's grade level in specific academic skills, such as reading, oral comprehension, math, written expression, and so on. Educational psychologists or school psychologists often carry out such testing. Another type of psychological test is called a *projective* test and it is designed to tap the child's inner thoughts and feelings. These tests are appropriate for children who are suspected of being emotionally disturbed, but are largely inappropriate for children being assessed for possible autism or PDD. (Sometimes, however, an older, higher functioning child—usually with PDD or Asperger's syndrome—may appear unusually depressed, anxious, or phobic. Then such tests may indeed be appropriate.)

The Role of the Child Psychiatrist. A child psychiatrist who is a physician trained in analyzing a child's behavior, may be the primary professional coordinating an evaluation for autism or PDD, or she may be the one who focuses on making recommendations about medications that could be helpful. These will be discussed in more detail in Chapter 14, on the medical management of autism. For now, it suffices to say that a fairly small proportion of very young autistic children are given medications, and that when they are, it is typically to treat specific symptoms, such as hyperactivity, rather than to treat the autism as a single entity. A child psychiatrist may either manage the use of medications directly or serve as a consultant to the child's pediatrician, who may be able to see the child more easily on a regular basis. Child psychiatrists tend to be more familiar with autism and PDD than the psychiatrist who sees adults primarily. Since all child psychiatrists need to complete adult psychiatry training before specializing in children, child psychiatrists tend to be a better resource for medication management in adult autistic individuals as well. Increasingly, some adult psychiatrists are becoming aware of Asperger's syndrome and are interested in how to treat it in adults, but up until now, psychiatric treatment of both children and adults with autism or PDD has primarily been the domain of child psychiatrists.

The Role of the Speech and Language Pathologist. Early on, autistic children have delays in both understanding and expressing ideas using language. Often the ability to express is more severely affected than the ability to understand. Difficulties in the development of communication skills were discussed in detail in Chapter 3, and treatment of communication difficulties is covered in Chapter 12. During an initial assessment of an autistic child, a speech and language pathologist may be brought in to decide how far along developmentally the child is in language understanding and language expression. Sometimes, especially if the child is not yet speaking at all, the language assessment is made more informally, through direct observations either by the speech and language pathologist or by other professionals involved in the evaluation. Speech and language pathologists can also evaluate "pre-language" skills. These include things like assessing how interested the child is in sounds, his spontaneous ability to comprehend and use gestures (like pointing), and the presence of language pragmatics—skills like taking turns, seeking attention, and sustaining an interaction nonverbally.

Speech and language pathologists often assign a child a receptive and an expressive language age. The *receptive language age* indicates how well the child understands language compared to normally developing children. The *expressive language age* is a measure of what the child can say, or for toddlers, what they can make known through the use of gesture. The results of such testing are important for treatment planning because they indicate the starting point for teaching language skills in the developmental sequence children usually follow.

The Role of Audiologists. Even before a speech and language assessment, a child who is not talking or whose ability to use language is greatly delayed is usually sent to an audiologist. With autistic children, parents often think the child is hard of hearing, but the hearing is somehow selective—clearly responding to certain TV commercials or the sound of the refrigerator opening, but acting seemingly deaf to the human voice. Such children virtually always have normal hearing. In young children, what appears to be voice deafness is sometimes an early indication of autism. The most common way to test the hearing of young children is sound field audiometry or play audiometry. This method of hearing test assumes that the child will tolerate head phones, sit more or less still (while being awake and alert), and will be interested in looking toward a sound if he learns a fun toy will appear after he responds. By and large, none of these assumptions are valid for young autistic children, and as a result, audiometric testing of this sort is often judged to be inconclusive. An alternate technique is to test brain function directly through the *auditory brain response* (ABR), which is also called *brain stem evoked response* (BSER), or *auditory evoked potential*. This form of hearing test requires sedating the child, but directly measures auditory nerve function, and the child need not cooperate. More recently, a third alternative has come into use—*otacoustic emission testing*, which only requires that the child hold still for about 20 to 30 seconds while tolerating a small ear plug (which is really a microphone). This can be a very good alternative for children with no interest in play audiometry, but a little capacity to hold still because the child need not be sedated for this procedure.

The Role of Child Neurologists and Pediatric Geneticists. "Rule-out" medical testing is primarily the domain of neurologists and pediatric geneticists. Neurologists take charge of brain studies, such as EEGs, CTs, and MRIs. Pediatric geneticists order and interpret studies of chromosomes and look for inborn errors of metabolism that are known to cause a variety of mental retardation syndromes.

Most parents are comfortable with the idea of a physical examination by a neurologist to rule out specific neurological signs that can be detected by examining the child's gait, reflexes, and senses. Sometimes, however, parents hesitate to pursue EEGs (which examine the electrical activity of the brain) or MRIs (which examine the structures of the brain) because it means the child will have to receive a sedative. Most autistic children do fine with the amount of sedation needed to fall asleep for an MRI or other test. However, a small proportion of young children will have paradoxical (reverse) reactions to a common sedative like chloral hydrate and become quite hyperactive or agitated. When this happens, the test has to be rescheduled, and sometimes parents are afraid to go through the same experience a second time. It may help to ask the neurologist how necessary the test is at this point (is it a routine "rule out," or is he looking for something in particular), and whether a different sedative or a different schedule of administration of the sedative might be used. It is an exceedingly poor idea to try to conduct such testing by physically immobilizing an autistic child, by strapping him down instead of sedating him, because it is cruel and he may injure himself. Autistic children will most often panic at such treatment, and I certainly know cases where children have broken thumbs or sprained wrists struggling to get free of such devices.

Often neurologists and geneticists are not directly part of an evaluation team, but are used as outside consultants whom the family is sent to see after (or before) the behavioral testing is completed. When neurologists or geneticists are brought in as consultants, they may be at the same center as the developmental evaluators, or if the developmental evaluation takes place at a specialized center fairly far from home, such referrals may be made to professionals closer to home. In the latter case, the doctors usually exchange reports when their workups are complete, or talk on the phone to clarify any differences or questions one another's findings have raised.

Assessment Methods in Developmental Evaluation of Autism and PDD

Developmental History

One essential component to making a diagnosis of autism is to obtain a history of the child's development up until the present time. When autism is suspected, the developmental history of the child will be quite different from that of children with other developmental disorders. The clinician needs to know exactly what to look for. Autistic children are not born with all of their symptoms of autism. In fact, the majority of autistic children appear quite normal at birth. The symptoms of autism emerge over time, and there are certain basic patterns into which symptoms evolve. These patterns are quite different from one another, so it can be quite puzzling as to how some children who start off the same as typically developing children end up being diagnosed as autistic.

When parents give histories of how their children have developed, different parents will have noticed different things. For one thing, when an autistic child is the first child, parents have no basis for comparison. In firstborns, come aspects of atypical development go unnoticed, and some things that are noticed seem not to be atypical. Sometimes after a second child is born, parents can look back and say, "I wasn't concerned about Jonathan when he was eighteen months old, but now that his baby sister is eighteen months old, I can see that Jonathan was very different from her, even by his first birthday."

Genetic History. Taking a developmental history also involves getting a picture of a family tree to determine whether there are family members with related disorders. Other cases of autism, PDD, or learning disabilities, especially language difficulties, occur more often in families that are likely to have an inherited form of autism. Some research suggests that 30 percent to 50 percent of cases of autism, PDD, and Asperger's syndrome may have an inherited component. Autism is seldom directly inherited, since it is rare for autistic adults to want to have children, but there is increasing evidence that partial forms of autism occur in many family trees where there is an autistic or PDD child. Along with certain diseases and other inherited characterstics (like eye colors), personality traits may also be inherited. In families with autistic children odd personality traits focusing on poor social skills seem prevalent. The presence of odd family members (like a forty-year-old uncle with two master's degrees who works as a plumber and who has always lived with his parents and has never really socialized) as well as very mathematically bright, but socially awkward relatives, are more frequent in families with an autistic child. Sometimes these family members are socially a bit awkward, but nonetheless very intelligent and accomplished, such as in the case of one autistic man whose father is a Nobel laureate. Autism seems to be a case of inheriting an extreme version of the trait of social isolativeness. There is some, but no real evidence that conditions like schizophrenia or major depression occur in families with autistic children. Physical disorders like heart disease or cancer have never been related to autism. A clinician taking a family history for possible genetic contributions to autism, PDD, or Asperger's syndrome will therefore focus on socially unusual relatives in addition to ones who may have actually had an autistic spectrum disorder.

Pregnancy History. During a developmental history, a doctor will want to know about the mother's pregnancy with the child, since certain pregnancy risk factors have been associated with autism. As covered earlier, research suggests that most of the risks in pregnancy related to autism are just that—risks, not causes. A generally accepted viewpoint is that pregnancy risks that occur to a somehow vulnerable fetus may combine to produce autism. Vulnerability may be something like the presence of an abnormal gene or the lack of a particular antigen to fight off a certain type of infection the fetus might be subject to. We do know that women with late first trimester viral infections of certain types (like rubella or cytomegalovirus) have more of a risk for having an autistic child. Also, children who may have been deprived of oxygen around the time of delivery may have a greater risk of autism. Prematurity has not been correlated with autism. More recently, some of the severely drug-exposed babies whose mothers have used crack or cocaine during pregnancy seem to have signs of PDD, especially when younger.

Sometimes by the time a parent gets to a specialized autism center, she has been asked the same questions about pregnancy and delivery two or three times. Providing the doctor with a written report from another doctor who has already asked these questions may spare the parent from going through this process again. Sometimes, however, an autism specialist may be looking for very specific things that other doctors haven't asked, so he or she may have different reasons for asking similar questions again. Parents shouldn't be afraid to ask why certain questions are being asked, or what responses indicate in terms of risks a child may have been exposed to.

Genetic Counseling. Once a history has been taken, complete with information about the pregnancy and your family's genetic history, you can ask your doctor whether you are at greater risk than most of having another autistic or PDD child. Studies of the risk of recurrence of autism in families with one autistic child suggest about a three percent risk. That means that among all families with an autistic child, three out of 100 will have another child with autism or PDD among all the other children the families end up having. Studies so far haven't really been able to take into account the fact that some familes may have a number of other fully or partly affected individuals (those with extreme social awkwardness, but who are not themselves autistic) while other families have none. In some cases, there are many risk factors associated with the pregnancy, but no family history of autism. All of these factors have to be weighed by a doctor who gives advice about risk recurrence for a particular family, taking into account research and counterbalancing the risk factors present in a particular case.

In about thirty to forty percent of cases of autism, neither a genetic nor pregnancy history will reveal any known risk factors. Such cases of autism may be due to a one-time gene mutation or to some kind of infection that the mother didn't even know she had during her pregnancy. Given the state of research, it is likely that in ten years we will know what causes at least some cases of autism and PDD, and also have a more precise and refined understanding of risk factors.

Behavioral Assessment

Behavioral assessment is the part of an autism evaluation that requires the most expertise. There are two main ways of collecting behavioral information. One is through informal or unstructured observation. The second is through structured or standardized observation. Some clinicians prefer a combination of the two. A doctor may try to get the child to play with various toys, which is an example of an unstructured observation. In such an unstructured assessment, the mother might be asked to get the child to play with the toys. An unstructured observation might take place in a waiting room, a doctor's office or playroom, in the child's home, or even in the child's classroom. One goal of an unstructured observation is to see how the child typically reacts when certain everyday things happen.

For example, we make natural, unstructured observations in our clinic when children are brought back from a testing room into the room where the parents are being interviewed. One thing I look for is what the child does upon reunion with the parents. It's a natural situation. Does the child spontaneously approach the parents? Does he make physical contact with the mother? Does he do this only if the mother guides and initiates the contact? How long is the contact sustained? Does the child make eye contact while approaching or being held by the mother? The answers to all these questions have very well-established norms for young non-autistic children, and a child who is being assessed for autism can be compared to those norms as a way of evaluating how well organized the social attachment to the mother is. Since in the course of our regular assessment procedures we have times when the child is separated from the parents, we can count on these reunions as a type of naturalistic mini-experiment in which to observe the child's attachment to his or her parents.

Usually, doctors keep a mental checklist of things they would like to see the child do. Although playing with the child may seem random to the parent, a variety of specific questions are being addressed, and the doctor can explain to you later what she was trying to learn.

Increasingly, however, clinicians are coming to rely on standardized methods of assessing children's behavior. This means putting the child through some set of tasks, activities, or situations in which other autistic or PDD children have been similarly rated. By doing this, clinicians can develop standards and correlate these standards to different diagnoses, levels of severity, developmental level, etc. There are an increasing number of standardized assessments that are used with autistic children, such as the ETHOS which we developed in our clinic, the ADOS and Play-DOS developed by Dr. Catherine Lord and colleagues, and the BOS, developed by Dr. B. J. Freeman.

The standardized play session we use in our clinic exemplifies how a standardized behavioral assessment works. Ours consists of nine two-minute episodes. First, the child and examiner are in the room together. It begins with the examiner directly interacting with the child—either talking or physically doing something, like tickling or bouncing. Starting with such an intrusive interaction "cold" with an autistic child often doesn't go over too well—and it isn't meant to. The procedure clarifies the child's diagnosis by helping us see how the autistic child is different from the language-delayed or mentally retarded child who isn't autistic and who generally will warm up to the examiner fairly readily. In the second two-minute session, the examiner goes off and suddenly starts playing alone. We look for whether the child notices the change in the examiner's behavior toward him, or whether the child just ignores him. The autistic child is usually happy to be finally left alone by this pesky person. Other non-autistic children usually continue to approach the examiner or show disappointment or anger that their new "playmate" has suddenly ignored them. In the third two-minute session, the examiner again approaches the child and begins to try to induce the child to play with a toy or object the examiner feels he might be interested in. By now, the child is a bit used to the examiner, and since this play doesn't require direct interaction, the child usually does a little better than the first time around. Then, these three two minute episodes are repeated, except this time the adult play partner is one of the parents rather than the examiner. Often, an autistic child does much better with the parent because the parent plays with the child in familiar ways that are more acceptable to him. Finally, in the third set of three two-minute episodes, the examiner goes back in and copies the parent as closely as possible. Some autistic children do better with the examiner when the activities are familiar, almost as well as with the parents, and so we learn that for these autistic children, a familiar routine can be very important to normalizing behavior. We are also able to make many observations about the child's social style—for example, how well he responds to words or gestures; whether he prefers to be directly involved in play, or to learn through observation; and how the child shows when he or she is feeling overstimulated by social contact. The whole point of doing a standardized play session like this one is to have an anchor for comparing children to one another behaviorally. When children are each put in the same situation, their differences and similarities can be directly compared.

Autism Ratings. Many centers for evaluating autistic children do not use standardized autism observations, but do use standardized autism rating scales. These are checklists that are completed by either formally or informally observing the child, interviewing parents or teachers, reviewing records, and so forth, and then answering a series of questions about the presence or absence of autistic symptoms and their severity. Rating scales provide a way of quantitatively adding up symptom scores, and then comparing them with norms that will classify the child as not autistic, mildly autistic, severely autistic, "classically" autistic, and so on.

The most detailed rating system is the Autism Diagnostic Interview (ADI), developed by Dr. Ann LeCouteur and colleagues, which contains hundreds of questions about past and present behavior. Each response is rated for the severity of autism it indicates. A mathematical formula is used to tally up the completed responses (which are administered by a trained examiner who has interviewed a parent). The formula produces a score that tells whether the individual should be considered autistic or not. Except in very specialized university-based clinics, or in assessments where the person being assessed might become part of a research study, the ADI is usually not used (or absolutely needed). It is mainly a way of assuring that diagnoses are made on the same pool of information about each child.

The most widely used autism rating scale is the Childhood Autism Rating Scale (CARS) developed by Dr. Eric Schopler and colleagues. The CARS has thirteen different areas that are rated, and include measures of all of the symptom areas associated with autism. Children are rated from 1 to 5 in each area, with "1" being normal behavior for the age, and "5" being highly atypical behavior. After the ratings are made, there is a way of weighing the responses to determine if the child is autistic, and how severe the autism is. Another frequently used autism rating scale is the ABC (Autism Behavior Checklist), which works in a way similar to the CARS. Like the CARS, it provides a good clinical description of what the child is like and does so in a standardized way. Both measures can be used after a clinician has observed the child in a clinic, at home, or at school. The CARS and ABC require a moderate amount of training to be used properly (nowhere near as much as the ADI), and most often are used by clinicians who specialize in developmental evaluations, though perhaps not autism.

The oldest autism rating scale is the E-2 Checklist, developed by Dr. Bernard Rimland, founder of the American National Society for Autistic Children. This scale measures how severely or "classically" autistic a child is, but it has its own standards rather than being tied to the ones generally in use in successive editions of the DSM (the main standard for diagnosing autistic children which was described in Chapter 1).

As far as parents and practitioners are concerned, probably the best use of rating scales is to use them to chart changes in a child's clinical profile over time. If you child's evaluation includes having one of the scales administered, make sure to get a copy, as it will be a good reference point for the future. Rating scales can be used to track progress in an educational program or in a drug trial. Some scales are global, however, and won't detect small improvements in behavior, but these scales can isolate large changes in certain symptoms of autism that interfere with the child's ability to learn and function in everyday tasks.

Intelligence Testing and Determining Degree of Mental Retardation

An essential component of an evaluation for any developmental disorder is intelligence testing. Some parents are apprehensive about intelligence testing because they are not sure whether or not they want to know their child's IQ (intelligence quotient), especially if their child is delayed and they are hoping things will get better. The reason that getting intelligence testing is important is that it tells you where a child is developmentally at a particular point in time.

Is My Child Retarded, Too? Parents often fear a diagnosis of mental retardation even more than a diagnosis of autism. For many parents, autism is somewhat of a black box at first. Mental retardation, on the other hand, is more widely understood as something that doesn't go away. About seventy percent of children with autism, and a somewhat smaller percentage of children with PDD, *do* have some degree of mental retardation along with their primary diagnosis of autism or PDD. When a young child is initially assessed, the exact *degree* of mental retardation may be hard to predict, but often, it is possible to tell if there *is* mental retardation or not. The presence of different degrees of mental retardation says something about how fast or slowly the child is likely to learn, and how far mental development will ultimately go.

At first, a diagnosis of mental retardation can feel like the doctor is saying that nothing about the child will ever change or get better. That's not true, of course. But children with mental retardation learn most things more slowly and according to degree of impairment, need different instructional strategies to develop their best potential. The purpose of IQ testing, therefore, is to determine the relative strengths and weaknesses of the child intellectually, to figure out how to tailor the teaching methods to the child's abilities and disabilities, and how much change can be expected, and how soon.

Sometimes the term "developmental delay" is used instead of "mental retardation." Some clinicians use these terms interchangeably. "Developmental delay" may sound less ominous than "mental retardation," as if the train is *delayed,* but will be here soon. In this sense, the term "developmental delay" is a misnomer that, in my opinion, gives some parents false hope; it can even be misleading. Although I must admit that I, too, find it easier to talk about "developmental delay" rather than "mental retardation" to parents, I try not to do it. At least, I try to explain that mental retardation means slow learning, and an ultimately less completely developed capacity to reason and act, so parents can be clear about the status of their child's development. In most cases, the degree of mental retardation present is possible to ascertain with good reliability by the time the child is five years old, and often sooner.

Many IQ tests for very young children (infants and children up to four years old) report results according to mental age. A *mental age* is an age at which the average child can do something. So, for example, the average mental age for saying one or two words (besides "momma" or "dada") is fourteen months. This means that fifty percent of fourteen-month-olds can do this. In addition, IQ tests have standards developed with each item, so the examiner can also know that by eighteen months, for example, eighty-five percent of children can now say at least two words. Therefore, IQ testing allows us to precisely measure where a particular child is relative to other children the same age. Most important, IQ testing allows us to measure the relative strengths and weaknesses of a child. If a chold has age-appropriate abilities with certain

nonverbal tasks (such as nesting cubes) but still has little language understanding, it may be possible to use the child's visual astuteness to get him to learn
pictures, to which words are eventually associated (more about this later in
Chapter 9 on early intervention).

Are IQ Tests for Autistic Children Accurate? A major concern of parents
whose child is undergoing IQ testing is the feeling that the child will be ill-
behaved for the tester and that the child's "true" intelligence will not be seen.
This concern may be warranted at times. In the jargon of people who develop
IQ tests, there is "true score," which we never can fully measure, and various
estimates of "true score." "True score" is the result that would be obtained if
all conditions for testing were perfect. In giving a child an IQ test, the examiner hopes (1) to come as close as possible to a "true score" and (2) to understand the factors that account for any differences between actual performance
and the "true score." How does the examiner know if he or she has come close
to "true score?" Cross-validation should always be used by checking with the
results of other testers who may have done earlier or overlapping tests. The
examiner should ask parents (and teachers, if possbile) whether little Joshua
really can sort by colors, even though he didn't appear to be able to sort by
colors today. Sometimes when a skill is "emergent," or just manifesting itself,
the child can do it in one place, with one familiar set of materials, but still not
do it all the time. In addition, many autistic and PDD children have difficulty
generalizing, meaning they get stuck on moving a skill learned in one place to
another place. For example, that might mean that Joshua is really good at
sorting one-inch colored foam balls into round white Tupperware bowls at
school, but couldn't sort colored cardboard chips into little colored boxes for
the IQ tester. In this case, "lack of ability to generalize" becomes a factor that
explains some of the difference between "true score" and performance, and it
means that we have to come up with some ways to help Joshua generalize
better. (This might start with something as simple as having the teacher give
Joshua colored cardboard chips to sort into the Tupperware *just after* he's
sorted the foam balls, and gradually changing the learning situation from then
on.)

In addition to the problem of generalizing, which can be a real learning
handicap, there is the problem of "virtual disability." Virtual disability can be
thought of as the degree to which the child may fall behind due to lack of
curiosity about new things, resistance to change, or time spent repeatedly
doing one thing rather than experimenting with new things. Over time, if a
child is untreated, this virtual disability can truly become a factor that limits
the development of intelligence.

Testing autistic children requires special expertise, training, and experience. A tester who does not work with autistic children on a regular basis, or
does not understand what the main features of the cognitive disabilities associated with autism are, is not likely to be able to do a good job. In our clinic, and
in others that specialize in testing autistic children, we use behavioral shaping

methods during the testing session. This means we will give the child M&M's, raisins, Cheerio's, or whatever works to motivate him. (We don't, however, advocate this as a full-time teaching strategy.) The testing session can be seen as a contract: We want the child to do something, and we have to give the child something *he* wants in return. A tester generally has no or little preexisting relationship with the child, and we want the child to be motivated. Since autistic children are seldom motivated to do something just to please a friendly stranger, we give the child something he does want instead. An IQ test is designed to measure cognitive ability, not lack of motivation: To see whether or not a child has motivational problems, we do not need something as elaborate as an IQ test.

Many very young autistic children scream and cry throughout attempts to test them—even if they are cooperating somewhat. They just don't accept the idea of being asked to do something on someone else's schedule. This is important information in itself. Even if the child cooperates on only a few tasks, a skilled examiner can sometimes make sense of where those tasks fit in developmentally and reach some conclusions about easier things the child can probably also do, as well as similar, more complex tasks he may be able to do soon.

In testing autistic children, it also helps to keep them in a confined space, and in a room with few visual distractions. Testing an autistic child where he can "escape" or make his own choice of activities is not likely to be very successful. Successful techniques for testing autistic children include starting with items they can do easily, and saving more difficult (and disagreeable) verbal tasks until things are really under control. Often having a parent in the room for testing is *not* helpful, because the child will have a whole bag of tricks he knows he can use on Mom or Dad to get away from doing what he doesn't want to do, and the bag is likely to get opened up right away if Mom or Dad is worried the child will have a tantrum, reject all the test materials, and therefore look very unskilled. Also, having parents out of the room gives the examiner a better analogue for a classroom situation, and how ready the child is to attend and conform in that type of instructional setting. Sometimes, however, having the parent present, in as passive a role as possible, is necessary, especially if the child is very young and has little experience being away from parents in an unfamiliar setting.

One thing about IQ testing that parents often ask about relates to the jargon involved. There are a number of widely used terms that are used repeatedly and can be defined briefly. To begin with, intelligence is often broken into two main areas—verbal and performance.

Verbal Intelligence. Verbal intelligence (VIQ) involves the ability to understand and use language for the purposes of communicating with others, and for building knowledge of the world around you. There are two main forms of VIQ: (1) *Receptive language*, which refers to the child's ability to understand what is said to him. It can be measured by showing a child pictures to see if he knows, for example, which of a series of four pictures is the dog. It also can be measured by documenting the complexity of commands a child can follow. (2) *Expressive language,* which refers to how the child uses spoken language. Expressive language refers to language that children use meaningfully. Many young autistic and especially PDD children talk (repeat things) a great deal, but don't really understand what they're saying yet. Most IQ tests do not directly measure such variations in expressive language. However, overall, almost all autisitc children test below their age in language expression abilities. In fact, VIQ is almost always impaired in autistic and PDD children. One exception is that some autistic and many PDD children have excellent auditory memory (which *is* a component of VIQ). While such children can recite from memory long segments gleaned from TV or videos, they still often have relatively little comprehension of what these recitations might mean. As was described in Chapter 1, one of the main things that distinguishes children with Asperger's syndrome from children with other autistic spectrum disorders is the fact that AS children have relatively normal VIQs.

Performance Intelligence. Performance intelligence (PIQ) involves reasoning that is reflected in the actions we planfully carry out. For young children, this can be measured by how well and how fast they can complete pegboards, form boards, and puzzles; how well they can stack blocks; and how well they can recognize visual features of objects. Autistic children tend to do much better on PIQ tasks, and PIQ skills that are normally learned in the first three years of life often develop on time, or nearly on time. Other terms associated with performance IQ testing include "visual-spatial" (meaning the ability to accurately perceive objects in space), "visual-motor" (meaning the ability to do something based on what you see), "gross-motor" (meaning large muscle activities, such as walking, running, or riding a trike), and "fine-motor" (meaning the ability to do small manipulations with the hands) abilities. In the first five years of life, autistic and PDD children tend to do quite well, some excellently, on PIQ tasks. However, after age five, even nonverbal reasoning often requires language (like arranging pictures to tell a story), and a child who still is not talking may be reassessed as having a lower PIQ than when he was younger.

So the important thing to remember is that when a very young child receives IQ testing, it's not the IQ score that tells us what to do in terms of treatment planning. Rather, it's what he *can* do compared to what he *can't* do, and why there seems to be a difference. The IQ score itself is mostly an indicator of long-term prognosis. In very young autistic children (under three-and-a-half-years), or in other autistic children who haven't yet received any special education, the IQ score is the most unstable. Even in those children, however, there is some global ability to predict the overall degree of mental retardation as explained earlier.

Kanner's Islets of Intact Ability. When Leo Kanner first described the syndrome of autism, his definition (which has since evolved) included "islets of intact ability." By this, Kanner meant areas of intellectual functioning where the child did much better than in other areas where the child was impaired. We now underatand that these islets of intact ability, or "splinter skills," primarily involve performance intelligence, and specifically often pertain to things the child can do by using a termendous rote memory—such as the memorization of dates through application of a basic formula, or memorization of factual information. Some older children and young adults, particularly those with PDD and Asperger's syndrome, succeed in higher math or games like chess—while still having social skills no better than a four-year-old. In Chapter 13, we'll discuss how to achieve a balance educationally and psychologically in these children who do so well in one area, but have persisting difficulties in others. As a general rule, the child is not helped overall, if attention is paid only to the splinter skills without equal efforts to bring the problem areas of development up to par.

Specific Tests of Intellectual and Adaptive Functioning

There are several intelligence tests that are used more frequently than others. Which test is used depends on the mental and chronological age of the child. There is no IQ test especially for children with autism or PDD, so no particular IQ test diagnoses the disorder. The following is to familiarize you with tests used at different ages. Among these tests, it doesn't matter so much *which* one is used; more important is that the examiner be able to make use of the findings based on her or his experience with the test, and be able to make recommendations about teaching your child. Most of the major standardized IQ tests that will be described here are highly correlated with each other in terms of overall score. A child who receives one of these tests probably doesn't need to get another one at the same time unless there is something specific that went wrong, or a specific question that was raised in the administration of the first test. The same IQ test should not be readministered more frequently than once every eighteen months. If IQ tests are repeated more frequently than this, the child will, to some extent, learn the tasks, and you will be measuring learning rather than intelligence. The exception to the eighteen-month rule is infant tests, which can be administered even once every four months or so, because infants change quickly, and the tasks mostly involve everyday activities (like putting an object in a cup), rather than use of materials developed especially for the test.

Tests of Infant Intelligence (Birth to Three Years). The most widely used infant tests are the *Bayley Scales of Infant Development.* The Bayley has been around since the 1960s and has recently been revamped as the Bayley-II, which has brought it up-to-date in a number of ways. There are two parts to the Bayley, the Mental Development Index (MDI) and the Performance Development Index (PDI). The MDI is the most useful of the two parts of this test for assessing autistic and PDD children. Mental development can be further broken down into expressive and receptive skills. The Bayley's MDI indicates a mental age equivalent for the child, as well as an MDI score, which can cautiously be interpreted as an IQ score. The overall age-equivalent score may tell you little about the child, and when reported to a parent, it won't ring true. For example, a thirty-two-month-old autistic child may get an age-equivalent score of fourteen months. Her parents can see that, in many ways, she is not like a fourteen-month-old—she is toilet trained, can put together fifteen-piece puzzles, and figure out all the child-proof locks on the kitchen cabinets. However, because she does not automatically smile in response to being spoken to, does not respond to her own image in a mirror, is unable to identify pictures of everyday objects by pointing, her age-equivalent score is severely marked down. In cases like these, it is most useful to know highest items passed and earliest items failed on the test, in order to make some sense of the level of a particular child in specific areas like receptive language, imitation, and social responsiveness. The Bayley's PDI is generally not needed in assessing autistic children because early motor development delays are usually not part of the picture, or are of minor concern. However, if a child has delays in motor coordination as well, the PDI will be a useful way of documenting them.

Other infant tests sometimes used are the Gessell Scales and the Cattell Scales. Both were developed in the 1940s and have undergone little revision since then. The Gessell is often used by pediatricians and has subscales that can form a useful basis for picturing relative delays in language compared to social-communicative development and motor development. A newer infant test is the *Mullens Scales of Early Learning*. This has very up-to-date norms and breaks development into areas we need to consider separately—like receptive and expressive language, visual-motor skills, and perceptual-motor organization. Like the Bayley, it gives mental age equivalents in each area of development.

There are also numerous educationally based scales used to describe functioning in children under three years old; these are primarily given in school settings. Although these are not IQ tests per se, most yield scores that describe level of mental development in various areas.

Tests for Preschool Age (Three to Six Years). At this age, selection of an IQ test is determined by the mental age range at which the child is functioning. Some four-year-olds may be mainly functioning like two-year-olds, and so infant tests will still be appropriate for them. Several tests are used for children in the three- to six-year developmental range. An older test, but one that is well suited for autistic children, is the *Merrill-Palmer Scales of Mental Development*. This is a test that most autistic children actually enjoy taking because it offers a wide variety of performance tasks (but is weak on verbal tasks). Since many autistic children in this age range still have very limited language use (below the eighteen-month "floor" of this test), it doesn't really matter that the language section is weak. However, having a variety of nonverbal measures of intelligence is helpful in identifying skills within the realm of things the child can do. This can include looking separately at things like spontaneous problem-solving (figuring out that round pegs go into round holes), versus imitation with an object (for example, building a tower by copying a model), versus body imitation (wiggling a thumb in imitation). Wherever the examiner finds the child is weak, that is where skills need to be built. A major limitation of the Merrill-Palmer is that the norms are very outdated and the "age-equivalent scores" come out higher than on better normed, more recently developed tests. This is important to know, because a child who looks like he has a "normal" IQ on the Merrill-Palmer at age three may score in the mildly mentally retarded range on another test at age five (and it won't be because he has begun to lose ground).

For children aged four to four-and-a-half years, a frequently used test is the *Weschler Preschool and Primary Scales of Intelligence—Revised* (WPPSI-R). The WPPSI-R is the first of three interlocking Weschler IQ tests that measure essentially the same things from age four through adulthood. Like all the Weschler tests, there is a Verbal IQ (VIQ) and a Performance IQ (PIQ), and a summary score called the Full Scale IQ (FSIQ), which is essentially the average. When there is a difference of more that fifteen points between the VIQ and the PIQ (which there almost always is in autistic children), the "split" or "splinter" is considered statistically and clinically significant. (The FSIQ also becomes an increasingly meaningless number, the greater the split.) Often autistic children can be administered the WPPSI performance subtests (there are six), but need a "younger" test to assess language, if language development is significantly behind PIQ.

Another test that is frequently used with children this age is the Kaufman ABC (K-ABC). The Kaufman can be partly reported by parents, and so in some situations can be more convenient for an examiner to administer. However, there are certain qualitative clinical observations a doctor will make when working directly with a child, and nothing can substitute for this. The K-ABC has several subscales and correlates will with other IQ tests that can be given to children of the same age.

The other test that is frequently used at all ages starting around age three is the Stanford-Binet III. This test breaks down results into three areas. Some testers prefer it to the Weschler series because it spans such a wide range that it is the single test that can handle the greatest splinter in abilities. For some children, the splinter can be so great that verbal ability may be at the two-and-a-half-year old level, while nonverbal abilities are at the ten-year-old level. In such cases, a SB-III may be particularly useful. The SB-III does not reflect the profile of autistic people as well as tests that make a distinction between verbal and performance IQ, and so it seems to be used less with autistic individuals.

Intelligence Tests for Children and Adolescents. Some of the tests already described—namely, the Kaufman and the Stanford-Binet—are used with preschool-age children and continue upward through the school-age period. The only additional test that is widely used with autistic children, and that is first used at school age (six years old and older), is the *Weschler Intelligence Scale* for Children–III (WISC-III). The WISC-R or WISC-III has essentially the same subtests as the WPPSI or WPPSI-R, only at a more difficult level. Given the VIQ/PIQ splinter in many autistic children, sometimes the WISC-III performance subtests can be used alongside the WPPSI verbal subtests. When this is done, the results on verbal IQ would not be reported as in "IQ" number, but rather as an age-equivalent score.

Intelligence Tests for Adults. Relatively little IQ testing is done on adults with autism, mainly because it has usually been done many times before, but also because after about ages ten to twelve the results tend to be nearly the same (plus or minus ten points), time after time. Sometimes IQ testing is done because some confusion exists about whether a "high-functioning" autistic adult is really mentally retarded or not. In that case, IQ testing is usually done simultaneously with testing of the level of adaptive functioning (see the next section), to see how capable the individual is of using his intelligence to get along. The Standard-Binet III is used for adults, as is the Weschler Adult Intelligence Scale—Revised (WAIS-R). The WAIS-R has the same subtests as the WISC-R and WISC-III, and usually the results of a WISC-R or WISC-III obtained around or after puberty (the time at which cognitive development is considered complete) will be essentially the same as those obtained on the WAIS-R. Since the WAIS-R can only be given at a mental age of seventeen or above, it is usually used only on the highest-functioning adults with autism, PDD, or Asperger's syndrome.

    In addition to intelligence tests for adults, there are another group of tests known as "neuropsychological tests," which include the Halstead-Reitan and Luria-Nebraska batteries. These tests have been designed mainly for detecting specific acquired brain damage in adults, but can sometimes be useful in differentiating adults with Asperger's syndrome from adults with unusual patterns of nonverbal learning disabilities. In my clinical experience, the use of neuropsychological batteries for children is not particularly informative for the majority of autistic and PDD children, but sometimes are used.

Test of Adaptive Functioning. In addition to intelligence tests of the type just described, tests of "adaptive functioning" or "functional skills" are also used. These tests measure how the individual is able to use the intelligence she has to get along in everyday life. Tests of adaptive functioning are especially important for identifying skill deficiencies in adult autistic people, because some of the brightest individuals accumulate a lot of knowledge that is only of limited interest to other people (such as knowing the distances between planets, or the number of elevator banks in certain prominent skyscrapers). For an autistic person, knowing many such esoteric facts does not necessarily mean that he or she can make change from ten dollars, figure out how to ride public transportation, or independently know when to change bed linens. Although the intellectual skill may be there—for example, to strip a bed and remake it—the desire to do it may not be there. Much of what we do to fit into society comes from observing and voluntarily wanting to emulate the standards of most people around us. Normally developing young children learn to wash their hands after using the toilet—not because they really understand the theory of germs, but because they are told to do so, and everyone else does it.

When adaptive functioning is measured, differences in adaptability that stem from a lack of social skill are evident even in young autistic children. However, as little ones, autistic children are usually relatively good at adaptive behaviors that don't involve pleasing someone else, but do involve pleasing themselves—feeding themselves, getting around physically, taking off clothes (when they don't want them on), and other adaptive milestones in the everyday functioning of toddlers.

The most widely used test of adaptive behavior is the *Vineland Adaptive Behavior Scales* (VABS). For young children, this test is usually administered by interviewing parents about skills the child has or has not yet achieved. For some teenagers and young adults, it may be completed by interviewing the patient, with some cross-checking for reliability with a parent or caregiver. The VABS gives separate scores (corresponding to levels of mental development) for communication, social skills, everyday living skills, motor skills (in children under five years), and maladaptive behavior. Two other adaptive behavior scales that are sometimes used, and that measure similar things, are the Alpern-Boll Scales and the AAMD Adaptive Behavior Scales. Administering the VABS or a comparable test can be especially helpful when trying to obtain services for a child or adult with high cognitive functioning who has a diagnosis of PDD or Asperger's syndrome, since a number of public agencies do not serve people based on these diagnoses alone. A VABS may show that such an individual is functioning with significant adaptive impairment, despite a normal IQ.

Early Diagnosis

Two remaining topics deserve special attention in this chapter on diagnosis. The first is the topic of early diagnosis. A major factor to be considered during the diagnostic procedures just described is how *early* the child get to see a professional for a diagnosis, since this will have a direct impact on how soon treatment is obtained, and what type of treatment is decided upon as most appropriate. The second remaining topic, which will be covered in the last section of this chapter, is that of *differential diagnosis*—deciding whether the child has autism or a closely related disorder.

At our clinic at the University of California, San Francisco, we've focused a number of years of research on the early diagnosis of autism. This has included annual followup and retesting of all the children we first see under age three, extensive research on a parent-reported questionnaire designed to screen for autism and PDD in children under three years old, and studies of home videotapes made of autistic children before age two. We have also studied issues that lead parents to recognize or fail to recognize signs of autism, as well as how our health-care system works in providing parents with information about their child's developmental problems.

How Does Autism Develop Over Time?

Not surprisingly, we have learned that autisitc children are not born with all (or maybe any) of their symptoms. The symptoms develop in a predictable way over time. We have studied these patterns of development to learn how early signs of autism can be recognized, and in which areas of development.

The first thing we learned is that, although parents typically state that problems with language development are their main (or only) concern, parents in fact realize that there is a juxtapositioning of language difficulties with an absence of imaginary play. It is often most difficult for parents to identify their child's difficulties with social development since these are more a matter of degree, while the language and play difficulties seem more easily quantifiable. A child who only says three words at age two-and-a-half, or a child who ignores new toys right from the beginning, is clearly different from siblings and friends' children at the same ages. Also, perhaps parents are so strongly "programmed" to both give and get love from their children, that as long as the child reciprocates in some contexts, they feel the need for mutual affection is being met, and no "alarm" about social development sounds as loudly as it does about absent language, or odd or absent play. With discussion, however, most parents can accurately describe atypical social development in their autistic children who are as young as eighteen months old.

In one study we did, we found that pediatricians, too, are helped by being made aware of the juxtapositioning of social and language deficits. Two developmental complaints—for example, about language development *and* odd play—were much more likely to be a red flag than any complaint presented singly.

Home Videos of Autistic Toddlers. From family videotapes made before autistic children turned two, we were alerted to several ways in which autistic toddlers were different. Quite prominently, they lacked social referencing—meaning they did not look toward an adult to "share" what they were doing when they had just succeeded (or failed) at a task, nor did they look to adults in a situation where a toddler might normally expect to be praised or punished.

Autistic toddlers had difficulty perceiving the social ambience. For example, many of the home videos were made at Christmas or birthdays or other family gatherings. When a birthday cake would be brought in the room, everyone would look at it—even babies as young as ten to twelve months. Typically, the autistic toddler just didn't know what all the excitement was about—or that there was excitement in the air. Even at his own second birthday party, an autistic toddler tends to look rather disconnected from what is going on.

Scenes of the autistic toddler among other children showed a child who seemed as if she was in her own invisible bubble, in a setting apart from others. Attempts by others to approach were generally ignored or shunned in an offhanded manner, by turning away or by wincing.

Autistic toddlers often seemed more serious about what they were doing, with less emotional expressiveness, and fewer interludes of distraction to check on something they might have just heard, unlike normal children who tend to love to be on camera. It was in fact hard to get an emotional reaction from autistic toddlers even when the videotaper (usually the father) would try to get them to "ham" for the camera. For reasons we do not yet understand well, some of our videos of autistic toddlers under one year of age show babies who are much more normally reactive to the camera than the same children a year later.

The Pervasive Developmental Disorders Screening Test (PDDST). Another way we have studied early forms of autism and PDD is through a parent questionnaire. Parents fill out the questionnaire for each age range, up to the current age of their child. The tables below show selected PDDST questions that parents are asked to answer about their child. All of the questions here are ones that at least half of the parents of autistic children respond to positively. Parents of children with PDD tend to endorse the same questions, but with slightly lower rates than those of children who meet the full diagnostic criteria for autistic disorder.

Just as we would not expect to see all the symptoms of autistic disorder in any one autistic child, neither would all the emergent symptoms of autism be present in any one child. The same rules apply for the diagnostician, who will need to be sure that the early signs present in any one child are in fact precursors of various "full-grown" signs of autism. In fact, most of the signs we found to be frequently positive in children three to four years old (see the last section of Table 3) are basically the same expressions of autism seen in younger children. The PDDST, therefore, is especially useful in describing early symptoms of autism and PDD, especially between eighteen months and three years. If you have a child in this age range, determining whether some of these PDD symptoms are present should provide some guidelines as to whether your child may be on the way to developing a full-blown case of autism of PDD.

In the next section, we'll consider other non-autistic PDDs as another approach to understanding diagnostically what is autism and what is not.

Table 3 Pervasive Developmental Disorders Screening Test

Age in Months	Questions rated "Mostly true" by 50 percent or more of parents of children with autism
Birth to Six	Does your infant seem unusually interested in moving objects, or moving lights (compared, for example, to his interest in looking at faces)?
Six to Twelve	Does your baby sometimes stare or tune out, making it hard to get his attention?
	Some babies show they want "up" by reaching, others cry or fuss; would you say your baby is the type to cry or fuss—and not reach up when he wants "up"?

(Continued)

Table 3 Pervasive Developmental Disorders Screening Test (*Continued*)

Age in Months	Questions rated "Mostly true" by 50 percent or more of parents of children with autism
Twelve to Eighteen	Does your baby ever seem bored or uninterested in conversation around him?
	Have you noticed that your baby can be very alert to some sounds and not to others?
	Does your baby either ignore toys most of the time, or almost all the time play with 1 or 2 things?
	Have you ever suspected that your child might have hearing difficulties?
	Do you wonder if your baby knows his name?
	Does your baby strongly prefer or strongly dislike particular foods?
Eighteen to Twenty-four	Does your baby seem uninterested in learning to talk?
	When you're trying to get your baby's attention, do you ever feel that your baby will avoid looking right at you?
	Does your child seem unafraid or unaware of things that are dangerous?
	Does your baby ever seem to be talking in his own language?
	Does your baby avoid playing with dolls and stuffed animals, or even seem to dislike them?
	Does your baby have a hard time getting used to playing with new toys, or playing new games, even though he may enjoy it when he gets used to it?
	Has your baby not yet begun to show what he wants, either by using words, pointing, or making a noise?
	At times do you feel that your baby doesn't care if you're there or not?
Twenty-four to Thirty	Does your child often seem to understand only part of what is said to him?
	Does your child only try to communicate when there is something he wants and can't get for himself?
	Does your child try to get away with using as few words as possible? For example, saying "juice" for anything he wants to eat?
	Will your child lead you to a desired object as a way of showing you what he wants?
	Does your child prefer things he can play with the same way, over and over, such as a "See-n-Say," or toys with buttons he can push?
	Does your child seem particularly fascinated by motion? For example, will he flip pages of a book, sift sand, spin objects, or watch running water just to see the movement?
	Can your child do some things so well that it surprises you when he can't do other things?
	Does it seem that your child can pretty much understand, but still usually does not follow directions?

(*Continued*)

Table 3 (*Continued*)

Age in Months	Questions rated "Mostly true" by 50 percent or more of parents of children with autism
	Does your child usually enjoy being tickled or chased, but does not usually enjoy playing patty-cake or peek-a-boo?
	Up to this age has your child ever gone through a period when he stopped using words he once used?
	Does your child understand most or all of what is said to him, but not yet say any or only a few words?
Thirty to Thirty-six	Have you worried that your child doesn't seem too interested in other children?
	Does your child not yet imagine make-believe people and actions when he plays?
	Does your child seem unusually interested in mechanical things, such as light switches, door latches, locks, fans, vacuums, or clocks?
	Does your child seem unable to learn through watching and copying others (like catching a ball or swinging)?
	Is your child uninterested in watching TV, or only watches things a child his age wouldn't usually watch—like MTV, or certain game shows?
	Does your child sometimes seem to learn a new word by its melody rather than by sounding it out?
	Does your child primarily enjoy hugging and physical contact when he wants it, and not when it's your idea?
	Have you sometimes worried whether your child feels pain as much as other kids? For example, will he fall down hard and not cry when you expect him to?
	Does your child show an ability to echo things exactly as he's heard them, or to imitate sounds better than real words?
	Has your child ever forgotten old words when he's learned new ones?
Thirty-six to Forty-eight	Does your child mostly echo things exactly as he's heard them before?
	Does your child play with toys in ways that really aren't the main way the toy was meant to be used?
	When excited, does your child flap his hands or fingers?
	Have you worried that your child's tone of voice is unusual? For example, does it sound monotonous, high-pitched, or sing-song?
	Do you feel that your child acts too upset when there are changes in routines or schedule?
	Does your child seem very concerned with order and neatness when he plays? For example, does he like to line things up, or sort things over and over, or insist on putting things away when finished?
	Does your child know which way you will go when you go in the car, and will he get upset if you go another way or somewhere he doesn't like?

Differential Diagnosis

By way of comparison, various non-autistic PDDs, particularly Asperger's syndrome and fragile X, have been referred to repeatedly. Earlier in this chapter, fragile X was again mentioned in the context of genetic testing and counseling. The term *differential diagnosis* refers to the act of differentiating among several related diagnoses that are considered in addition to the one that is ultimately made. In this section, we look at Asperger's snydrome in more detail since it is often the diagnosis considered when a child is suspected of having PDD or autism but does not have significant mental retardation.

The section that follows is intended as a "stand alone" section. If Asperger's syndrome is being considered as the appropriate diagnosis for your child, especially if your child appears to have little or no cognitive delay, and was not recognized as developmentally different until three or four years of age, this section will be helpful in understanding how Asperger's syndrome differs from autism and PDD. A parent with a younger child or a professional working with younger children might want to skip this section. The second differential diagnosis that will be discussed here is fragile X syndrome, which I would recommend skipping unless your child or a child you know definitely has fragile X syndrome.

Asperger's Syndrome

Along with the diagnostic labels of autistic disorder and PDD,NOS, there is another diagnosis that is increasingly being used to describe children who have signs of autism, but who are less severely affected overall. This diagnosis is Asperger's syndrome or AS. As we discussed in Chapter 1, with the publication of DSM-IV and ICD-10, Asperger's syndrome (or Asperger's disorder, as it is offically entitled) became a separate diagnostic category for the first time. In this section we will discuss what AS is and is not, how it is distinguished from autism, and the ways in which AS is thought to be similar to *and* different from autism. The difference is that those with AS tend to have symptoms that impair them less overall. Children with AS will display some symptoms of autism in quite a pronounced way, while certain other symptoms are not present at all. There is increasingly good evidence that AS is very closely related to autism in terms of brain function and probably has the same or similar genetic basis, but is generally associated with less mental retardation. Autism and AS may be *etiologically* the same entity—that is, have the same origin in many cases—but the reason there has been a push to distinguish AS as a separate diagnosis is that it seems *prognostically* different from autism.

One study done of all children under sixteen years old in one section of London estimated that AS was half as common as autism and included some children who started out looking autistic, but more closely fit the description of AS as they got older. Another study in Sweden showed that AS was even more predominately a male disorder than autism—affecting about ten boys for each girl.

Asperger's syndrome is considered a disorder, but there is some evidence that mild forms of AS may be expressed in a way that might be described more as a personality style. Such cases may be so mild that a diagnosis of AS is not warranted. Such children are socially immature and loners, but do not have the eccentricities that characterize individuals with AS. As school-age children, such individuals may have seemed quite normal around adults, but different from other children in the context of a peer group. Some research has suggested that this type of "personality style" may be quite prevalent among siblings of autistic children who are thus suspected of having a genetic form of autism. Those with Asperger's syndrome have described themselves as social loners; they may find it hard to look at people when they speak to them, and others may see them as perceiving the world in black and white. We can imagine a continuum, where AS is manifested as a clear disorder at one extreme and a personality style at the other extreme—with all the variations in between.

Origins of the Asperger's Syndrome Diagnosis

Asperger's syndrome is so named because it was first described in 1944 by Hans Asperger, a Viennese pediatrician interested in finding ways to treat children with learning and emotional problems. Although he first published his work in 1944, and Kanner published his original account of autism in 1943, the two were unaware of each other's work. The children described by each were very similar, although a few of Asperger's cases were more mild types, and a few of Kanner's cases were more severe. There was little to no scientific exchange between Americans and Germans at that time because of World War II, and so when these studies were initially published, there were no opportunities for Asperger, Kanner, or others to systematically work out the similarities and differences between the cases each had described. After the war, the diagnosis of AS came into use in European psychiatry, but not in America. During this period, the use of the term AS took on increasingly specific connotations for European psychiatrists, as they saw more cases. Similarly, as American psychiatrists saw more cases of "Kanner's syndrome," the definition of autism became increasingly specific in the United States. Although Asperger and Kanner had started out describing groups of children who were more similar than different from one another, the elaborated European and American definitions moved further apart because Americans read little European research. Finally in 1981, Lorna Wing, a well-known British child psychiatrist who has studied autism for many years, brought Asperger's work into the English-language literature. For the past ten years or so, the appearance of Asperger's syndrome as a concept in American and English psychiatry has stimulated a great deal of research and led to support for including AS as an "autistic spectrum disorder" in the diagnostic manuals used by psychiatrists for diagnoses. Interestingly, an English translation of Asperger's original paper has only recently appeared (1991) in the form of a well-annotated translation by Uta Frith, who has included Asperger's paper in her excellent edited volume titled *Autism and Asperger Syndrome*, which is the single best reference for the reader who is primarily interested in learning about Asperger's syndrome.

What Were Children with Asperger's Syndrome Called in the Past?

Because Asperger's Syndrome has recently been introduced as a diagnosis, the symptoms that make up AS are just being recognized as a distinct diagnostic entity. Many professionals are beginning to read about AS in the literature for the first time. Many doctors feel that some of the patients they've seen in the past probably had AS, but at the time, the problem was described as mild autism, PDD,NOS, schizoid personality disorder, a severe expressive language disorder, or even childhood schizophrenia.

The *Diagnostic and Statistical Manual* of the American Psychiatric Association lists the following criteria for AS:

A. A lack of any clinically significant general delay in language or cognitive development. Diagnosis requires that single words should have developed by two years of age or earlier and that communicative phrases be used by three years of age or earlier. Self-help skills, adaptive behavior, and curiosity about the environment during the first three years should be at a level consistent with normal intellectual development. However, motor milestones may be somewhat delayed and motor clumsiness is usual (although not necessarily a diagnostic feature). Isolated special skills, often related to abnormal preoccupations, are common, but are not required for the diagnosis.

B. Qualitative impairments in reciprocal social interaction. Diagnosis requires demonstrable impairments in at least three out of five areas:

1. Failure to use eye to eye gaze, facial expression, body posture, and gesture to regulate social interaction.
2. Failure to develop (in a manner appropriate to mental age, and despite ample opportunities) peer relationships that involve a mutual sharing of interests, activities, and emotions.
3. Rarely seeking or using other people for comfort and affection at times of distress, and/or offering comfort and affection to others when they are showing distress or unhappiness.
4. Lack of shared enjoyment in terms of vicarious pleasure in other people's happiness, and/or a spontaneous seeking to share enjoyment through joint involvement with others.
5. A lack of social-emotional reciprocity as shown by an impaired or deviant response to other people's emotions; and/or lack of modulation of behavior according to social context, and/or a weak integration of social, emotional, and communicative behaviors.

C. Restricted, repetitive, and stereotypical pattern of interests and activities (however, it would be less usual for these to include either motor mannerisms or preoccupations with part-objects or nonfunctional elements of play materials).

The recency of AS as a diagnostic category explains why many ten-year-olds, twenty-year-olds, and even forty-year-olds who had never been diagnosed as having AS before are now receiving this diagnosis for the first time.

Main Features of Asperger's Syndrome

The best way of understanding what AS is is to contrast it with autism. Asperger's syndrome is on the same "spectrum" of neurologically-based social dysfunction as autism—meaning that there is some overlap between the two diagnoses. There are a substantial number of individuals who meet DSM criteria for autistic disorder who also can be diagnosed as having AS, especially below age ten. However, most AS individuals have more mild overall impairment, higher IQs, (especially higher verbal IQs), and a better ability to adapt than most autistic people. It can even be said that between an autistic and an AS individual of the same chronological and mental age, the AS person typically will appear less impaired overall. Some children who were diagnosed as autistic when younger develop in ways that make AS a better diagnosis for them when they are older. IQ is one way in which those diagnosed with autism and AS tend to differ: It should be noted, though, that not all autistic people with higher IQs should be labeled with AS—many have all the symptoms of autism, just higher IQs. Less often, AS individuals can display mild retardation. In addition to different profiles of intellectual ability, individuals with autism and AS differ in the quality of their social relatedness and in activities and interests.

Social Impairments in Asperger's Syndrome. Probably the most noticeable thing about individuals with AS is the social difficulties they have. For a teacher or other person familiar with children with very specific learning disabilities, AS can be characterized as a specific and severe inability of social understanding. Just as a deaf person may end up with a distorted idea of what is going on because one of his senses in "turned off," an AS individual can be thought of as selectively "people-deaf" or at least "people hard-of-hearing." The combined information we normally integrate from the juxtaposition of words, gestures, and timing in conversation is poorly comprehended by an AS person. People with AS are very literal and tend not to comprehend aspects of social interaction that vary in meaning depending upon context. People with AS are rule-oriented; they can learn by rote basic social rules, like "stand at least three feet away from someone you are talking to," or "look at the person you are talking to," but tend to apply the rule inflexibly, standing three feet away when the arrangement of furniture would make five feet more natural, or staring *too* fixedly while talking.

As an example, I remember one patient whose parents had difficulty because once their ten-year-old son was taught to kiss, he wanted to kiss family members and strangers alike. So, they taught him the rule "You can only kiss people at our house." This worked fine—until one day a UPS man had to come inside to get a signature on a parcel delivery!

A puzzling feature of individuals with Asperger's syndrome is their inability to comprehend what friendships are about. Most are either indifferent to the idea of friendships, or have no idea how to make a friend. If one asks a young person with AS, "Do you have a best friend?" you may get one of two rather odd types of responses. The first may be "No, I don't have any friends." This statement can be delivered with the same lack of emotion as if you had asked "Do you have any non-fat milk at home in your refrigerator?" and been told, "No, I don't have any non-fat milk." The second type of response is the type given by individuals with AS who have learned that one *should* have friends, and/or believe they *do* have friends. On probing, you might discover the "friend" is someone that hasn't been seen or heard from in three years, and that, at the time, was known only slightly. More poignantly, a "best friend" is often a nonaffected adult who works for their county's social service agency or residential living facility, and who comes by once a week to take them shopping for personal items, or to McDonald's for lunch. Again, in that rule-oriented way, a best friend may be identified as someone who is seen each day or someone with whom greetings are always exchanged—like the local bus driver.

Some young adults with AS really seem to want friends but aren't able to cope with all the things they need to do right to make a friend. On the other hand, if anyone (say at work) shows an interest in being friendly, they may overreact and begin to call that person on the phone frequently, holding one-sided conversations about their own particular interest. Nedless to say, this flags the recipient of such calls that the AS person is a little beyond just odd, or eccentric, and people tend to pull away after these one-sided initial contacts.

Other people with AS, particularly younger, preteen children, tend to express little or no desire for friendships. They may rebuff what few attempts classmates make to be friends, or be actively hostile but in an impersonal, self-centered sort of way. One nine-year-old AS boy, J.R., whom I met in Los Angeles, had a IQ in the 130s (well above average), but was in an LH (learning handicapped) class at school because of his poor social skills, behavioral problems, and lack of interest in following the curriculum. His mother said J.R. had no friends in his class because he persisted in referring to other students jointly and individually as "stupid" when they gave wrong answers to easy questions. J.R.'s classmates, though the same age chronologically, were about four years behind him academically, and he knew it. Therefore, J.R. told me, he did not see why he should desist in using the adjective "stupid," if, in essence, it was an accurate descriptor. For the higher functioning AS individual, being right is always much more important than being conciliatory or gracious. This approach to social interactions has sometimes been aptly described as "active but odd." The individual with AS may actively make contact with others, but the nature of the contact in no way reflects the qualities or responses of the other person.

For those of us who recognize AS as a severe disability in understanding social cues, insensitive behavior can often be seen as a discrepancy between what one needs to do to be accepted socially, and what an individual might do if no one else was there. In this light, many of the social faux pas committed by individuals with AS can appear amusing—much like watching a 10-year-old boy trying to act like a tough, macho 16-year-old because he has an older friend he wishes to impress. However, day-to-day living with such an unusual personality can be a challenge. In Chapter 13, we'll say more about interventions related to social skills development.

The Preoccupying, Narrow Interests of the Person with Asperger's Syndrome. There are many, many special interests of people with AS. Having one or more peculiar, intense interests is considered part of the definition of AS. There are some peculiar interests that strike the rest of us as particularly fascinating, and that are seen over and over again in a number of AS and high-functioning autistic individuals. These include rote memorization of bus and train schedules, memorization of calendar days and dates for years into the future and past (as in the movie *Rain Man*), extensive knowledge about the weather or aspects of astronomy, and classifications of plants and animals, especially big animals like whales, bears, and dinosaurs. There has been some speculation about how such topics get picked; perhaps they take hold at a time when the individual is especially impressionable—a brief "open window," when there is a period of imprintability. It has been suggested that these open windows may occur around transition times (like moving to a new house) when old routines are no longer available, and there may be some sort of urge to quickly make new routines (meaningful or not) to fill the old void. For a topic of special interest to imprint itself, however, it seems to have to have certain features. One is that it contain some class of elements that can be subject to rote memorization. Second, the topic is usually one that can be learned from books, TV, or computers, rather than from interpersonal communication. Third, the topic usually lends itself to list-making or some other classification exercises.

When trying to make conversation with someone with AS, it usually doesn't take long for them to initiate their topic of special interest, even if the transition to the topic isn't particularly smooth. Paul, a 24-year-old with AS, retains facts about giants. A casual conversation with Paul can go from: Me: "What did you do today?" Paul: "Watch TV." / Me: "Do you ever watch sports?" Paul: "Basketball. . . . Do you know who the tallest person ever in the NBA was?" Me: "Kareem Abdul-Jabar? (wild guess)." Paul: "No!! (Gives correct answer)." Paul: "Do you know who the tallest Scottish giant was? Do you know how tall he was?" Then, despite the fact that I didn't even know the tallest basketball player, Paul's conversation continues with queries about the tallest men re-

corded in each of several nations. After a while, it is hard for even an empathetic listener to continue to show interest, but the person with AS does not
read either subtle or not-so-subtle cues to change the topic or desist. The urge
to go on with the topic is usually quite strong once started. Despite many
attempts I've made to find out, the person with AS is pretty much at a loss to
explain why he considers giants, calendars, bus schedules, or whatever, so
fascinating although one girl with AS I know will tell her mother that she has
"lost the love" of a topic whenever she moves on to a new one (which is only
once every few years).

If you are around a person like this daily, it certainly isn't necessary to
"partake" in this one-sided conversation constantly. It is quite possible, and
not harmful to them, to impose limits on repetitious talk. In fact, doing so is a
helpful way of modeling more appropriate conversation. For example, if a
young man with AS asks you about the highest elevation in India, and then the
highest elevation in Pakistan, you can interrupt and say "You know, Byron, I'd
like to talk to you more about geography, but right now I need to go to the
grocery store." Of course, it sometimes takes two or three repetitions to get
your point across; and when you return from the grocery store you can be
assured that a continuing discourse on "elevations" will be waiting for you. The
most successful way to curtail repetitive conversation around favorite topics is
to constrict the time, place, and duration of when such "conversations" may be
held. The goal is to have the use of the conversational topic appear more
normal. So, for example, Byron might be instructed that after the dinner
dishes are done, we can go in the living room, take out an atlas, and discuss
elevations of mountain ranges on the Indian subcontinent for fifteen minutes.

Asperger's Syndrome in the Younger Child

Despite what is known about Asperger's syndrome in school-age children and
in adults, little is known about how to tell the difference between very young
children with AS versus those with autism. As was already mentioned, there
are a number of individuals who meet criteria for autism when younger, but as
they mature, the picture of AS emerges more and more clearly. On average,
AS is detected later than autism, because the absence of early language development, which is initially striking in virtually all autistic children, is not so
prominent in those with AS. While language may be delayed, it may not go
through an "immediate echolalia" phase. Eye contact may be poor, but the
child can be seen as serious or independent. The social need for others may be
diminished, but a relatively better relationship with the mother may mask
that.

There may be limited topics of interest, but parents tend to be impressed
with the child's intelligence because at an early age, the child memorized vast
tracts from videotapes, or book after book of Dr. Seuss. Reasoning ability may
seem unusual, but this can be seen as divergent, creative thinking, rather than
a disturbance in social understanding. For example, J.R., the boy mentioned
earlier, had come up with his own classification of plants: "Those that grow

from the top down—like grass" and "Those that grow from the bottom up—like trees". (It wasn't easy to get him to explain this further, or for him to see why this explanation was not sufficiently complete for me.) Similarly, there was Leon, who built a "gravity/ anti-gravity machine" out of Leggos: the "gravity" part rotated on a horizontal axis, the "anti-gravity" part rotated on a vertical axis. (Leon was also very interested in migrating polar bears.)

Despite displaying precocity in certain ways, even the highest functioning AS children are recognized as very different by the time they enter kindergarten, when their lack of social skills sets them apart from peers in a very marked way—even if they are academically excellent. Sometimes such children are first diagnosed as "aphasic" or "dysphasic" or "language disordered," meaning that they are seen as having difficulty processing language the same way as the rest of us even though they may use language exceptionally well. The idea that such children may be aphasic comes from observations that little of what they say incorporates verbal feedback they have just been given. For example, David, age five, came to our clinic recently—full of questions about heaters, how they were set, what the numbers on them meant, how the numbers corresponded to the outside temperature, and soon. Despite repeated (albeit basic) explanations of how our heating worked, the same questions repeatedly and enthusiastically reappeared every forty-five minutes or so. How early the social deficits of AS are noticed depends partly on whether there are older siblings to be compared with and how much exposure to peers the child gets in the first few years. In years past, many parents of AS children were subjected to years of psychodynamic explanations for their child's condition, followed by years of play therapy designed to help the child express his inner conflicts, along with, of course, collateral parent visits to help the parents resolve their alleged ambivalent, hostile, or otherwise unhelpful conscious or unconscious feelings toward the child. Whenever I read through records of AS cases with such previous treatment histories, I am saddened by the fact that if you look closely, it can be seen that these childrens' problems also were recognized to have a developmental basis; not knowing what to call it, however, doctors often will have diagnosed and treated them for an emotional disorder instead.

Longer Term Prognosis and Adults with Asperger's Syndrome. How do children diagnosed with AS turn out as adults? That is the question many parents ask when their child receives a diagnosis of AS. In the beginning of this section, a point was made that those with Asperger's syndrome tend to have a better prognosis than those with autism. More can live independently. Others live near their families, who do a certain amount of checking in. One big factor in degree of independence is the ability to attain some degree of economic self-sufficiency. The biggest obstacle to economic self-sufficiency is finding the right job and work situation, and motivating the individual with AS to want to work. In later chapters, we will address treatment issues in detail, both for individuals with AS and individuals with autism. For now, the focus will be on the results of studies and case reports of people with AS as they have become adults.

Part of the generally better prognosis for those with AS is that they have less mental retardation, on average, than those with autism. Individual outcomes vary with a number of factors, intelligence being one and social support another. Generally, people with AS do better in supportive settings where those around them are aware they are in some way disabled and are willing to make some kind of accommodation to that. AS people can do relatively well if they work at a job that complements their narrow range of interests. For example, Vincent, now in his early forties, is preoccupied with Mozart, and listens to Mozart in much of his free time. He was able to get a janitorial job in a large university's music library. Although this was not a very high level job, he was happy to be around the music. He also benefitted from a job that was highly routine, and that didn't require being around other people who spoke to him frequently.

Probably the most difficult thing for familes to accept is that despite having a possibly in-depth knowledge of a particular subject, the individuals with AS generally end up functioning at a lower level than their IQ alone would pre-dict. For Vincent, the Mozart man, being a janitor was all the pressure and responsibility he could adequately handle. Also, the peculiar interests of those with AS tend to be so narrow that the knowledge may generalize poorly to all aspects of what is needed to do a more complex job. For example, even if you know all the train arrivals and departures out of Manhattan on Amtrak, in order to work at the ticket window, you also need to know how to operate a cash register, run credit cards, and answer phones—all at the same time. As a rough rule of thumb, higher functioning autistic and AS people seem to do better in more rural, less complex towns than in big cities, where life is faster paced.

Working in a family business where you are protected by your connections can help too. One young man, Barton, whom I first saw about a year ago, was in his mid-twenties, had an above-average IQ, and has AS. He came from a rather well-off family, and they had helped him adjust by getting him a job *L.A. Law*-style, doing filing and photocopying in a large law firm where his father was a partner. (*L.A. Law* for the uninitiated, was a television program in which one of the main characters was an office assistant with mental retarda-tion.) Although Barton could have his bad days, he was protected by his relationship to the boss—and from what I could tell, pretty well accepted there. Barton aspired to learn word-processing and databases, but realized that because of his "difficulties" this was harder for him than for most people. Another teenager, Steven, was very interested in the Latin names of plants, and at age fourteen carried an umbrella, trench coat, and attache case filled with magazine and newpaper clippings about plants (which he would readily show you if you asked). As he got a little older, he was given a job at a small local newspaper published by his grandfather. His job was to clip out "classi-fied" ads, count the words, and attach it to a corresponding invoice. Not all success stories about AS adults come from families with bountiful financial resources. Some AS people end up doing gardening, maintenance work, or stockroom work. What is usually most important to them is that they have an outlet to express their special interest, and some measure of independence.

The downside of the relatively better prognosis for individuals with AS is their vulnerability to a variety of psychiatric disorders. A number of psychiatric conditions occur more frequently. This is probably a combination of constitutional, inborn or genetic risk factors in combination with the fact that AS individuals often have the feeling that they are *not* like everyone else (since they are not). A study done in England showed that thirty-five percent of adults with AS had some psychiatric disorder, including ten percent who had some sort of severe manic and/or manic-depressive psychosis; thirteen percent with some other psychosis; and fifteen percent with depression, anxiety, or obsessive compulsive disorder. Manic-depressive psychosis was three times more common than schizophrenia. Depression was the most common psychiatric diagnosis. In my own clinical experience, psychiatric disorders in young adults with AS are caused mainly by their being pushed too hard, and not protected enough. In other young people with AS, incipient psychiatric disorders seem to be just off-stage from a very early age, and as a clinician, you find yourself a fairly helpless bystander with a strong hunch that a particular child or adolescent with AS is on the road to developing a psychotic disorder. In some individuals, the vulnerability seems so strong, that the course of the development of other psychiatric disorders along with the AS seems almost inevitable. In other cases, the outcome seems more malleable. As we discuss treatments, there will be suggestions for deciding how much to challenge, train, and teach a person with AS without causing so much stress that development of a psychiatric disorder seems more likely.

Fragile X Syndrome

Fragile X syndrome involves an abnormality of the X chromosome, which can be detected in a blood test. As discussed in Chapter 1, fragile X is inherited by boys from their mothers, who may have no problems themselves or may have certain mild learning disabilities. Sometimes fragile X can cause PDD and, very occasionally, autism in girls, but most often affects males. Males with the fragile X syndrome sometimes meet criteria for autism but more often meet criteria for PDD. Children with fragile X syndrome who also have symptoms of autism or PDD most often have the specific symptoms of poor eye contact, sing-songy tone of voice, echolalia, and hand-flapping. Many also have difficulties in social relatedness; however, children with fragile X syndrome often have less severe problems with social relatedness than other autistic children.

Most physicians will suggest a blood test for the fragile X syndrome as part of an initial diagnostic workup. Although only about three to five percent of males with autism have the fragile X syndrome, it is worthwhile to have the test done: If a child does have fragile X, the mother's future pregnancies can be monitored, and fragile X can be detected by amniocentesis. Even if parents plan no further children, identification of an autistic or PDD child as having fragile X may have implications for family planning for relatives of the mother (especially the mother's sisters), or for sisters of the autistic child, all of whom may be "silent" carriers of the fragile X chromosome. At present, however, knowing a child has fragile X syndrome does not alter treatment. The child's treatment plan is developed symptom-by-symptom, the way it is for any other autistic or PDD child.

Chapter Summary

After clinical visits, medical tests, and psychological tests have been completed, the clinician or team of clinicians who have conducted the assessment typically meet with a child's parents to present and explain the diagnosis, results of testing, and treatment recommendations. Sometimes, all of the doctors and clinicians who have been involved in the assessment are present for the debriefing; sometimes just the lead doctor. Some parents attend debriefings with their child's teacher, speech therapist, or caseworker. This can be really helpful: The parents have someone on their "side" who can ask more technical questions and, later, can explain things that may have been missed or misunderstood.

The diagnostic debriefing is an emotionally traumatic time. Parents are often hearing what they fear most. It is, in fact, very difficult for many doctors to give bad news well, and sometimes the doctor may "fuzz the edges" of what he or she has to say in order to soften the psychological impact of the information being given. The information that has been accumulated about the child is only useful if the people to whom the information is disseminated understand it. The psychological defenses that both parents and doctors can construct to deal with the painful process of learning about a child's disability can impede understanding, and therefore, later, treatment of the disorder. In the next chapter, we will discuss the psychological issues that surround a diagnosis of autism or PDD, and how parents work through the distress and, often, outright grief that follows a diagnosis of autism.

◆ ◆ ◆

CHAPTER 6

After the Diagnosis:
Coping with a Sense of Loss

Natural Defenses and Grief

When a couple plan to have a baby, the one thing they hope will not happen to them is having a child with a disability. If a couple is particularly worried, the mother undergoes amniocentesis; if the results are normal, parents are generally reassured. When the baby is born, if the delivery has gone well and the baby comes out healthy, everyone is joyous. A large percentage of physical and developmental anomalies are detected around the time of birth, so if the baby appears normal then, everyone stops worrying about having a baby with a disability. Almost always, at birth, the autistic baby is believed to be normal. Although a very small number of mothers felt there was something odd about their autistic baby from birth, most feel that there was nothing wrong.

Sometime later, however, concern begins to grow that the baby *does* have some sort of a problem. In the last chapter, we talked about developmental screening and how children get tracked into the process of successive evaluations that eventually leads to the diagnosis of autism or PDD. In this chapter we will focus on what the diagnosis of autism feels like to parents and how parents cope.

There are several stages at which parents of autistic or PDD children begin to realize that their child may have a problem. At first, the concern is subconscious. In fact all parents experience some degree of subconscious worry—they may notice something in their child's behavior that makes them worry that their baby or toddler will be late to talk, not very coordinated, or not as intelligent as others in the family. At some point, both parents may discover that each is worrying about the same things and this tends to make the worry more real. Sometimes, an aunt or grandmother will come over and make an off-handed (or pointed) observation that suddenly brings the subconscious worry a parent has into full consciousness. At this point some parents just wait and watch the problem for a while. Others call their pediatrician instantly, even though it's Saturday. From the beginning of the realization that there is a problem, some parents cope by hanging back, keeping themselves calm, and trying to keep distance and objectivity in their analysis of what might be going wrong. Other parents feel the drive to take action immediately, do *something*, and get answers as soon as possible. There are many different coping styles. There is no completely right way to cope, no completely wrong way to cope. Some ways of coping tend to be more helpful than others. The goal here is to understand your own coping strategies, and how your coping may currently be helping or hindering your ability to deal with your child's autism, the rest of your family, and other important aspects of your life.

In addition to coping with their own feelings about a child's disability, most parents are also trying to communicate with a spouse who may or may not be perceiving the child's problems similarly. Parents need to work through their feelings about a child's diagnosis of autism or PDD, and there are stages that most parents pass through and questions that are often asked. Knowing how other parents think and reason when they are faced with their child's diagnosis may reassure you that you are not alone in having confused, angry, sad, or uncontrollable thoughts and feelings when you child is diagnosed with autism or PDD. Other people's solutions and reactions to learning their child is autistic may give you insight into your own situation. I certainly have met many wonderfully altruistic parents who would like to feel that their own working-through can serve as some sort of a guide to families coping with the same sense of loss.

Autism and Bereavement.   Many aspects of coping with the diagnosis of autism are similar to the stages of grief that are experienced when a beloved family member dies. The stages in grieving associated with bereavement have been well-studied and shed some light on what happens when parents have a child diagnosed with a lifetime disability.

The "death" that the parent experiences is the death of the idealized child. Parents have beliefs and feelings, albeit amorphous ones, of who they want their child to be as he grows. As suspicions of the child's disability grow, it is as if a terminal illness was progressing; a diagnosis of autism seals the fate of that idealized child who "dies" with the acceptance of the diagnosis. Of course, the physical child lives, and in some ways, his presence, and perhaps even some of his actions, keeps alive some of the fantasies about the idealized child being resurrected some day.

All parents, whether their child is handicapped or not, deal simultaneously with the reality of who their child is, and who they would ideally like their child to be. For parents of autistic children, the discrepancy is much larger— and harder to reconcile.

In coping with a diagnosis of autism or PDD, parents experience a particular burden that is unique to autistic spectrum disorders: the child is selectively impaired in social reciprocity. Although autistic children may love their parents in their own ways, they express need and affection differently from other children; this keeps parents reaching across some chasm to try and bridge the difference. The mother of one of my patients wrote a powerful and touching poem about her son's diagnosis with autism, and the loss of her idealized child:

Finding Out
Broken sleep / And broken dreams / Surround the chaos
Of diagnostic evaluations and / Brain scans and / The silent drives home.
Where is that far away place / Your big blue eyes so often go? / Can I follow you
there, / And then just once / We could read a Sesame Street book together.
It took me so long to say it. / That word. / Autism. / Autistic. / My little boy / Who was
supposed to play baseball with Daddy, / To be excited when the fire truck went by,
And now all I do / Is thirst for you to say, / "Mommy, can I have some juice?"
                                    (*Connie Post, 'Seasons of Loss' 1992*)

Initial Reactions to the Diagnosis of Autism

Two to four times a week, I sit with parents of young children and explain that their child is autistic, and what they will need to do about it. I live at the end of the long road of diagnostic evaluations. As many times as I've given a diagnosis of autism, PDD, or mental retardation, it is still very painful for me to do. It is very hard to train new doctors to do it (although that is part of my job, too). Whatever pain I experience in *giving* the diagnosis, it has to be a pinprick in comparison to *receiving* the diagnosis.

Some parents intuitively understand their child is autistic before the doctor actually uses the word "autism." Some parents need to hear the diagnosis of autism from several different sources before it can be fully accepted. Sometimes parents don't tell me that their child's been diagnosed autistic before, or don't tell me the previous diagnosis—just to be sure that my opinion is independent. Parents come for second, third, and fourth opinions or however many their insurance policy will tolerate. Parents with twenty-five-year-olds show up just to see if we *still* think it's autism. Acceptance of the child's disability is a gradual and never-ending process for many families.

There are different ways that parents can find out that their child is autistic. Sometimes they discover it themselves while reading or talking with others. Sometimes a teacher, speech therapist, or school psychologist off-handedly, hurriedly, or nervously tosses the term "autistic-like" or "autistic features" with respect to some difficulty the child is having. Sometimes the word "autism" is first suggested by a busy pediatrician who tells the mother he is ordering a brain stem evoked response (BSER) test to rule out hearing loss, and then also writes "possible autism" on the bottom of the lab slip that he hands the mother to take to the audiology department along with her child. I have met immigrant parents, whose first language is not English, who think the doctor has said their child's problem is due to the fact he is "artistic"—even though, they tell me, the child doesn't paint or even hold a crayon properly. In such cases it is certainly clear that no one has made the effort to give parents the needed facts. On the other hand, there are big multidisciplinary diagnostic centers where parents come back week after week for fifty-minute sessions to discuss how they feel about their child's diagnosis of autism, and are coached to get "through" the acceptance of the diagnosis before worrying about treatment.

My strongly held position is that starting with treatment is the best way to begin to work through the acceptance of the diagnosis. I see treatment planning as the single most powerful resource in coping with a diagnosis of autism. The sooner the treatment begins, the sooner there will be some positive change in the child and the parents can begin to see that the child's situation is not hopeless.

Observations about the Child That Are Contradictory to the Diagnosis

In talking about a diagnosis of autism with parents, it is important for a doctor to know what the parents think their child's problem is and what they understand autism to be. A common vocabulary and a common knowledge base is necessary before any new information can be added. As was described in Chapter 1, a diagnosis of autism is based on one of the existing diagnostic standards, like the DSM-IV or ICD-10 criteria. As the doctor describes how your child's behavior fits the diagnostic criteria for autism or PDD, be sure to ask about anything that seems unclear or inconsistent with other observations you've made about your child. After the meeting about the diagnosis you will probably be able to come up with examples of behavior that run counter to the types of things that the doctor "counted" as part of the autism. A diagnosis is a professional judgment about the predominant form of a behavior. No child ever meets any one diagnostic criterion 100 percent of the time. If your child sometimes does things that seem to run counter to the diagnosis, it's important to bring them up to understand how the doctor sees them, or to get insight into how the more positive behaviors can be shaped so that they can be expressed more often. Another reason it is important to thoroughly discuss any contradictory observations that you and your child's doctor may have is that if you save them, and *don't* discuss them, you'll probably find yourself using them later to talk yourself out of believing the diagnosis. It is better that you air your concerns, and have an opportunity to fit the doctor's responses to your questions.

Needless to say, doctors aren't perfect, and most children aren't textbook cases of whatever diagnosis they receive. Even the most experienced doctors see some cases of autism or PDD that are irregular in certain unusual ways. This is because the diagnostic criteria are really just descriptions—a "best guess" that describes a majority of children with similar problems. There are definitely children who are the proverbial square pegs. As a diagnostician I can unequivocally say that there is no point in trying to fit square pegs into round holes. Instead, it is important for the doctor to let parents and treatment professionals in on his or her views about what the diagnostic ambiguity ("square pen-ness") may mean for future development, treatment, and possible diagnostic changes. One way to do this is to assign a percentage of certainty to a diagnosis. There are definitely 100-percent autistic children, but there are also "50-50's" out there. A forthright professional opinion on diagnostic certainty is extremely important if parents are to trust the person giving the diagnosis. Parents are experts on their own kids too, and are in an excellent position to detect rubbish.

Stages of Coping

Dissociation, Disbelief, Numbness, and Saturation. It is incredibly difficult to sit and listen to a litany of what is wrong with your child when you already know there is a problem. Diagnostic debriefing is a painful but necessary process. As the doctors talk about what is wrong with your child, you may be feeling more and more bombarded and helpless. All the while you keep hearing more bad news. After a while, you may even feel as if this isn't really happening to you. Feelings of disbelief or dissociation from what is being said are natural ways in which our psyches cope with emotional trauma. Looking back on the day you received the diagnosis, you may feel as if you weren't really there, but somehow got all the details by watching the diagnostic debriefing on TV or by some other remote means.

For some parents, the diagnostic debriefing is necessary to assure them that all the observations they have made of their child's unusual behavior fit together and constitute a real entity. In a way, such parents react to a diagnostic debriefing much the way some people react to news of the death of a loved one—by wanting to know all the details that led up to the final illness or accident.

Some parents react to the diagnosis of autism with disbelief, another way our coping mechanisms have of keeping bad news at an emotional distance from our most inner core. Parents will say "Well, I knew something was wrong, but I didn't expect to hear he was autistic!" Or, "This can't be right, no one in our family has ever had any sort of problem like this before!" Or, "If he was autistic, his nursery school teacher wouldn't have said 'he's definitely *not* autistic.'"

For some parents the initial news of the diagnosis is such a blow that it is experienced in an almost physical way as a kind of numbness. New information ceases to penetrate. It is no longer possible to ask questions. It is as if your ability to comprehend what is being said has reached a saturation point. Parents find themselves saying "I'm sure I have questions, I just can't think of what they are right now."

Outcry and Hopelessness. Once the diagnosis of autism begins to penetrate, the first reaction is often an outcry: "Why me? Why my child?" Unfortunately, autism is a disorder with no easy answers to that question. (At least none that science can provide right now.) As we discussed earlier, the overall odds of having a child with an autistic spectrum disorder are probably around one in 750 to one in 1000. One feels unlucky, hopeless, and defeated by the odds. The sense that such a misfortune befell you although you did nothing particularly wrong can make you worry that any future actions might somehow precipitate even further bad fortune. Although many parents can consciously dismiss this type of reasoning as irrational, it can certainly reinforce a pessimistic perspective on the future.

Understanding the Causes of Autism as a Way to Promote Coping. One effective way to counteract feelings of hopelessness about the diagnosis is to understand as well as possible what may have caused a particular case of autism or PDD. In Chapter 5, we discussed the genetics of autism and genetic counseling for parents. Getting a basic understanding about the genetics of autism at the time of diagnosis can be helpful. Roughly thirty to fifty percent of cases of autistic spectrum disorders are believed to have some genetic basis. Some believe that perhaps half of the genetic defects are inherited, and the other half may be caused by new mutations. Autism, PDD, and Asperger's syndrome all seem to be genetic variants of the same or similar disorders. Families that have a member, even a distantly related one, with an autistic spectrum disorder very likely have a higher chance of having a child with an autistic spectrum disorder than a family with no relatives affected with any type of developmental disorder. If you have an affected family member, you took a certain risk (probably quite small—unless the affected member was the autistic child's sibling), and lost. At least you know you are at risk, and you can consider this in planning other children. Although no one wants to be at risk for having children with a serious genetic defect, having some knowledge of cause tends to restore some sense of control over the situation—at least in terms of future family planning. Similarly, if your child's autism may someday prove to be caused by a new mutation, you were very unlucky, but you can feel relatively better about the fact that if you have another child, the exact same mutation would be exceedingly unlikely to happen again.

Other cases of autism are probably exacerbated, if not largely caused, by suboptimal events during pregnancy and delivery. No factors are absolutely causative, although some, like having rubella during pregnancy, would have put you at very high risk. If there seems to have been a serious known risk factor in your pregnancy, at least you can feel somewhat assured that a subsequent child would not be autistic (unless the suboptimal condition of the pregnancy was likely to recur).

Blame and Guilt. While it may help to have some kind of explanation for your child's autism, and it may help you feel more in control of future family planning, understanding it does not cure the child in any way, nor indicate anything, one way or another, about the child's treatment. Knowledge of what likely went wrong cannot change the past, however, and dwelling on the past never helps the present. Sometimes, as hopelessness about the child's diagnosis turns to externalized anger, blame arises.

Telling parents about possible causes of autism or PDD is a double-edged sword as far as coping goes. On one hand, knowing about possible causes may give some context for what has happened and may allow for regrouping in terms of future family plans. On the other hand, some couples begin to use the information as ammunition to distance themselves from guilt and self-blame about the child's disability.

The type of parents who tend to cope with their rage at their child's autism by blaming one another usually have drawn their battle lines before stepping into our clinic. If we sense a minefield, we try to tread carefully. Usually it begins with the mother quietly coaxing the father to "Tell about your Uncle Henry from Detroit's boy," or "What did your mother say about that cousin of yours back in the Philippines who died when he was nine?" Sometimes the father has a similar return volley. If the desire to place genetic blame is strong enough, I hear about all kinds of non-developmental disorders—including everyone who died of heart attacks and which side had the most alcoholics— despite my attempts to explain that there is no evidence that these disorders increase the risk that autism will occur.

A husband's strategy for distancing himself from blame may be to ask pointed questions about his wife's pregnancy: "What about the antihistamine you took after your allergy attack from your sister's cats?" Or, "Tell the doctor about the wine you drank at your baby shower." Some mothers also ask anxiously about the most minor violations of their health regimes during pregnancy—even ones they have discussed repeatedly with their obstetrician. On a rational level, most parents recognize that neither an antihistamine or a wine spritzer is likely to have caused something as severe as autism. But there's a lot of free-floating guilt out there looking for a place to land, and if one is anxious enough, guilt can come to rest on any small infraction.

Hopelessness. "How much difference can treatment make (anyway)?" This question is often asked in the first few moments after completing the description of the child's diagnosis. The answer is, a great deal. All the difference in the world. The core emotional fear that parents experience when first given the diagnosis of autism is that the child will always remain as we see him presently. Perhaps the helpful effects of treatment for autism and PDD are initially difficult for parents to recognize because they don't know anything about it yet. A large number of parents may feel that the child will never grow past the way he is at the moment of diagnosis. Having a developmental disorder is not like becoming paralyzed from the waist down and never being able to walk again. Although the child is likely to have autism or PDD always, he *will* continue to change, grow, and develop new abilities. Even people who face major permanent physical handicaps such as being paralyzed adapt so they can do many of the things they wish. Autistic children also adapt.

Bargaining. Another coping strategy is *bargaining.* As if the diagnosis were negotiable and the doctor had the power to make a deal, some parents try to cope by "asking for a reduced sentence." It is a coping response that says "I can deal with this, if only I didn't have to deal with so much." It would be nice if this could be true and doctors, like judges, had the ability to give out a reduced sentence. Bargaining happens most often as parents try to deal simultaneously with the diagnosis of autism and also with a diagnosis of mild or moderate mental retardation. Parents will say "I knew there was something wrong. I guess I expected you to say she was autistic. I didn't expect to hear she had mental retardation, too." A doctor can explain that about fifty percent of children diagnosed with autism also have mild to moderate mental retardation. If a diagnosis exists, it exists. It may be hard for some parents to realize, but in terms of the reality of the child's condition, the doctors are in as helpless a position as the parents. Another form of bargaining is attempted when parents try to argue a diagnosis of autism "down" to a diagnosis of PDD,NOS. Since many clinicians hedge on giving a diagnosis of autism, they will have given a preliminary diagnosis of PDD,NOS pending a more complete workup for autism. This makes it all the harder for parents not to feel the diagnosis of autism is being dealt out as a punitive act.

Psychological Defenses and Accepting the Diagnosis

Denial. A few parents, upon receiving the diagnosis of autism, ask "What if you're wrong?" Fair enough question. There are certainly cases of autism that clinicians diagnose with more or less certainty. Usually the more experienced the clinician is with autism and PDD, the more certain the diagnosis. Some clinicians are more experienced in diagnosing young children, others feel much less certain about diagnoses made in younger children. Sometimes a doctor *is* wrong. It is important for a parent to examine his or her feelings that a diagnosis of autism or PDD may be wrong, and determine whether this feeling originated from the *wish* that the doctor be wrong, or from a belief that the diagnosis is faulty because something he said might be viewed as incompletely reasoned or contradictory. Denial is a defense mechanism that protects us from painful aspects of reality. Denial per se is not wrong. However, when denial prevents parents from appreciating the need to find help for their child, then the denial may have harmful effects.

Denial may have deleterious effects if it means that the child's behaviors that may be harmful to himself or others are not recognized. For example, Keri, a six-year-old boy with PDD, began waving a real hammer in close proximity to the head of his infant brother. His mother panicked. His father, however, stated that the only thing Keri had ever done with a hammer was to hammer nails—he was not worried. The father's denial of the real danger to the infant was not helpful in training Keri to behave more appropriately with a hammer, or in removing the real danger of injury to the infant. Denial can prevent a parent from responding judiciously to a particular situation and often hinders the initiation of appropriate timely treatment.

The most frequently encountered form of denial in parents of autistic children is holding on to the belief that the child will grow out of his problems. If the autistic child is an only child it is easier to hold on to this belief than if there are siblings, particularly younger siblings with whom the child's rate of development can be compared. Sometimes it is possible to "forget" (deny) how rapidly an older sibling developed. However, when a younger sibling begins to surpass certain aspects of the autistic child's development, it is harder to fail to observe the differences. Also, having a normally developing younger sibling lessens the personal psychological injury that parents can't help but feel when they have produced a disabled child first. Once another, normally developing child comes along, it may be less personally hurtful to acknowledge the disabilities of the first child.

Denial of a child's disability through the belief that the child will grow out his problems is more common among parents of children with the diagnosis of PDD than with autism because PDD children usually have more moments of close to normal behavior. Parents of PDD children sometimes suspend themselves in an "only if" world, feeling "only if" their child would be different in some subtle way, no one would notice that anything was wrong. "Only if's" can include things like "only if he wouldn't flap," "only if he wouldn't say the same repetitive thing over and over," and "only if he just would look at people who talk to him." In addition, the early emerging special abilities of some PDD children, like their enormous rote auditory memories or the ability to do complex puzzles at an early age, help parents of PDD children and some autistic children to feel they are seeing the eccentricities of genius rather than the symptoms of a disability. For example, sometimes the PDD child's lack of interest in peers is seen as his being "bored" with them because they can't do puzzles as big, or do them as fast, or concentrate as long at producing complex geometric arrangements of Leggos.

Denial can be expressed in the form of feeling that there is something wrong with people who comment on the child's problems as opposed to admitting that there may actually be something wrong with the child. A typical scenario for this type of denial is parents who move their autistic children from a first, to a second, to a third pre-school—all within a few months—before pursuing the possibility that there is a basis for teachers' comments that the child seems quite different from other children in the program and is unprepared to participate in the requirements of the school day.

Another form of denial is believing that differences in development are expressions of individuality. Some parents believe that their child's refusals to comply are an early expression of a strong-willed, creative person who needs to do things his own way. One very educated parent who had read widely about autism, and had read that autistic children often line things up, insisted that *her* son lined up Matchbox cars, not because he was autistic, but because he found pushing them on the floor too mundane and traditional an application.

Expressions of these types of beliefs are not fatuous constructions, but a way of becoming comfortable with who the child is, in a way that does not assign pejorative significance to a behavior that is the result of "brain damage." The mother of the boy who lined up cars made fairly adaptive use of denial for coping (she didn't have to worry that her son's behavior with toy cars was abnormal), *but* her way of going about it nevertheless does raise concerns about whether she might not generalize this response so widely as to avoid taking action on other symptoms of her son's autism as well.

Emotional Coping with Ambiguous Diagnoses. One of the things that can make it really difficult to cope with a diagnosis of autism or PDD is being told the diagnosis in an ambiguous way. It is especially hard to know how to feel when a doctor says "Yes, something's definitely wrong; it might be autism, it might be PDD; we just can't be sure. Come back in six months and we'll have another look." To many parents who have been subjected to such ambiguous diagnoses, the uncertainty may seem almost as unbearable as the diagnosis itself. For example, if you had a lump in your neck and the doctor said "It might be lymphoma, I'm not sure, come back in two weeks and we'll have another look," it would be a hard two weeks. If you did have a malignancy, you would certainly want to begin treatment. You might be afraid that anything you might do in the meantime might make your condition worse. You might feel that any little thing that went wrong was confirmation that you *did* have cancer. Emotionally, this is how many parents feel when they've received a tentative "soft" diagnosis of autism or PDD.

Some parents have never had anyone explain that autism is a more fully expressed form of PDD; if their child who was initially diagnosed as "at least meeting criteria for PDD" is later diagnosed as having "autistic disorder," they may be shocked and confused, rather than understanding that they are really having the same diagnosis reconfirmed. It is important to try to get a clear answer from a diagnostician (or have him or her refer you to someone who can give you a clear answer) so that you can effectively begin to cope with whatever it is that is holding back your child's development. Ambiguity naturally makes many people anxious, promotes denial for others, and often results in post-ponement of appropriate interventions.

Killing the Messenger. Sometimes parents get angry and frustrated with doctors because they feel the doctors are giving them the runaround, or not giving the parents the whole story, or trying to cover up one another's mistakes. Other parents feel, in some irrational way, that if the doctor hadn't said the child was autistic then it wouldn't be true. Even though a parent may consciously *realize* that such thinking is irrational, the anger toward the doctor can well up and the need to strike out at *someone* can become overpowering. A couple of years ago, I sat in on a parent conference between a very fine psychologist on my staff and a very angry, very tense mother whose recently estranged husband had refused to come along to his son's evaluation. The psychologist told the mother that we felt her son had PDD and mild mental retardation and explained why we thought this was so. The mother did not comment on the diagnosis, but said angrily to the psychologist "You must get your jollies from telling people their kids are retarded!" The psychologist could barely hold back her tears. What this mother said was very hurtful to a fine professional trying to do a difficult job as humanely as possible. In this situation, it is likely that the mother was acting out her feelings of abandonment by the father by daring the psychologist to reject and abandon her also. It is natural to feel abandoned and disconsolate at the time of diagnosis. Luck has abandoned you, and you have been let down by all the faith you put in how good prenatal care and being a good parent would ensure a healthy child. But the professional is your link to getting help. The diagnosis is not given as a personal insult (although it may feel that way). It is very sad to me when parents maladaptively cope with their child's diagnosis by "killing the messenger"—trying to discredit or reject the doctor as if, magically, such an action will also undo the child's disability.

Grasping at Straws. Sometimes parents cope with their child's diagnosis in a way that is a passive-aggressive form of killing the messenger. By this I mean that some parents act out their anger at the doctor by looking for treatments that doctors say are unscientific or unproven or don't make sense. It is as if some parents feel they are actively doing more for their child if they keep their child away from recommended treatments, and instead invest time, money, and energy in "cures" with no apparent rationale. (In Chapter 15 we'll talk about some current non-mainstream treatments such as these.) Most parents consider and reject this way of coping with their child's diagnosis right off. Many parents who have read various things in the popular press about autism before receiving their child's diagnosis will say: "I think I know what you're going to say, but I feel I just have to ask: How do you feel about . . . the role of food preservatives, rotation diets, cerebral milk allergies, etc." My concern about people who follow unproven treatments for their children is that they go into it with a belief in miracles. When the miracle never comes, they must feel all the more let down and abandoned—and no further along in realistically coping with their child's diagnosis, or in initiating effective treatment than when they started.

Cultural Beliefs about Disability in Children

There are certain characteristic ways of coping with a diagnosis of a disability in a child that are fairly distinct in different cultural groups. At our clinic in San Francisco, we see a very culturally diverse population and have an opportunity to try to understand and work with many culturally different beliefs about disability. Nationally, our system of services and supports for families with autistic children is basically set up to serve the needs of white, American, middle and upper middle class families. Families from other cultures, however, may have different feelings about why they have a handicapped child, what they perceive as social support, and how they feel the child should best be cared for. In trying to help all families, it is important to understand cultural differences, and to work within a family's cultural background to give help they want and can appreciate.

In our experience, the families that probably have the most difficulty handling a diagnosis of a handicap in a child are Asian families, particularly those of Chinese origin. A relative of a Chinese autistic child once explained to me that the reason there is so much shame attached to having a handicapped child for Chinese families is the cultural belief that if you do something immoral, and it goes undetected, you will eventually be punished in the form of a handicapped child. Then everyone will be aware of your misdeed. This certainly would explain why Chinese families seem to seek treatment at later ages, resist settings with other disabled children more strongly, and why some Chinese mothers take on a martyred role in relation to their child while the father remains remote. Chinese families often have less interest in attending support groups or meeting other parents of autistic children compared with white American families who have the same level of education. Less public forms of social support, such as individual parenting sessions or reading about autism extensively, may be more acceptable.

A diagnosis of autism in a child is particularly difficult for Latino families if the handicapped child is a son, and especially hard if the son is the firstborn. Latino fathers often regard the handicapped child as a personal insult to their machismo and say so. Such fathers can be eager to find a way to blame the child's disability on the mother, or to insist on seeking a physical cure (like brain surgery). Latino women, on the other hand, are often very religious and more easily accept the child's disability as some pre-ordained aspect of fate that they don't really expect to change much, one way or the other. Overall, however, Latino families often cope better than families from other cultures, especially if the family size is large. Siblings usually provide substantial help with care, and there more often is extended family with children who are at a similar developmental level as the autistic child with whom the autistic child can play side by side.

Among African-American families we see, there is often a relatively accepting attitude toward handicaps. This may be due to the fact that more African-American families have close-by extended family support than do some of the families we see from other cultures. The autistic child tends to spend more time with siblings and peers in child-governed activities, and so the parents tend to get less stressed out in caring for the autistic child than in white American culture, where the mother typically sees child care as mainly her responsibility. However, some of the older African-American grandmothers (and also Chinese grandmothers) espouse a "bad blood" theory of developmental disabilities, and can be harsh and unsupportive of their daughters if they feel the child was the result of a poor choice of father. (I've never really decided whether this is a genetic theory, a racist theory, or both, but it usually comes up if the father is of another race from the mother, or has completely disappeared.)

Some families, particularly more religious families (irrespective of which religion it is), have a strong sense that their autistic child should always be cared for in the context of the family, rather than in some sort of a group home or residential facility when he grows up. Sometimes, parents with strong religious faith are the most concerned about having a number of other children so that the future care of the autistic child will be distributed. In general, religious families seem to cope better with the diagnosis of autism than more agnostic families, and seem to see some larger moral purpose in having a disabled child than other families do; therefore, such families are often more accepting.

Concerns about Prognosis

After parents ask lots of questions about the diagnosis of their autistic or PDD child, there is often a pause. Then, one of the parents (usually the father) says "I know this must be hard to predict, but what will my son be like when he grows up? Will he be able to have children? Marry? Live independently?" The answer (and the precision of the answer) is different for each child; it depends on his degree of disability, how old he is, and how much treatment he's already had. The interesting thing is how many parents feel compelled to ask this question.

Why do parents feel the need to ask about the adult future for a toddler? How often do we think about whether non-autistic two-and-a-half-year-olds will get married? One possibility is that the question is a way of recasting and downscaling the "idealized child" whom we discussed at the beginning of this chapter. This is a realistic thing to do. It is important as a parent to have some notion of how far your child might be expected to go. There is no reason for a doctor to say "There's no way to know." Or "The sky's the limit!" *if* that's not true. (It's just an easy out for him or her.)

As we discussed in the last chapter, one reason for testing IQ is to determine the degree of mental retardation that may be present along with the autism. As a very general rule, I tend to "add" autism to the degree of mental retardation to determine how well an autistic child is likely to function as an adult. By this formula, if an autistic adult has a normal IQ, he or she will tend to fit into society as a mildly mentally retarded person might. If an autistic adult has mild mental retardation, he generally comes to function like a moderately retarded adult; and so on. By the time a child is five or six years old, it is usually possible to broadly determine the degree of mental retardation, although such information must be tempered by many factors, such as how fast the child has learned so far and under what types of teaching circumstances, whether or not the child has developed spoken language and how much, and whether those around the child help him make progress.

It is really important for parents to have at least some broad parameters for what they can expect of their child's development because if they don't, they may unrealistically expect far too much. Then, some time down the road, they will turn around, note the lack of fantasized progress, and feel they have failed their child. It is hard enough to parent an autistic child without taking on the burden of personal responsibility and failure for circumstances beyond their control.

Fear That the Child Will Never Grow Up. Some parents are overwhelmed by the sense that their autistic or PDD child will never grow up. They are worried about who will be willing to parent the child when they are no longer able to. In some cultures (for instance, in Asian families) this is rarely a concern, because parents automatically think in terms of siblings taking responsibility for one another. In reality, there are all kinds of social service support systems that help care for very mildly to very severely disabled adults. When a toddler or pre-school aged child is just diagnosed, it doesn't do much good to spend time learning too much about these systems (they are discussed further in Chapter 13), but it can promote coping just to know such help exists.

Biology versus Psychology. Often, I think it's ironic to look and see where our understanding of autism has come in the last twenty-five years. Twenty-five years ago, autism was blamed on cold, rejecting parents, "refrigerator parents" who supposedly caused their children to withdraw into their own worlds. Today, we have a more enlightened, neurobiological model that no longer lays blame on the parents. This should make parents feel better. But, interestingly, the construction of the "refrigerator mother" theory held out more hope for a cure than the neurobiological theories of today. Twenty-five years ago, a parent was led to believe that if only she could "warm up" to her child (with endless psychotherapy all around), the child would come back into the parents' world. If only it were that simple! Psychoanalytic treatments for autism failed miserably. Neurobiological theories imply the existence of brain difference on the molecular and/or neural levels. These are things we can't fix today, or any time in the near future. We can't grow new parts of the brain any more than we can grow missing fingers. So parents today are left to put their faith in rehabilitative treatments that are the equivalent of learning how to use your hand well despite a missing finger.

Some parents explicitly understand that autism is a physical problem that can't be undone, only adapted to. The degree of realism with which parents face the biology of autism helps take parents further down the road to the acceptance of their child's disability. Often, accepting autism as a permanent disability comes in large part from comprehending the biological nature of the disorder.

One of the things that is most wonderful and amazing to see during the process of giving a child's diagnosis of autism to his parents is the way many parents immediately react to their child. Often parents reach out and take their child on their lap, hug him, and touch him tenderly while they cry, or look like they are about to cry. The bad news seems to elicit some type of counteracting, protective response. It is as if the bad news itself had hurt the child like a bang on the head, and the parent has an urgent instinct to provide comfort. This always reminds me that autistic children are children first and autistic second.

Fantasies about the Child's Death. Great feelings of protection for the child are not necessarily incompatible with intrusive, irrational fantasies of harm coming to the child. It is not uncommon for parents of handicapped children to imagine a tragic death befalling the child, or even the parent somehow acting in a way that brings about the child's death. These fantasies are unconscious attempts to control what feels so out of control. One may feel very guilty for entertaining such fantasies, but guilt at imagining harm befalling the child should be tempered by the realization that such fantasies are not pathological. Your spouse may have the same feelings too, even though you may never be able to share these feelings fully with one another. One family I followed had a four-year-old severely retarded autistic boy with tuberous sclerosis (a brain tumor disorder that accompanies a small proportion of cases of autism). In this family, the father was the one who always called the clinic and came to appointments, while the mother became more remote. On one visit the father told me that his son had recently undergone a nine-hour neurosurgery because of an unusual complication of his tuberous sclerosis; the tumor had been growing rapidly. The father spoke of his anxious wait during the surgery. I imagined that he had probably been waiting to hear that the child had survived—while possibly, the mother had been waiting to hear that the boy had died. Neither parent in this case can be called good or bad. Each coped in a different way.

We once did a study at a state hospital that involved drawing blood from vegatively mentally retarded adults (that is, the type of individuals who are sometimes pejoratively called "vegetables"). The medical director at the hospital was required to call parents for oral consent to have their children be in the studies. We sat while she made some calls, each of which began thusly: "Mrs. Jones, this is Dr. Hooper, Johnny is still alive. I'm calling to ask . . ." She explained matter-of-factly that this group of parents had such strong fantasies and wishes for their children's death that she needed to tell them that the child was *not* dead at the beginning of every call in order to calm them.

Chapter Summary

For most parents, an extreme emotional response to the diagnosis of autism is a transitional stage. Full acceptance and understanding is a lifetime process that depends partly on how successfully the child responds to treatment. In Chapter 7 we will discuss the impact of the autistic or PDD child on family functioning; also, how families can get help for themselves if grief and adjustment reactions to the child's disorder become prolonged or immobilizing.

CHAPTER 7

◆ ◆ ◆

Family Issues

The Impact of Autism on Parents

Before parents of an autistic child were parents of an autistic child, they were a couple. Before they met, they were individuals with their own separate identities. In the process of meeting the extraordinary demands of raising an autistic child, it is very possible for the husband and wife to lose each other, and for each parent to begin to lose his or her identity separate from the child. In this chapter we'll discuss family issues. This will include how feelings and expectations about parenting are different when the child is autistic, and how having an autistic child in the family can affect siblings. Families have available to them various types of social support, and in this chapter we'll discuss the roles of relatives and friends. Finally, we'll discuss what is often the most difficult issue for families with an autistic child—deciding when and why a residential placement might provide better care than keeping a child at home.

Influences on Parenting the Autistic or PDD Child

Many factors influence how a family adapts to the added demands of having a child with autism or PDD. Compared with other developmental handicaps, autism and PDD can be an even more difficult challenge for families because children with these disabilities do not "give back" in the same way that other children do. Although autistic children may be affectionate and responsive in their own ways, the ways are still different from what parents with older children have come to expect, and what parents of firstborns may have imagined a parent-child relationship would be like.

A basic dynamic that gets set up very early in some families centers on the fear that the autistic child will experience any form of discipline or restriction as rejection. Some mothers and fathers feel that their child's aloofness is a personal rejection of them rather than an incapacity to relate. They reason that if the child is thwarted in any way, he will become still more aloof in response to future parental behavior. So, in some families, the autistic child really rules the roost. He does whatever he wants to parents and siblings, and destroys all sorts of household items in his regular course of "play." This type of family dynamic is not good for the autistic child's ultimate growth and development; it is not good for his siblings; and it's not good for the husband and wife as a couple. In this chapter, we will discuss the kinds of concerns and conflicts that arise in many families with autistic children. The purpose is to help parents (and therapists working with families) recognize these kinds of situations and deal with them. There will be examples of how families meet challenges; we will identify stressors that make a family's ability to function grow worse, and also identify protective factors that help families cope.

Every couple, and every family, can be described in terms of its strengths and weaknesses. As a family grows and changes, there will be natural points at which the family will function better and other times that it will function worse. This is true whether or not there is an autistic child in the family. Family functioning is influenced by many things relating to how in control of circumstances the family members feel themselves to be. Do the parents feel they are earning as good a living as they should be able to? How much work pressure are they experiencing? Is work pressure made worse by having to take time off to help care for the autistic child? Does the child's presence affect the career paths of the parents—for example, by limiting the amount of traveling either is willing to do for the job? If the mother is staying at home, is it her "free" choice, or a "forced" choice on account of the autistic child? Is family income being limited by changing work patterns? Does the couple feel they are living in a house or apartment that provides adequate space for raising this child or having another child? Are future family plans being endangered by their child's diagnosis of a disability? What kind of social supports for their lifestyle does the couple receive from relatives and friends? Is the couple at a stage of life when friends and relatives are having children too? How well do the mother and father get along? How well did they get along before the autistic child was born?

Families with the best functioning prior to the birth or diagnosis of an autistic or PDD child usually do better than families who did poorly before the added stress of a child with special needs. Finding yourself the parent of an autistic child does not make your life easier. For some families, the added stress of an autistic child magnifies existing problems; for other families, it creates new areas of conflict. It can be helpful to examine what goes wrong with some families, but it is also helpful to examine the ways in which some families manage to adapt as well as possible.

Length and Strength of the Parents' Relationship. Statistics on divorce and separation among parents of autistic and PDD children are hard to come by, but some studies show that up to fifty percent of children with a handicap have experienced the divorce or separation of their parents. In some cases the parents were never married, and in some cases, the parents split before the child's disability was identified. Even including such cases, the high rate of divorce and separation in families with a disabled child testifies to the additional stress. (Population statistics show that about one-third of American marriages now end in divorce—indicating that for families with disabled children the rate is about 20% higher.)

The preexisting stability of the parental relationship is a big factor in how well parents can work together in raising an autistic child. On the most basic level, "stability" can refer to how long the couple has been together or how long they have been married. As a general principle, couples that seem to cope best are those who have already been together for some time before the birth of their autistic child. Taking numerous pregnancy histories (as I have), it soon becomes clear that a not insignificant number of American marriages are initiated shortly *after* conception of the first child. Usually these are couples who already have a steady relationship and are old enough to start a family. However, if the pregnancy was the basis for the marriage, there may be an assumption that one partner was somehow "responsible" for it. If the resulting child then turns out to be autistic, the parent who feels the pregnancy was "caused" by the partner may consciously or unconsciously place blame on the partner. Subsequently, if the "more responsible" parent does not live up to his or her obligations, the other parent feels all the more wronged by the difficulties imposed by the presence of the child.

The "Planned Child," the "Unplanned, but Desired Child," and the "Unwanted Child." A closely related issue to who is "the more responsible parent" is the issue of where the disabled child fits into the family planning pattern. Many children are both wanted and planned. At other times, the pregnancy is not explicitly planned or avoided, but when pregnancy occurs, the child is desired. Some children are not really planned and come at a time that clearly increases life stress, but are "had" anyway. How well the family copes is often related to which of these groups a child falls into.

When a pregnancy is unplanned, one or both parents may have strongly felt that an abortion was not a possibility. Close family members may have encouraged continuing the pregnancy even though neither parent really wanted a child. Sometimes it is these family members who end up parenting the child, especially mothers of teen daughters. Sometimes the pregnancy is unwanted because the parent has been on a binge of drinking or drug abuse early in the pregnancy, and the mother fears the fetus is already damaged (which it may be). Sometimes denial of the severity of the substance abuse problem takes the form of continuing the pregnancy, even though a child is not really wanted. While some relatives or parents may briefly harbor the romantic notion that having to care for a child with special needs may inspire a dysfunctional adult to "straighten up and fly right," get clean and sober, or take antipsychotic medication regularly, it seldom happens; usually, the child is neglected, or worse, and often ends up unexpectedly in the care of an aunt, uncle, grandparent, or the other biological parent. The care of these children always presents major challenges to whatever social support system the dysfunctional parent has near her.

Many parents report that pregnancies were unplanned, but desired. Sometimes, though, such pregnancies occur when family circumstances are not as optimal as they might be. For example, one parent might still be a student; or there may have been a plan to move to a larger place that now has to be deferred; or a grandparent may have just died or be ill, requiring that extra attention be spent on the surviving grandparent; or the father might be in the military on a tour of duty away from the base where his wife is living. Most families do not see such circumstances as stressful enough to avoid a new pregnancy, but if they are coupled with the birth of a child who requires special attention, such minor stressors can have a more serious impact.

For families who have carefully planned the arrival of their baby, having a baby who turns out to have special needs can be especially painful. Such families have usually consciously considered the whole matter of social supports available to their family and decided that the time was right, and that other stressors were manageable. Typically, many precautions were taken to prevent anything from going wrong. Such mothers get in shape before their child is conceived; they quit smoking and stop drinking even occasional glasses of wine while trying to get pregnant. Before the pregnancy is confirmed, these women even avoid an aspirin or an antihistamine; afterwards, they follow the most careful prenatal care regimen, and any comments made by the obstetrician are dissected for all possible implications. So when the child's autism is diagnosed, these parents may review everything they've done and feel guilty for not having "prevented" this outcome. Families who have planned their children very carefully often experience a greater sense of "unfairness" at having an autistic or PDD child, especially when they compare themselves to relatives and friends who live their lives in a less planful fashion.

Single Parents of Autistic Children. Without a doubt, perhaps the most difficult situation to be in is parenting an autistic or PDD child as a single parent. It is in this situation that the mother (it *is* the mother in the vast majority of cases) and any nonaffected siblings probably feel the most stress. These single parents are faced with the myriad of problems that have been well described for all single parents, multiplied by the extra time and other social and emotional costs of having an autistic child.

A major concern in single-parent families with an autistic child is how "parentified" siblings can become. In the absence of an adult helpmate, mothers, often without realizing it, depend a great deal on help from the autistic child's brothers and sisters. Seeing a three-year-old take her autistic five-year-old brother firmly by the hand as they are about to cross a busy street gives a picture of how much the life of the three-year-old can be affected by having an autistic sibling. Later in this chapter, we'll discuss the characteristic ways in which siblings cope with an autistic brother or sister.

Divorce and Joint Custody with Autistic Children.   One obvious factor in how well single mothers cope is the degree to which the child's father is involved in the family. Joint custody can be very helpful in many circumstances, as it gives both parents an opportunity to have a strong and steady relationship with their child, and gives respite to both parents. Unfortunately, most autistic and PDD children do best in an environment with a high degree of unvarying structure. I have seen some parents provide this by leaving the child at one house and moving themselves every week or two. Even with this type of arrangement, it is almost impossible for two parents who have little contact with one another to be consistent in the behavior they expect or won't accept from the child. Sometimes the child develops behavior problems in one home and not the other. Sometimes, the need to provide consistency and continuity falls upon the sibling, especially an older sibling. The Stark family is an example. Amid a hostile and seemingly never-ending child custody dispute, Angela, age 8, and her autistic brother Jake, age 5, go back and forth from their single mother Linda's laissez-faire, unstructured sixties-style Berkeley home, to the more highly organized home of their remarried attorney father. Since Jake is autistic, if certain things are not just so, he can become quite difficult indeed. So it falls upon Angela to make sure cowboy pajamas go with Jake from house to house lest all hell break loose in the house with no cowboy pajamas. She ends up in the role of interpreter for all the obscured and unconnected things that Jake has to say, since she has a more continuous view of his experience than anyone else, and speaking with other people's perspectives in mind is not something that Jake does well.

Parental Age.   Among the families we see, there is a broad range—from younger couples in their early twenties to older couples in their mid-forties—all of whom are trying to first understand and accept their child's diagnosis. While there are many individual differences, the younger couples often appear to be able to cope somewhat better than the older couples, possibly because younger parents have more physical energy, their lifestyle patterns are not as fixed, they are young enough to decide to have more children, and even to wait a number of years until they do so. Perhaps for younger couples, there have not been so many years to develop idealized fantasies of what family life should be like, and instead things are taken more as they come. One extreme, and rather wonderful, example of this is a mother of a profoundly retarded autistic boy, who was fifteen and unmarried when he was born. Now, at nineteen, she has gotten her high school equivalency degree, gone with her son to all his infant stimulation classes, and has qualified to begin working as a special education teacher's aide. She can cogently discuss various aspects of her son's concomitant neurological problems, and pretty much accepts her son for who he is.

For the older couples, especially when one or both have been married before, the drive to have a child is usually less. When these couples undertake late child-bearing or a "second" generation of children, an autistic child can seem even more devastating, and a bitter reminder of all the reasons they may have hesitated. Perhaps the most poignant example of this I can think of is an upper-class South American couple, the wife in her early forties and the husband in his early fifties. He had grown children; she had never had a child. They adopted a baby from an orphanage in their country of origin, but by age three, it was clear that the child was autistic and severely mentally retarded. The marriage had begun to fail. She had begged for a child and now was crushed because she had never envisioned motherhood could be so difficult, hating herself in her role as mother. In this particular case, we suggested that the child be returned to the orphanage, and that they try to recapture the positive aspects of their marriage. The father was tearful, but tried to remain stoic. The mother cried. A few months later, we heard through another member of a support group they had attended that the child *had* gone back, and for them, it had been the right decision.

Some couples are older when they have their autistic child because child-rearing was simply put off for a number of years, either because the couple married late or spent many years establishing their careers before having children. Such couples often seem to have a certain attitude of melancholy about their child's disability, but nonetheless cope fairly well. It can seem as if these couples have decided that the child is their just deserts for all the years they spent pursuing other endeavors when they 'should' have been getting down to the business of having children. Sometimes these couples feel that having waited until the eleventh hour on the biological clock, they are glad to have a child at all, and may be so inexperienced with young children that they do not readily understand the dimensions of their child's disability. One such couple seen in our clinic, the Ardales, are computer company managers in their early forties who both described themselves as "computer jocks." They had been together for eighteen years before the birth of their son Eddy. Both worked long hours, often leaving four-year-old Eddy, who was rather bright but clearly autistic, in the care of his maternal grandparents, who lived with them for this purpose. Both parents confessed to knowing little about child development; they had no friends with young children; there were no children in the neighborhood; and they did not have time during the day to visit Eddy's school. Although Eddy had marked problems in socially relating to peers and adults, peculiar language use, and many rituals, the parents seemed only concerned about learning appropriate disciplinary strategies. It was not until he reached age four that Eddy was sent for an autism evaluation by their pediatrician. Although the Ardales now feel they might have been able to do more for Eddy earlier if they had been aware of his autism, they accepted his difficulties as if they were a typical aspect of parenting faced by all parents.

Parenting Style: More Permissive versus More Authoritarian. One of the most often replicated findings in child development is that more educated parents tend to be more permissive with their children, and that less educated parents tend to be more restrictive. *Permissive* parenting consists of allowing the child to make many of his own choices and, hopefully, learn from his own actions. Such parents generally feel that it is best for the child to figure out what to do and when he wants to do it, in order to foster a sense of creativity and independent thinking. The *authoritative* parenting style is one in which parents define stricter limits for behavior, such as when and where a child definitely can and cannot do certain things, but allows the child to make choices within those limits of acceptability. More restrictive or authoritarian parents set firm limits for behavior they deem appropriate and do not feel it is necessary for the child to understand why the parent has made those limits, only that the rules must be followed readily and willingly. All other things being equal, these methods of parenting produce approximately the desired results. However, when the child has a developmental disorder, especially autism or PDD, the premises on which these philosophies are based become much less accurate. Parents with a permissive style often have the hardest time adapting to the methods that are generally more suitable in raising an autistic or PDD child. By virtue of being autistic, cognitively handicapped, or both, the autistic child's exploration tends to be more limited—more brief, more repetitive, or more unidimensional than would be the case with another child of the same age. Therefore, the philosophy of allowing the child to learn through his own choices works less well, and the opportunities to exhibit inappropriate behavior are greater.

If the parent takes the child's inappropriate behavior as "his own style," this further reduces the child's opportunities to move on. For example, Jeremy, a four-year-old autistic boy, had parents who both had graduate degrees. His mother had an art-related import business. When Jeremy started lining up and otherwise arranging crayons, she refused to intervene, even if he stared and flapped his hands at the crayons for very prolonged periods. She felt his activity was part of a unique creative process he was experimenting with. Despite being told that many little autistic children line up sets of like objects, and that such repeated behavior interferes with being exposed to broader forms of stimulation, she felt it would be unfair to him to interfere with the behavior. Other examples can be less benign: Ansel, a six-year-old boy (an only child of older parents), was brought to be evaluated by his impeccably-suited, erudite publisher father, and his mother, the director of an art gallery. One reported problem was that Ansel would frequently choke his father, which we saw for ourselves when Ansel abruptly approached his father, grabbed his beautifully made silk tie, and pulled at the knot until his father's face began to redden. Another problem was that when aggravated, Ansel would pull down his pants and threaten to urinate on the floor, which he sometimes did. Much to my amazement, Ansel's parents made no attempts to stop either of these behaviors, but rather, attended to him urgently and gently; they took these behaviors to mean that he was quite unhappy about something, and that the onus was on them to figure out what—right away. As we worked with these parents to implement some behavioral methods that would be effective in stopping these behaviors, and redirecting Ansel into more appropriate ways of requesting attention and help, it became clear how counter-intuitive a more restrictive approach to child-rearing was to them. Had this couple had a son whose level of intelligence matched their own— rather than a boy with PDD and severe receptive and expressive language impairments—their methods probably *would* have fostered the development of a creative, independent child cast in their own images. The very permissive, laissez-faire method of child-rearing goes against the grain of the more structured interventions that benefit many autistic spectrum children.

Educators and psychologists often think that less educated, more authoritarian parents are not as "optimal" as more permissive parents at structuring learning experiences for their children. However, when it comes to providing a highly structured, routinized, "do it over 'till you get it right" environment that can benefit autistic children, authoritarian parents do this quite naturally. We have seen a number of military families. In these families, both fathers and mothers have no trouble understanding or accepting the fact that their child needs to learn to follow narrowly defined directives when requested. Drill and repetition is okay with them, too, and this can be very helpful since autistic children need repetition to learn many sorts of things that don't come naturally to them.

A relevant case here is that of the single-parent father of a mute, severely retarded autistic boy, Roy, whom we followed for a number of years. His father, Mr. Naylor, was a very large man with a bushy beard who had a Harley-Davidson motorcycle repair business and a large tattoo on his upper arm signifying membership in the Northern California Hell's Angels. On one visit, when Roy was nine, the conversation began to be interrupted by Roy banging loudly on a toy xylophone. In frustration, because he could not hear me well over the sound of the xylophone, Mr. Naylor roughly yanked the xylophone away from Roy, shouting "Cut the shit!" About a minute later, Mr. Naylor returned the xylophone to Roy. A minute after that, Roy was banging again (but not quite so loudly). His father again removed the xylophone and repeated his admonition. On the third time with the xylophone, Roy tinkled quietly and appropriately on the keys with nothing further said. Although a behavior therapist would not have recommended exactly the same procedure, Mr. Naylor's natural style of parenting bore a striking resemblance both in methodology and results to what might have been developed as a plan to reduce Roy's tendency to produce overly loud sounds.

Parent Interaction Around the Topic of the Autistic Child

The mettle of parental mutual support is tested at several points along the road of parenting an autistic child. The first, as we discussed in Chapter 5, is in getting the diagnosis. Getting the child in the door for diagnostic assessment and treatment is a process that works best with cooperation of both parents.

The next stage, as we discussed in Chapter 6, is working through the emotional feelings around the diagnosis and avoiding the pitfalls of pointing the finger of blame at one another. Some couples get fixated at the blaming stage and can't begin to cope with raising the child until they realize that it doesn't help the child one way or another to "resolve" the blame issue. Until the couple can put the blame issue aside, they continue to be adversaries instead of a team working together to help the child. When blame is not set aside, an adversarial relationship develops and often results in overall polarization of the spouses. The conflict between spouses is usually soon translated into a successive series of adversarial positions on how to help the disabled child—how to teach him, how to discipline him, what to expect that he can or can't do, and how efficacious or hindering the other spouse's efforts are in getting the child better. Siblings can be recruited into this adversarial positioning, and as a result have to cope with conflicting loyalties between parents, and a poor understanding of what they really should be doing when they want to help their handicapped brother or sister. The reality of this situation is that because we know so little about what causes a particular case of autism or PDD, each parent will always hold theories that, at least for the present, can't be fully substantiated (or negated) with scientific findings.

The families who cope the best around unresolved issues of etiology are ones that believe fervently in equal time for the opposing points of view. Both spouses can accept the fact they don't see things the same way, but respect the right of the other parent to have his own point of view. When interviewing such parents, a mother might say "I know my husband sees this differently, and I think it's important that you hear what he has to say too." The key is that open discussion leads to a deferral of blame or a need to be proven right. In turn, the model of having an open discussion about the origin of the child's problems leads such couples to be able to depend upon one another and utilize one another as sounding boards for the issues that arise in parenting their autistic child. When parents can constructively discuss the behavior or difficulties of their autistic child, siblings adapt better too, because mention of their autistic brother or sister's problems by either parent does not mean that the stage is being set for parental conflict in which they may be a pawn.

Child Abuse and Autistic Children.   In the worst-case scenarios, parental lack of understanding about the autistic child's disability and conflict about how the autistic child should be raised result in physical abuse or neglect of the child. How often are autistic children abused? There are no good statistics. The methodologies used to detect abuse in other groups of children are less reliable in autistic children. Many are either mute or have language that is limited in such a way that self-report is unlikely. Since a number of autistic children have diminished pain reactions, especially when younger, the appearance of bruises and cuts does not mean the same thing as it does in other, more normally cautious, children of the same age. Excessive avoidance of the abuser is also hard to gauge in an autistic child. Autistic children can be anxious and avoidant around anyone who intrudes on their space—with ill intentions or good.

What we do know is that developmentally disabled children as a group are more frequently abused than non-developmentally disabled children. A variety of studies have estimated that the prevalence of child abuse in developmentally disabled children is significantly higher than for other children. It is quite possible that autistic children are abused at even higher rates than many other developmentally disabled children. Most at risk are children whose parents overestimate their receptive language. In these cases, parents will report that the child understands exactly what he is being told but is just pretending not to hear, care, or notice. It is easy to imagine how parents who have made such a fallacious assumption about their children could soon become angry at what they view as high levels of noncompliance—and react violently. Other parents react emotionally and may suddenly find they have unintentionally hit their autistic child when they see him or her doing something that could endanger himself or a sibling (like opening the front door and running out into the street). Other parents transfer their anger at the child's existence onto the child as if the "badness" could be beat out of him.

There are many good parents—who have never laid a hand on their other children—who find they have, without planning it, hit their autistic child hard enough to worry that he has been injured. This may have happened when the child was in a self-endangering situation, or it might just have been when the mother was completely frazzled from several hours of keeping up with a hyperactive three-year-old with no language and no judgment. In my opinion, such an episode does not make you a child abuser. It means you really need help better managing your child. You may also need some personal help examining your feelings about your child, and support in making plans to get some respite.

Psychotherapy for Families with Autistic and PDD Children

What role does psychotherapy have in the treatment of autistic children and their families? This is an often-asked question; there are a variety of answers.

Psychotherapy for Children with PDD and Autism. For some clinicians, especially behavior therapists, psychotherapy for autistic children harkens back to the days of the refrigerator mother hypothesis, when unresponsive mothers were blamed for autism. Neither the research literature nor my own experience impresses me with the value of dynamically oriented psychotherapy for autistic children. There *are* some autistic children who have had psychotherapy. And there are some points in certain autistic children's development when he or she *may* benefit from what some psychotherapists do. The non-cognitively impaired PDD child and the higher-functioning autistic child may benefit to some extent from play-oriented therapy. Psychodynamically oriented play therapy for emotionally disturbed children from two to about ten years old is designed to help the child work through his conflicts by reenacting them during play. For the higher-functioning PDD or autistic child, this same treatment milieu may be helpful in learning *how* to play. The therapist can provide an opportunity for one-to-one interaction at the child's pace. Parents who undertake such treatment should understand, however, that while such therapy may be *educational* it is not, strictly speaking, psychotherapeutic. At best, psychotherapy for a young autistic child may make him less resistant to social contact, and more willing to explore and play appropriately with a variety of toys—especially if the techniques used in therapy are carried over to home and school. What psychotherapy will *not* do is allow the child to suddenly one day "step out" of his own world. Beware of therapists who tell you it will.

Psychotherapy for the Higher Functioning Teenager and Young Adult with Autism or PDD. Higher functioning teenagers and young adults with autism, PDD, or Asperger's syndrome may benefit from psychotherapy for a couple of reasons. First, as it does for similarly affected younger children, psychotherapy may be able to serve as an educational setting for rehearsing and learning scripts and rules for appropriate kinds of social interactions. This type of work comes under the heading of social skills training and is sometimes done in groups as well as individually. A major limitation to this kind of work for autistic young adults is that they learn what to say, but have no drive toward social conformity, and therefore, little motivation to implement what they learn. For example, Randall, whom I've followed for the last eight years, has been very interested in girls since age fifteen. The problem is, he doesn't know how to express his interest. Now age twenty, Randall recently left a classroom where his social skills training group was being held to go to the restroom. Randall saw a very nice young lady (who turned out to be attending a rape recovery program), and followed her into the ladies' room to tell her that he wanted to kiss her. Randall meant no harm. He just had no social judgment, and his desire to kiss the young lady was greater than his desire to please the social skills group instructor (or his mother, who has repeatedly explained to him why he shouldn't do such things).

On the other hand, another young man of about the same age whom I referred for psychotherapy seems to have derived more benefit. The idea behind his twice-monthly sessions was for the therapist to keep an eye on him, try to work on some social skills, and make sure he wasn't getting into any bizarre patterns of behavior or becoming depressed (both of which he was prone to do). The therapy sessions became a major organizing aspect of this young man's routine, although he often didn't have much to say after he had consistently and punctually arrived. In fact, he enjoyed the routine of the sessions so much that he had great difficulty when his increasingly pregnant psychiatrist explained she would be transferring his case while she took a maternity leave. The sessions served to maintain the even keel of his life, as each week he could repeat the same routine of activities to his therapist.

On the whole, however, psychotherapy in any form tends to have limited usefulness for people with autism or PDD because they have very limited insight and very limited ability to take into account how others feel and think, even when they are smart in other ways. Furthermore, they almost always lack motivation for self-change. In teenagers and young adults, psychiatric disorders that may co-occur with autism, PDD, or Asperger's syndrome, like depression or manic episodes, can be monitored, but when they do occur, are most likely to remit as a result of psychotropic medications rather than as the result of insight-oriented therapy. (There will be more on psychopharmacology for autistic children and adults in Chapter 14.) The potential use of psychotherapy for autistic children needs to be considered carefully beforehand and on an individual basis. If it is to be used, the goals in terms of expectations for specific behavioral changes need to be planned in advance and reevaluated frequently to determine whether benefit is being accrued.

Individual Therapy for Parents of Autistic Children. There clearly are times when psychotherapy is needed for the mother or father of an autistic child. As we discussed earlier in this chapter, sometimes the added stress of a child who has special needs is the proverbial straw that breaks the camel's back. For others, bringing untoward fantasies about the child into consciousness may make parents feel they are losing control and going crazy.

It can be particularly helpful to have a therapist who has some understanding about what it is like to raise a child who is somehow different. The therapist may be someone who has personal experience with this, or has had a chance to work with developmentally disabled children and their families as part of his or her training. Sometimes I worry about parents who go into therapy with a therapist who hasn't read anything new about autism in the last twenty-five years. Such a therapist may imply that the parent must have unconscious rejection of the child that at least partially explains the child's symptoms. Autism is a biological disorder. It is certainly true that one may wish, consciously or unconsciously, not to have to face it. However, the disorder does not get worse because of a wish. Autism only gets worse if the wish is translated into very inadequate, inconsistent parenting that thwarts the child's ability to grow and learn.

Often, brief psychotherapy for parents—for example, five or fewer visits around the time of the diagnosis—may be helpful. Everybody is different, however; whether and how much individual psychotherapy a particular individual may benefit from will depend on how he or she feels about other issues in his or her life as well as the feelings about the autistic child.

Couples Therapy for Parents of Autistic Children. For some families, the psychological crisis that may be caused by raising an autistic child is more of an interpersonal issue than an individual one. As we have discussed, when coping with an autistic child *doesn't* go well, parents tend to become polarized, taking increasingly opposite views of the child. These couples often can benefit from conjoint therapy, where there is an opportunity for disparate views to be aired before a neutral third party who may be helpful at separating fact from fiction and examining why each parent works so hard at holding onto his or her own point of view to the exclusion of the other parent's point of view. Sometimes parents just need an arbitrator, someone in front of whom they can make agreements about what they will do if their autistic child hits the six-month-old again, escapes from the backyard, or tries to eat from other people's plates. Other parents can benefit from therapy because they lose each other as husband and wife. Just *going* to therapy carves out some time alone, and can be a first step toward negotiating other ways of making time, so that they won't have to give up their own relationship for the sake of the child.

Another issue that therapy can help with is a discussion of whether to have more children. This can be an emotionally volatile subject, with both parents feeling strongly ambivalent. While a genetic counselor or autism specialist can give the facts, working through the feelings about those facts can take a lot of soul-searching.

Family Therapy for Parents and Nonaffected Siblings. Sometimes it can be beneficial for the parents and siblings of the autistic child to have family therapy. Siblings may feel that they have extra rules to follow and extra difficulties to tolerate, and fewer opportunities to have good times with their parents. These things may all be true and may all be unavoidable. It may be helpful for a family to be able to discuss this explicitly and in front of one another. Family therapy can be an opportunity to negotiate specific contracts as to what family members must promise to do for one another—and what each will get in return. Like couples therapy, just going to family therapy with siblings can be a positive signal to the brothers and sisters of autistic children that their parents care about their emotional well-being too.

There are many specific kinds of adaptations and maladaptations that siblings make when they live with a brother or sister who has a disability. In the next section, we'll discuss some of these to further clarify some of the family dynamics that create difficulties for parents trying to balance the needs of their autistic child with the needs of their other children.

The Impact of Autism on Brothers and Sisters

Explaining Autism or PDD to Siblings

A watershed for many parents is the point at which they realize that they must say something to their other children about what is wrong with their autistic brother or sister. With autism, unlike a developmental disorder where there is an obvious physical defect, parents often have a hard time deciding *what* to tell their nonaffected children, as well as *when* to tell them. Often, parents defer this moment as long as possible, perhaps because "telling" adds another layer of reality and finality to the autistic child's status, or perhaps they feel the sibling will begin to stigmatize and reject the brother or sister if he or she has a "label" for what is wrong. In fact, most children *know*, implicitly or explicitly, that something is different about their autistic sibling before they are ever told anything. Kate, the six-year-old sister of autistic two-and-a-half-year-old Brandon, let her parents know this by presenting them with a picture she had drawn of her brother entitled "I hope you learn how to talk."

Sometimes the "time to tell" comes when the sibling begins to have contact with other children the same age as the autistic brother or sister. Mrs. Chen, mother of six-year-old Jessica and an autistic son who was three years old, told me about Jessica going over to play at her friend Amanda's house. Jessica came home and said that Amanda had a three-year-old brother too—only Amanda's brother talks a blue streak, builds trains with Leggos, and can drink from a cup. When Jessica asked her mom why *her* brother couldn't do those things yet, Mrs. Chen realized it was time to explain something more to Jessica. Until then, he was just her baby brother—and that's how babies were supposed to be.

Parents often express fear of telling their child about a label or diagnosis for the autistic brother or sister. Instead of thinking of the label as a stigma (although it is clear why parents have that fear), I encourage parents to let the unaffected sibling think of the label as an empty box into which all the observations about how their brother or sister is different can be placed. The word "autism" has no intrinsic meaning to a seven-year-old. When the sibling does something autistic, like flap his hands, the nonaffected sibling can be told he's doing that because he's autistic (or for an older child—that he's upset, and that's what autistic children do when they're upset). Then, atypical behavior can be seen as "something" rather than as unexplained, possibly evil, or magical, or even—as some younger brothers and sisters might believe—caused by their own misdeeds and unseen, unkind acts, thoughts, and feelings about their disabled sibling. Although I don't feel I learned much about autism from one of my late teachers, Bruno Bettleheim, I did learn many things about children. One is that you should never negate what they observe. If a child observes a behavior that is in some way odd or emotionally charged for him, you should try to help the child understand what he is experiencing. Dr. Bettleheim's axiom is especially important when you think of all the things that siblings experience with their autistic siblings that they experience in no other context.

Needing Different Standards of Behavior for the Autistic Child and for Siblings.

If parents follow the advice of a doctor or teacher and set more limits for their autistic child, and are able to do it in such a way that the results are desirable, they tend to adhere to a more limit-setting method of parenting for that child. Some parents, in order to be consistent, become stricter with all the children so that the autistic child doesn't feel separated out for more restrictive treatment. Either process can set into motion a pervasive sense of injustice on the part of nondisabled siblings.

Patterns of Sibling Coping

There are several prototypical ways that siblings cope with the special demands of having an autistic brother or sister. Most siblings evidence a combination of these various means of coping. To some extent, each prototypic method of coping has both advantages and disadvantages. Research suggests that about fifty percent of siblings of developmentally disabled brothers and sisters look back on their childhoods as compromised in some substantial way by the stresses associated with the presence of their sibling. The other fifty percent, however, end up feeling more neutral about the experience, or believe that it in fact helped them develop into a better person.

The Parentified *Child.* A common adaptation to being the sibling of a developmentally disabled child is to become *parentified:* this means acting more like a parent than like a sibling in relation to your brother or sister. The risk of becoming parentified for siblings of autistic children is really substantial whether they are younger or older than the disabled child. Older sisters are most likely to be cast into the role of acting like a third parent for their autistic sibling. Often parents will say things like their ten-year-old son is the "big brother" of his twelve-year-old autistic sister. While the ten-year-old may be more advanced mentally, he still has to deal with the incongruity of being "big" in relation to someone physically larger (and maybe stronger) than he.

Typically, the parentified sibling is assigned specific responsibilities for his or her brother or sister, which usually include things like physically guarding the other child's movements so he doesn't do anything dangerous. Despite the fact that the nonhandicapped sibling may be of an age where *he* might be expected to be watched for such behaviors, he becomes the "keeper" instead of the "kept." Amazingly, most siblings can rise to these occasions well, and I've seen numerous pieces of chalk, Leggos, and Fisher-Price Peg People being removed from the mouths of little autistic children by five-, six-, and seven-year-old brothers and sisters. When policing tasks like these go well, the sibling feels good to have done his job, and certainly has found a way to earn attention and appreciation from his overwhelmed mother. More worrisome is when the mission fails, and the autistic child begins to gag, or breaks something, and the seven-year-old feels like an abject failure.

To some extent, a sibling who learns to behave helpfully to someone less able is probably learning to be a more altruistic, caring person. The difficulty is in drawing the line between helpfulness as a good life lesson for the sibling and as an undue burden. Parentification can deprive a child of his own childhood. I have watched many second graders in a playroom full of toys sit quietly, acting like little adults while their parents talk about their brothers and sisters. They too are concerned about their sibling, and their occasional comments usually bear out the old adage that "little pitchers have big ears." Because they are siblings, children naturally have a strong identification with one another, and focus on the similarities between themselves and their brothers and sisters.

This makes the differences all the more apparent. Young children may feel they have to act super-good or else the "bad" behaviors they see in their autistic brother or sister may befall them. Because young children are very egocentric (self-centered), they may also feel that their own "badness" may have caused the "bad" behavior in their brother or sister. Often, during evaluations, parents hush their nonaffected children repeatedly for very small interruptions. I wonder how they manage to stay as still and quiet as they do. Maybe they feel that acting especially good in front of the doctor who is seeing their brother or sister will somehow help him or her.

On a more purely behavioral level it is clear that almost all parents of autistic children heavily reinforce parentified behavior. They need all the help they can get. Parentification in moderation is not likely to be harmful to a sibling. The situation is more worrisome when acting parentified becomes the only way to get parental approval, or when "helping" activities take so much time and psychic energy that the child has no time or place to be a child him- or herself.

For the parentified child, it is important that there be opportunities for him or her to *be* a child. This can include having a big birthday party with all the trimmings (while someone else takes his autistic sibling for the day), or it can be an opportunity to do another more routine activity like baking, gardening, or house repair with mom or dad without having to "help" the autistic sibling "help" at the same time.

The Withdrawn Child. Some siblings of autistic children do not try to earn parental attention by helping. They simply withdraw. The behaviors of their autistic sibling may drive them away, or parental demands for help may overwhelm them. The classic example I always think of is Raymond, the thirteen-year-old brother of Darren, a 275-pound, six-foot, aggressive, severely retarded, autistic sixteen-year-old. By the time I met the family, Darren had kicked holes in many walls and frequently hit others and banged on furniture to get what he wanted. His mother indulged him totally and, to hear her talk, you would have thought her son was an ornery thirty-pound three-year-old having the occasional temper tantrum. Then we discovered that Raymond, Darren's thirteen-year-old brother, had moved into the garage earlier in the year. Apparently, after years of being physically attacked, having his homework torn up, and having food taken off his plate, Raymond had had enough. Darren's parents thought this was a good arrangement. Knowing that they wouldn't have thought it a good arrangement if Darren was the one living in the garage, we suggested that it might be time they considered an out-of-home placement for Darren.

Other withdrawn siblings come to our evaluations and spend two out of three hours standing behind the draperies so they can't see us and we can't see them. Others build forts. These siblings create as much of an "autistic" wall between themselves and their autistic sibling as their sibling puts up to keep them out. They too live in their own universe, but it is self-imposed. A number of these children seem clinically depressed, and probably most of them are at risk for developing depressions as they grow older, if no one makes an effort to draw them out. It seems that, most often, withdrawn siblings are younger siblings—children who have never had a period of development where they have been the primary focus of their parent's attention. Mostly these are children who would never have been the most gregarious children anyway; the kind of children who are slow to warm up in a new situation. With the added stress of minimally available parenting, they psychologically "give up."

The withdrawn child may be the sibling most in need of his or her own psychotherapy around issues of coping with an autistic brother or sister. A withdrawn child is also very likely to benefit from a special relationship with a therapist that is just for him or her, and a therapy setting where the dominating actions of the sibling do not have to be included in the play, or can be gradually included as the child learns to understand and master his or her feelings toward the situation at home. One therapist who runs a group for siblings of children with various developmental disorders reports that one consensual rule of her group is that they won't have to talk about their brothers and sisters—they have enough of that the rest of the time. It's definitely healthy to encourage a withdrawn child to feel safe enough, somewhere, that he or she can be temporarily freed of constraints imposed by the autistic sibling.

It is also important that the withdrawn child have individual time to spend with his or her parents. This can be a one-on-one trip somewhere (even regular trips to the grocery store), or a special family outing where the withdrawn child has made the choice of destination and activities. For a child who feels depressed or powerless, having an opportunity to make choices that positively affect other family members can help restore a sense of self-worth, and a sense that he or she really exists psychologically as an operative family member and not just as an appendage.

The Super-Achiever or Family Mascot. Some siblings who are more extroverted adapt by compensating for the loss that everyone else in the family is experiencing. There are a couple of main variations. One is the child who can be described as the super-achiever. When parents find they have an autistic child, it is very reassuring to see the sibling develop normally. It definitely helps put the autistic child's problems into perspective. It helps even more if the nonaffected sibling is an exceptional achiever. If you have one child in special education, it feels particularly good to have another in a gifted education program. Some parents are able to make a positive adaptation to their autistic child's handicap by nurturing another child. This may be a transfer of parental aspirations or fantasies. Generally it is a good means of coping as long as the demands for achievement on the non-affected sibling are ones he can reasonably meet. The super-achieving child, just like the parentified child, comes to realize that succeeding in activities that adults value (like school, athletics, music) are ways of garnering parental attention. Of course, the types of sibling coping being described here are not mutually exclusive. Many parentified siblings are also very high achievers and serve as their family's "mascot."

Allowing this type of adaptation is, by and large, quite healthy, as long as the child is not pushed to achieve beyond his or her talents. It also provides natural opportunities for the nonaffected sibling to have undivided attention from parents—like when Dad coaches the Little League team, or both parents come (alone) to piano recitals. A pediatrician colleague of mine who is the older sibling of an autistic brother (and with whom I have written another book about siblings of disabled children) fits this category. He tried for years to obtain undivided parental attention and to be the center of attention by being funny. Now, he also has a growing career as a stand-up comedian. Going to medical school was among his attempts to "super-achieve" to get undivided parental attention. Hoping to be the center of attention for once, he asked his parents to come alone (that is, not with his twenty-three-year-old autistic brother) to his medical school graduation. (They brought his brother.) Even into adulthood, siblings of autistic children continue to fight the same battles around identity and how their identities are affected by competition with a sibling that may have been a "black hole" of all parental efforts.

The "mascot" version of sibling coping is the brother or sister who may lack the specific talents of a super-achiever, but tries hard to establish an identity that parents can't help paying attention to. This may be a child who acts funny or goofy or is a big show-off. Some mascot children may sometimes be testing the limits of what their parents can endure, but persist because they have fairly resilient personalities.

The child who adapts by creating a stir may also be the one in the family that tries hard to cheer parents up when they look glum. There is usually a combination of age-appropriate self-centeredness mixed with a bit of altruism that fuels the mascot child's engine. What she may really want to do is divert attention to her: I have a videotape of an autistic child beginning an intensive one-on-one therapy program; first is fifteen minutes of a screaming, resistant, autistic three-year-old, followed by a break in which the three-year-old's seat is left briefly empty—but soon reoccupied by his two-year-old sister, who fluffs her dress and sits down, seemingly eager to receive this focused attention herself.

The Withdrawn Child. Overall, withdrawal from family life is probably the most maladaptive response on the part of siblings. A very withdrawn child should be seen by a therapist who can assess the situation and suggest interventions that may be helpful. Parentified children can be worrisome too, because they subjugate their own needs so easily. Their behavior is similar to the pattern sometimes described as "co-dependency" in the literature on adult children of alcoholics. Co-dependents don't feel like worthwhile human beings unless they are helping someone who is helpless or out of control. On the positive side, parentified children grow up to be special education teachers, pediatricians, and social workers in disproprotionate numbers. On the less positive side, they get into relationships with spouses who abuse drugs or alcohol, or who are chronically unemployed—in this way they continue to have someone dysfunctional to take care of. The super-achieving and mascot children probably have the healthiest adaptations because they operate with an intact sense of self that derives either from achievements outside the home or from a certain ability to view family dysfunction at a distance as reflected by their ability to use humor to describe their own difficult situations.

Acceptance of the Autistic Child Outside the Home

Extended Family Support

Social support is what you perceive it to be. Helpful and helping relatives, friends and public agencies need to be *perceived* as helpful for a parent to feel they are really getting some relief. As parents face their child's diagnosis and begin to plan treatment, they do so within the context of an extended family system that can possibly provide help. Extended family support is a very complicated matter. It involves not only the geographic availability of family members, but also the quality of preexisting relationships.

A Role for Grandparents. In some of the best situations, parents receive substantial support from their families. We've had many grandmothers, and some grandfathers, come to our clinic with their grandchildren to lend support to their son or daughter. Grandmothers in particular can be ideal supports because they tend to know more about how children develop and somehow seem to more easily accept a child, despite limitations, than a parent sometimes can. In general, grandparents seem less often unable to take action because of denial of a child's disability, and are more often ready to undertake a pragmatic approach to treatment. Maybe it's because older people come from a generation in which less educated people were more common. The idea that their autistic grandson might never graduate from high school, or learn to read or write, and maybe "just" be able to be a gardener, may be acceptable to them. Grandparents take the diagnosis of autism less "personally" than parents, who are more often flooded with waves of conflicting emotions of grief, shame, and guilt. Maybe grandparents can be more objective because they don't feel they'll have to worry what will happen to the child when he's an adult, or when *his* parents are too old to care for him.

Younger single mothers in particular seem willing to accept their mothers as authorities on child-rearing in these situations, and therefore experience it as supportive when their mothers take active roles in making decisions about their child's special needs. Other parents rely on grandparents because of the demands on their own lives. I have a patient with two busy physician parents and a retired school psychologist grandmother. From the beginning, the grandmother became her grandson's educational expert and eventually had his home certified as a non-public school so that she could have access to resources for teaching him with a program she managed.

More often than not, grandparents are supportive and helpful. But, if there are preexisting unresolved issues between the grandparent and the parent of the autistic child, they may surface in grandparental perceptions of how their child's flaws are causing or worsening the grandchild's autism. Sometimes getting the grandparent to know more about autism by reading a book or an article helps. Sometimes having the grandparent try to care for the child for a weekend helps the reality of the situation sink in.

A Role for Aunts and Uncles. We have already discussed how grandparents are often welcomed as a source of social support. The relationship between parents of autistic children and their own brothers and sisters can be more complex when it comes to understanding and acceptance of the autistic child. Mothers of autistic children often get very good social support from sisters. It can be really helpful when there is an older sister who is a more experienced parent and who can help put things into perspective. Sometimes when parents of an autistic child are around their young nieces and nephews, they begin to make comparisons about development; at that point they may ask their brother or sister whether they too have concerns about their autistic child's development. Some brothers and sisters wait until they are asked before sharing their observations. Others offer their opinion sooner.

Siblings usually intend to be helpful when they suggest to a brother or sister that their child may have a problem. But siblings can be competitive too. And sometimes sincere efforts to help are taken as criticism. Brothers and sisters with older children are often able to realize, before the parents do, that their nephew or niece is developing differently. If a brother or sister chooses to point this out, the sibling runs the chance of alienating the brother or sister— and also not getting the message across. One example is that of Kathleen, whose four-and-a-half-year-old son, Eric, was severely language delayed and mute. Kathleeen came from a high-achieving family—her parents were wealthy, her two siblings were physicians, and she herself was well-edu-cated—but she was an unemployed, agoraphobic alcoholic married to an un-successful businessman who was almost her parents' ages. Kathleen could at least feel superior to her psychiatrist sister on the count that she was married and had a child. When Eric was two-and-a-half, and her psychiatrist sister began to point out Eric's developmental problems, Kathleen took this as jealous competitive hostility (which it may have been) and ignored the truthful component of her sister's observations for two years. Eventually, with heavy grandmaternal intervention, Kathleen did seek treatment for Eric.

On the other hand, family support can help break through a couple's denial about their child's disability. Another family we follow, the Johns, had three children, eight-year-old Robert and twin four-year-olds, David and Clara. David was autistic, but not diagnosed until age four because his mother,

Martha, had a history of chronic and debilitating depressions which had been made much worse by the recent diagnosis of David. In the course of evaluating and planning for David, we received letters explaining Martha's own psychiatric status, concerns about David's development, and general family concern about how the Johns could learn to cope better, as well as great willingness to help from aunts on both sides of the family, including one who flew out from New York to help organize the family. Eventually, the maternal grandparents took David to live with them in the Midwest for a time because of fear that Martha would have to be hospitalized if not separated from the child by another means. With David out of the home, Martha recovered a little, got treatment for herself, and achieved some acceptance of David's condition. Clearly, without family support in getting to and accepting David's diagnosis, Martha's denial would have continued, David would have remained untreated, and Robert and Clara would have continued to be neglected, as Martha would have spent increasing amounts of time isolating herself from the realities of her children's needs.

Parental Friendships. Friends can be another form of social support when dealing with an autistic child. At first, parents may feel at a loss to know what to tell friends about their autistic child. It may not be clear to them that their friends know that something is even wrong with their child. Their friends may not know anything more about autism than the fact that Dustin Hoffman played an autistic man in the movie *Rain Man*. It can be hard to know where to start explaining the problem. One father of an autistic boy told me that for the first year after his son was diagnosed, he began to cry whenever he tried to tell a friend about his son's autism. He went on to say that although he would cry in the first minutes after he said the word autism, he would be able to recompose himself; after that, it felt very good to be able to talk about it openly.

Some parents feel that their social group changes after their child is diagnosed with autism. Sometimes the child is hard to take to anyone else's house. Sometimes parents feel that friends are subtly rejecting them. Some friends reach out more strongly than before, recognizing the additional stress. Families who are very involved in their churches often find good support there.

Something we frequently do in our clinic is to pair parents together. Friendships are based on common interests, and when dealing with autism becomes a major focus, meeting new people in the same situation is very appealing for some people. We usually pair mothers who have similar children, arranging it so that one mother's child is slightly older than the other's child; in this way, the mother of the younger child can benefit from the experience of the mother of the older child. The mother of the older child benefits because she feels that the knowledge she has accumulated is of value not just to her but to others. Other parents become friends because their children are in the same special education classes. Some meet through the Autism Society or other support group. Whether or not you have friends with autistic children, it *is* important to feel that autism is something that can be talked about and that doesn't have to be hidden away. A great deal of psychological stress comes from compartmentalizing a major emotional part of one's life away from other parts, and that's what happens if talking about autism becomes a taboo topic. Although friends may not know what to say or do at first, most want to help and be supportive but may not know what to say, especially if they've haven't known anyone with a disabled child before.

Going Out in Public

Today, Americans are supposed to know it is "politically correct" to display an accepting attitude toward handicapped persons, but this is not always what families with autistic children experience. A child's "bad" behavior in the absence of "looking handicapped" can result in people in public places automatically faulting the parent for the child's bad behavior. In some ways, parents of children with Down syndrome have it the easiest. Their children have an appearance that is widely recognized as "retarded" by most Americans, even if they can't remember what it is called. If you go to the grocery store with your four-year-old Down girl in the grocery cart, and she pulls six boxes of Cherrios off the shelf, people will look at you sympathetically and help you put back the fallen boxes. If you go to the market with your little boy (who looks normal but is in the same special education class as that little girl) and *he* pulls down the Cheerios, people will look at you like you are a rotten parent who can't control her wild kid. This is to say that much of the stigma that is attached to parents of autistic children comes from the fact that their child's handicapping condition is not readily visible and therefore is assumed not to exist. Since badly behaved children are more common than developmentally disabled ones, the public tends to make the more likely attribution, and this can stigmatize parents of autistic children as "bad" parents.

Being made to feel like a bad parent because your autistic child acts badly is hard to counteract. Probably the most damaging aspect is that parents begin to wonder if they really *are* bad parents; whether if they *were* more adequate parents, their child *wouldn't* pull down cereal boxes in the market, and so on. On one level, it is enticing to believe that you, as the parent, *are* at fault, because the belief implies that if you change your behavior, the child's inappropriate behavior can be made to go away. There are many behaviors that a well-informed parent of an autistic child can be helped to deal with, but, realistically, if the child is ten, and has a mental age of three, it is only reasonable to expect the child to act like a well-behaved three-year-old when he is on his best behavior. This is not something that the people at the next table at a restaurant are going to realize.

People may stare at or avoid a child in a wheelchair, but an autistic child does not call attention to himself until he acts "weird" or "bad." Family members who are around the child all the time find it difficult to know just how normal their child does or does not appear to others. As families get more used to the atypical behavior of the autistic or PDD child, they are likely to resent people who stare at their child or show disapproval when the child, in the family member's opinion, is still acting fairly normally (like lining up all the silverware at the table in the restaurant end to end). Some families successfully cope with this form of stigma by actually marking the child in some way as handicapped, so that people will hopefully be more generous in their evaluations of the child. Forms of self-imposed markers for the autistic child include putting the child in an extra-large stroller (the kind that fits a child up to seven or eights years old), or putting a medical alert bracelet on the child to subtly indicate that this child has some sort of "condition." One mother I met a number of years ago carried brochures from the National Society for Autistic Children with her. Most people who stare or look disapprovingly at an autistic child out in public are not consciously reacting in a negative way *because* the child has a disability. Taking this into account, and thinking of occasions when you may have unknowingly done the same thing, may make you feel better.

Spending Time Outside the Home Without the Autistic Child. An important goal for all families with an autistic or PDD child is to go out without the added responsibility of the child. In talking about siblings and their special needs, we have already discussed the importance of planning family outings where the siblings get to choose the activity and get to have events focus on them—without having to worry about whether or not their autistic sibling can join in, tolerate the wait, or pay attention long enough without being disruptive. It is equally important that parents go out together on their own. Various public agencies provide respite care for just this purpose. If the family falls apart because the parents can't remember anything they like about each other anymore, then the autistic child is not ultimately being helped. For a couple to function well together, they must have shared pleasure as well as shared responsibility.

Many parents say that they would like to go out alone but are afraid the child will fall apart or be impossible for anyone else to manage. There is usually more than one grain of truth in this. With some planning, a short parental absence will not be harmful to any child.

Many autistic children are sensitive to routine and sameness and so will do better if a babysitter comes to their home rather than if they are taken somewhere. It may be possible to get a babysitter who is a classroom aide in the child's school program, or in an adjacent class where the child is generally known. Sometimes having a sitter who "sits" one or two times with the parents at home, before going out, will help the transition to being left without the parents. For some families, having a sitter in the house while company comes over is almost like being alone as a couple. There definitely are autistic children who cry for extended periods when their parents go out. But in the same way a baby learns to sleep through the night, there may have to be a period that is uncomfortable for the child: when he is allowed to cry it out so that he can experience the new rules—that he is alone for a while, but that eventually it will end. A sitter left with an autistic or PDD child should be someone who understands that talking, carrying, bouncing, or otherwise distracting the upset autistic child may make him even more overstimulated and agitated.

As an autistic child gets older, parents may want to—and need to—take vacations alone. These may be short weekend vacations, or longer ones. I am in the camp that says parental sanity comes first, and only after that, can good parenting follow. For families of teenage autistic or PDD children who are looking toward some sort of residential placement in the next three to five years, getting away for a couple of weeks allows both the parent and child to learn how it feels to become a little less enmeshed—and for the child, how it feels to be a little more independent.

The Psychology of Choosing Residential Treatment

The final topic for this chapter is the issue of residential treatment. It's here in this chapter as a family issue, because it is mainly that. Usually there are educational programs that can serve a child appropriately whether he is at home or at a residential program. The decision of when and why to opt for residential treatment is one that is different for every combination of child and family characteristics. It is an issue where there are no rights or wrongs. What is right for one family may feel horrible to another family and vice versa.

The first and very important thing that needs to be said about this topic is that no one is ever going to force a parent to put an autistic child in an out-of-home placement. A diagnosis of autism or PDD does not mean a child cannot or should not live with his parents. Gone are the days when children were wrenched from their families by coercive doctors claiming to know what is best for everyone. It just doesn't happen to families with children diagnosed with autism or PDD. The fact is that today such prescriptions are virtually never made, except for profoundly retarded, medically fragile babies, and there is a significant trend to keep even those babies at home.

Mainstream American Culture and Changing Attitudes Toward Developmental Disabilities. In American culture, we've seen some very positive changes in the last 30 years in how the developmentally disabled are viewed. Through the 1950s there was very little available in the way of compensatory education for the cognitively handicapped. Children recognized to have more severe handicaps, such as children who were obviously dysmorphic or deformed at birth, were assumed to be severely retarded also. The quality standard of medical practice at that time was to help families with the decision to place such a baby in an institution, to forget the baby as much as possible, and to get on with their lives—that is, have another baby soon. Many parents did as they were told, and probably, if they believed strongly enough in the infallibility of doctors, were able to live with their decisions relatively well. Other families parted with their children and never got over the trauma.

As the field of special education developed, and as earlier and more intensive interventions were tried, some developmentally disabled children made greater progress than had been predicted. There was growing awareness that many developmentally disabled children including some autistic children, did better if they had exposure to more normal role models, and had some pressure to conform to rules of everyday living. Over time, the professional trend became one of recommending special education while the child lived at home, rather than placing the child out of the home. Residential programs *are* still available, and sometimes they are the right choice.

Types of Out-of-Home Care. The nature of out-of-home residential care, when it is used, has changed dramatically. There are very few "institutions" left. Institutional care for the developmentally disabled refers to large programs with hundreds of residents living on hospital-like wards of ten or more patients. Most of these programs—for all but the most severely retarded—have closed. Mainly, such programs have been replaced by smaller facilities than provide care for ten to forty residents, or group homes that provide care for six or fewer residents. These programs are community based, and residents attend school and other programs used by developmentally disabled children and adults who still live at home in the same community.

Most autistic or PDD children who go into out-of-home placements go into group home programs; some go into small residential schools that provide both a home-based training component and a schooling component. Group homes are in fact homes—houses in any residential neighborhood, in any community, where the children served by the group home usually share a bedroom with one other resident, and where a small group of staff provide care in shifts. Sometimes group homes are in fact a version of foster care in which an autistic child lives with one set of parents plus one or more other foster children, and/ or one or more children of the foster parents.

When Parents Choose Out-of-Home Care. Right at the time that their children are diagnosed, parents often ask about options for the adult care of a person with autism or with PDD. Of course, no one is making specific plans at that point, and prognosis has a great deal of variability. Still, many families seem to need a rough outline of the future, some brackets, to grasp the changed sense of reality they experience when they realize that their child has a lifetime disability.

All other things being equal, I most often encourage parents to begin thinking of out-of-home care for their autistic or PDD child when he or she is the same age at which siblings will be leaving the nest. Most families are fairly comfortable with this. In some cultures were extended families live together though, there is more of a hope and expectation that the autistic or PDD child will, as an adult, be able to stay in the same home with the rest of the family. Most families do look toward out-of-home placement as the high school years end (age 18 or 19) or when school district funding ends (age 22).

Reaching semi-independent status is a form of developing autonomy, and a developmental task that should be considered for everyone, but adjusted to the developmental level of independence that can be achieved. For some young adults who have autism and also have severe to moderate mental retardation, this may mean a group home and a day treatment program where they work on self-help skills. For young autistic adults with mild mental retardation, it may mean a group home and work in a sheltered work environment. For higher functioning autistic young people and many young people with PDD, a group home plus training to work in a supported employment environment (a job with a job coach) may be an appropriate placement. (Some of these concepts are discussed in more detail in Chapter 13.)

For some families, however, residential placement may be necessary when their child is younger. One set of criteria that I hold to strongly is that a child should be put in residential placement if he is a danger to himself or to others, especially siblings in the home. If various behavioral measures have been sincerely tried, and various medication trials have failed to cause significant behavioral change, *and* the child is still really in danger of hurting himself or others, then a residential placement should be seriously considered. Most often, these cases involve autistic children who are severely to moderately mentally retarded and who are also very, very active. No two parents can monitor a child who has no judgment or impulse control for 24 hours a day, especially if the child sleeps briefly, irregularly, or almost not at all. The wear and tear on the whole family can be enormous. My criterion is that if a child does something to a sibling that would be considered child abuse if the parent did it, and this happens more than once, despite supervision, an out-of-home program should be considered. A recent news report alleged that a severely retarded autistic man had killed his infant nephew by throwing him out a third-story window. It is easy to understand this scenario when one considers that the autistic person involved may have been very irritated by the baby's cries, and that he could not have been expected to understand that the baby was really another human being like himself.

I encourage parents to consider residential placement before a child's behavioral problems reach crisis proportions. A much more appropriate and high-quality placement is likely to be found if a search is begun before a last-minute decision has to be made. Some autistic children just require a degree of structure, routine, predictability, and limit-setting that cannot reasonably be provided in a normal home environment. With the added structure of good quality out-of-home care, many children who were terrors in their homes settle into more manageable human beings.

Sometimes residential placement is needed because family circumstances are overwhelming. There may be more than one developmentally disabled child in the home, or an elderly grandparent who requires chronic care. The parent him- or herself may have a poorly managed psychiatric disorder that is made much worse by the child's presence. Young single mothers with no good social support may be unable to cope with an autistic child. Some parents who are borderline mentally retarded or mildly retarded themselves really can't comprehend the special needs of their autistic child. Sometimes, after years of assiduously exploring every possible intervention, some parents simply burn out from the requirements of implementing many different therapeutic approaches. Some parents feel afraid they may begin to abuse their child out of frustration. Some parents simply feel they are not prepared to handle the child or the situation.

In any of these cases, a residential placement in conjunction with an appropriate school placement is very likely to be in the best interest of the child, the parents, and the rest of the family. With perseverance, a good caseworker, and an understanding of the various agencies involved, such a placement is usually obtainable, although it could take, one, two, or occasionally even three years. Families with greater economic resources usually have more choices and can make things happen more quickly.

No matter why a family chooses residential placement, the choice is never easy. There are always left-over ambivalent feelings. Parents may have to do a lot of talking to give each other permission to make the decision for residential placement. Contact with a therapist or professional who works with autistic children may provide support for the choice.

When a child first moves out of the home, there is bound to be a sense of loss. Anyone who monopolizes attention is going to be missed. It can help to think of how the child can benefit from more consistent structured care than that provided in a home environment. Thinking about a new home routine without the child helps too. Often, residential schools recommend, and I strongly endorse, that the child not come home for the first month or more. Not only does it give the child time to learn a new routine, it gives his family time to learn a new routine, also.

Chapter Summary

In this chapter, we discussed how families can gain support to deal with living with a child who has autism or PDD. Some of the support comes from within the family itself. Other support comes from outside the family—from relatives and friends, and also from agencies and schools that can alleviate strain and promote coping so crises can be avoided. In the next part of this book, we'll discuss specific aspects of the educational system, as this is the largest single resource for helping children with autism and PDD to develop.

PART II

Treatment Resources

There is no *one* way to educate a child who has autism or PDD, any more than there is only one right way to educate a nondisabled child. There *are* some general principles that apply, and different philosophies supported by different groups of educators. Rather than designating an educational philosophy as "right" or "wrong" (for example, being "for" or "against" mainstreaming), we'll go through the pros and cons of each issue and try to place you, as a parent or as a professional planning for the education of an autistic child, in the position of being able to weigh what will best meet appropriate goals for your child.

When speaking of children with developmental disabilities, the term "education" is often used more broadly than it is with nonhandicapped children. Usually, it is interpreted to include early skills that usually *don't* first emerge in school—like learning to talk—and can also include adaptive behaviors such as becoming toilet-trained or learning to eat with utensils or, for older students, learning to ride a bus or hold a job. Academic subjects are, of course, included too, and can be taught either in the usual way, or with more of a functional focus. (In Chapter 13, we'll discuss guidelines for selecting appropriate content for a particular child's educational program.)

Each year, parents are faced with negotiating a new individual educational program (IEP) for their child (as will be discussed in Chapter 8). Another critical point occurs each September, whenever a new teacher is introduced and/or the child moves to a new classroom. Having a good IEP is one thing, having it implemented as planned is another. Parents are basically put in the default position of being the consumer watchdogs of their child's special education. Therefore, as a parent, it's a worthy goal to understand what your child will need to promote his learning and why. Knowing how to observe in a classroom and assess program characteristics allows parents to monitor intelligently the educational process as implemented by teachers and school administrators. (In Chapter 10, we'll discuss how to be an educated consumer of classrooms and special education teachers.)

As an autistic child matures, parents are faced with a couple of critical points when educational goals may need to be scrutinized with particular care. The first occasion is the child's first IEP. After that, many children progress more or less smoothly through a system of teachers and school staff who provide continuity in planning and goals. Other times when it is important to examine closely a child's educational progress and future goals are when a child moves from a preschool to an elementary school program, or from an elementary to a middle school, or from middle school to high school. Children grow at different rates, too—partly as a function of their capacity, partly as a function of their teaching. So there are times when a child's educational progress in his current program seems stalled, and parents and school personnel will have to consider carefully whether a change in curriculum focus is needed. There are points at which a child may need to shift from a more academic to more functional skills focus, or from more verbal to a more nonverbal focus. These are really sensitive periods, when all involved have to look carefully at objective measures to feel justified that "downsizing" a child's long-term objectives is not read by parents as a lack of interest on the school's part in trying to help the student achieve more.

In the next five chapters, we'll discuss how you know when you've reached critical turning points in educational planning, and what you need to know to make decisions about how to proceed. Most of the focus in this part of this book will be on specific educational recommendations, including initial goals of early intervention (Chapter 9), help in developing attentional skills and behavioral control (Chapter 11), language skills (Chapter 12), as well as pre-academic and academic skills, and everyday living skills (Chapter 13). We'll also cover the structural aspects of classroom life; for example, how to determine how many children should be in a class, what kind of training and support teachers and aides should have, and different instructional methods (Chapter 10).

In the last two chapters of the book, we'll cover other approaches to treating autism. In Chapter 14, we'll discuss how autistic spectrum disorders are sometimes treated with psychoactive medications, along with special education. We will focus on what medications can be expected to do—and what they can't be expected to do. Finally, in Chapter 15, we'll address some of the more controversial treatments for autism that have emerged over the past several years. Some of these nonmainstream treatments become popularized after they appear to have worked for just one child (or for a small number of children), but not for most, and it's important to become an educated consumer of such approaches.

The flowchart in Chapter 8 outlines the various sorts of services and programs we'll discuss in the second half of this book. As we go on, you can refer back to it to see how various educational and developmental services fit together.

CHAPTER 8

♦ ♦ ♦

Finding Resources

The first hurdle for parents of autistic and PDD children is realizing that their child has a problem. The second hurdle is finding out what the problem is. The third is planning what to do about it. In this chapter, we discuss how to find educational and other resources for your child, and how to act as an advocate for your child's best interests. Basically, as a parent, you need to know what resources are available to you, and who can help you get them. This includes infant stimulation programs, special education programs, state-funded services for the developmentally disabled, and additional therapy for language, physical, or social skills development. Available resources also include other books on autism or parenting special-needs children, and parent support organizations such as the Autism Society of America. Depending on your child and the resources available in your area, you may also find that you need to become your child's legal advocate or even your child's special education teacher. Figure 6 is a flowchart of the agencies, services, and treatment available for autistic children in the United States. As we go along, we'll discuss each box in the flowchart and explain how and when children are eligible for these services, and how various services interrelate.

The Rules of the Game

Getting your child into a good program, or getting funding for other needed services shouldn't have to be difficult, but sometimes it is. By and large, people who work in the educational or developmental disabilities systems are not bad people. I believe that ninety-nine percent of them are good people. They certainly are not in this line of work just to make a lot of money. These people do their jobs because they feel that what they do can make a difference. The problem is that resources are scarce. Special education is a fairly expensive commodity, and it has seldom been a high "social agenda" priority for

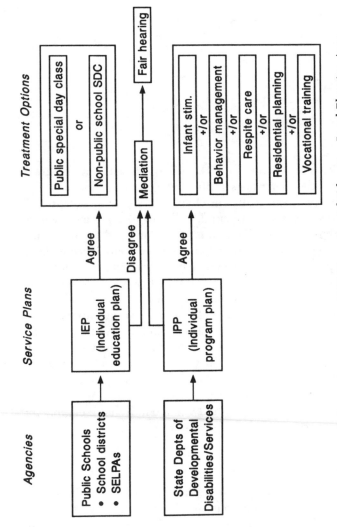

Figure 6 Treatment resources. (SELPA = Special Education Local Planning Area; SDC = Special Day Class)

politicians or fundraisers unless they themselves have direct experience with disabled people. Basically good people who must act as gatekeepers of developmental services are put in a position of having to prioritize the allocation of resources based on complicated written rules, as well as informal criteria that usually are not (and cannot) be made totally explicit. Parents are faced with two tasks: getting to know the written rules—the special education, developmental disabilities, and insurance laws—and also figuring out how the unwritten part of the system in their locale works. In this chapter, we'll cover the written rules that generally pertain across America, and how to make them work to the greatest benefit for your child. For readers outside of the United States, this section may be helpful strategically in getting services, but the specific "ins" and "outs" of laws and agencies can be skipped. As for the unwritten rules for obtaining help, no matter where you live, it certainly bears repeating that being pragmatic, and remembering that you attract more flies with honey than with vinegar, will smooth your path when you are looking for help for your child.

Eligibility for Developmental Disabilities Services

To receive any kind of developmental services, a child must first go through an intake process and become qualified. The two main types of agencies through which your child may qualify for services are the special education system and the developmental disabilities system. Once qualified, the child may be periodically reviewed, but initial eligibility is the more difficult and time-consuming process.

In the United States, each state has a Department of Developmental Services (DDS), or some equivalent. In many states, developmental services are proffered through a system of *regional centers,* nonprofit agencies chartered by the state agency to serve some specific geographic area's population of developmentally disabled people. In California, for example, there are twenty-three regional centers, each of which serves about three to six counties. Any pediatrician or developmental specialist will know the name and phone number of the local regional center or county DDS office. While each state may follow slightly different procedures for delivering services, all within a state are subject to the same rules as to who is eligible for services and who is not.

A Diagnosis as a Ticket to Services

In many states, children with a diagnosis of autistic disorder or autism *are* eligible, while children diagnosed as having pervasive developmental disorder (PDD, NOS) are *not* eligible for developmental services. If the child also has a diagnosis of mental retardation, the child will be eligible for developmental services regardless of whether he or she is also diagnosed autistic or PDD. The regional centers/DDSs are designated to serve some, but not *all* children with developmental disorders. For example, children with learning disabilities are not served by most DDSs or regional centers, although such children may clearly be eligible for special education. Many clinicians and researchers believe that the distinction drawn between autism and PDD by the regional centers/DDSs is not meaningful and deprives PDD children of needed services. The counterargument is that the line must be drawn somewhere, just as it is drawn between mental retardation and learning disabilities. One of the main advantages of the broadening use of the label of "autism" or "autistic disorder" since the publication of DSM-III-R (1987) has been that more children more easily qualify for services now than in the past. Sometimes a clinician may feel that "PDD" more accurately describes the profile and severity of a particular child's autistic symptoms, but will go ahead and label the problem "autism" so as to ensure that the child gets as much help as possible. In these situations, it is important to remember that one main reason for obtaining a diagnosis in the first place is to obtain needed services, and if the parent understands the difference between what the doctor is writing down, and what the doctor can really say about the child's prognosis, that's what's really important.

Waiting Beyond School Age to Obtain Developmental Services. Most autistic children are first identified as eligible for developmental services between the ages of two and five. However, some autistic children who have relatively less cognitive impairment don't get signed up for developmental services at that stage. Sometimes it's because the parents don't really accept the diagnosis of autism, or they see the child's symptoms as so mild as to not need the kind of services mainly designed for children who have mental retardation as well. Some wealthier families don't bother to qualify for services because they would just as soon pick and choose among specialists for their child, rather than receive services off a roster of publically funded therapists of various sorts. In these cases, state developmental services might not be sought until the child is much older. In our clinic we see a number of such patients who are between twenty-two and twenty-four years old—the twenty-second birthday being the latest date at which the public schools terminate special education services. Sometimes these individuals clearly and easily qualify as autistic or as having some degree of mental retardation. More often, they are individuals who more clearly meet the diagnostic description of Asperger's syndrome (see Chapter 5) or are considered to have PDD,NOS, but seem too mildly affected to be described as autistic. Nevertheless, these individuals often experience problems in becoming independent from their families, getting jobs, or continuing into higher education. Therefore, they too can sometimes be eligible for services designed for people with autism based on their having a condition that can technically be described as "similar to" autism, and causing significant adaptive impairments in everyday functioning.

In the cases of these young adults with AS or PDD, the DDS/regional centers will inevitably ask "If this individual is so substantially handicapped, why didn't he show up sooner?" and then try to deny services. It is therefore advisable to qualify an autistic or PDD child, even a higher functioning child, (even a child for whom there is no immediate need for services), when he is younger. By young adulthood, the need for services may have to be proved more circuitously—for example, by arguing that the young person has significant adaptive impairments, meaning that he cannot use the intelligence he *does* have to function independently. (Tests for measuring adaptive functioning were discussed in Chapter 5.) Sometimes first-time service reviews that are done on young adults mean going back through years of records and trying to reinterpret observations and diagnoses given long ago when different sets of diagnostic descriptions were in use. Parents pursuing such a strategy may eventually prevail, but go through an anxiety-provoking process, and usually end up spending a significant sum on advocates or attorneys and on independent evaluations.

Help Provided Through Developmental Services Agencies

The developmental services agencies basically pick up where the schools leave off in terms of providing help for families with developmentally disabled children. Services provided through developmental service agencies usually include case management, developmental assessment, infant stimulation programs, behavioral intervention services, respite care, vocation training, sheltered workshops placement, day treatment programs, residential placement and, most importantly, funding for all of the above (under certain circumstances). Sometimes funding may also be provided for speech and language therapy, legal advocacy, or transportation, depending upon whether there are or are not other agencies or insurance that may pay for those things. Eligible and appropriate developmental services are enumerated in a document referred to as the child's IPP (Individual Program Plan), which is negotiated between parents and the agency and is based on the child's diagnosis, age, and needs.

Case Management. Most developmental services agencies assign each child a representative who may be referred to as a case manager, caseworker, social worker, client program coordinator, or so on, depending on what that person's qualifications and duties are. As a parent, you should consider this person your child's advocate. The caseworker is someone who knows the system that you need help from; if you form an alliance with her or him, the caseworker can help you leverage the most out of the system. A case manager comes to know you and your child usually through yearly reviews and more frequent contacts, as needed. The typical limitations to good case management are case managers who are assigned too many clients; who are constantly having their caseload changed by administrators; or who burn out of their low-paying jobs at astonishingly high rates, leaving parents unsure who their current case manager is. Unfortunately, because of high turnover in some agencies, case managers can be young and inexperienced and know less than the parents of the clients they serve. If you feel your child has been assigned to an ineffective case manager, you should ask who the case manager's supervisor is and request someone in a position to be more helpful. The squeaky wheel gets the grease, etc. A case worker can be a bridge to the educational system too, and help you through that process as well, so it's important to find someone you can work with.

Developmental Assessment. Some developmental services agencies provide families with funding for developmental assessment or actually do developmental assessment in-house. At the very least, a thorough developmental assessment should be provided at the time of initial intake to determine eligibility for various sorts of services. Many agencies provide periodic reassessment, especially when eligibility or appropriateness for further services come into question.

Infant Stimulation Programs. The first service that many families benefit from after their child becomes a client of their regional center or DDS is payment for an infant stimulation program. Despite the name, "infant stim" programs are special education services for all children up to three years old. Then, at age three, in most states, special educational responsibility is transferred to the school district. (More details about what infant stimulation programs can provide is described in detail in Chapter 9.) It suffices here to say that the infant stimulation programs need to be reimbursed for each child they serve, and that developmental services agencies pay for much of this. What also needs to be clear here is that the state developmental services agencies themselves usually do not directly provide services; rather, they contract with other agencies that do. For example, many infant stimulation programs are actually run by organizations like the Easter Seals Society, March of Dimes, larger hospitals, and the like. Many parents are initially confused by this because an agency with a name like "Golden Gate Regional Center" seems to imply that there is a "center" (an actual place with children) somewhere.

Behavior Intervention Services. Developmental agencies sometimes provide therapists or pay for therapists who are specially trained to use behavioral methods to address behavioral problems the parents may be having with the child at home. (Behavior therapy principles will be discussed further in Chapter 11.) For younger children, problems that behavior therapists can help with may include throwing tantrums, toilet-training, self-injurious behavior, or "self-stimulation" behaviors. Sometimes behaviorists work on helping the child develop better means of communication as a way of reducing tantrums. In school-aged children, behaviorists may help with issues of compliance, table manners, and grooming. For adolescents, behaviorists are often called in to help the adolescent learn socially acceptable ways of expressing sexual desires. Other behaviorists work specifically with young adults around skills needed for living in the mainstream, like travel training, having responsible work habits, and social skills development. Typically, developmental services agencies have a standard number of hours of behaviorist time they are allowed to allocate to one family for work on a specific set of behavioral goals. If some satisfactory progress has been made toward the behavioral goals at the end of the allotted time, it may be possible to receive further authorizations for more help if the therapist thinks further significant progress is likely. It can be very helpful to know what the rules are ahead of time. An advantage to working with a behavior therapist is that he or she is someone who can come into your home and demonstrate techniques for behavior change in context, thus providing both parent and child with a lesson on how better to function. Sometimes it is possible for behavior therapists to work with teachers also in order to provide continuity between what the child is learning to do at home and at school. More often, however, the developmental disabilities and educational systems are unfortunately rather territorial and proprietary, and hesitate to allow therapists to cross boundaries.

Respite Care. Another big help that developmental service agencies may provide parents is respite care. This means experienced care providers that can care for your child while you get time off for yourself or to be with your spouse or with your other children. Sometimes respite care is offered in your own home, and in other cases, involves taking the child to the care provider's house. Generally, families are allocated a certain number of respite hours per month (for example, in California it's hypothetically sixteen hours), and these can be used on a regular basis—like one afternoon a week—or the hours can be saved up so that parents or parents plus other siblings can get away for a couple of days a few times a year. Because some agencies are so overwhelmed, there is sometimes more demand for respite than there are care providers or funds for respite care. Sometimes it's possible to have a friend or relative who is good at caring for your child become authorized to receive respite payments for taking care of him. In some locales, respite care is a free service, and in other places, it is provided as a sliding scale subsidy.

At first, many parents hesitate to use respite care, even though they may desperately want a break from the full-time extra-heavy demands of caring for an autistic child. Usually the parent is reluctant because of fears that the child will have a tantrum and completely fall apart if left with an unfamiliar caregiver. While your child may tolerate separations very poorly, more likely than not, a distressing separation won't occur more than a couple of times before the child gets an idea of what's happening and begins to accept the situation. (For very separation-anxious, change-sensitive autistic children an in-home respite worker will probably work out best, at least at first.) It *is* very important for parents to take some care of themselves as well as their autistic children and to get a break occasionally. An experienced respite worker has seen tantrums before and has been trained to handle them. A good respite worker will be available to talk with you the first time you leave your child and be willing to discuss what reactions the child might have, and how separation distress will be handled.

Vocational Training. Many families find that they don't really want much contact with developmental service agencies until their autistic child is beyond school age. Parents with large extended families tend to use respite care less, and when the child is in a really good school system, less case management or advocacy is needed. However, when the child is twenty-two and school services cease, families are faced with deciding what to do next, and this usually involves obtaining job training, supported or sheltered job placement, supervised group living settings, or, for individuals who are lower functioning, a day treatment setting where there is a safe environment and recreational opportunities. Most states have departments of vocational training and/or rehabilitation that assess handicapped individuals to help identify potential job skills. After a vocational assessment and vocational recommendations are made, developmental service agencies are usually key in identifying and funding placements where job experience or supervision can be obtained.

Job Coaching and Supported Employment. One type of job support for autistic people with relatively better skills (usually those autistic people with either no or only mild mental retardation) is some form of supported employment. This means working at a regular job site under the supervision of a job coach, who may either be an individual who works exclusively as a job coach, or is a specially trained supervisor from the place of employment. Some job coaching is funded by developmental services agencies, but in some cases particular employers will agree to provide extra training and oversight in exchange for giving a reduced salary (or no salary) to the autistic worker—depending on how many hours he can work and how much he can do independently.

Sheltered Workshops. Some individuals with autism or PDD need more on-the-job supervision, or have interfering behaviors that make it quite difficult to work at a regular job site. For individuals with PDD in particular, the difficulty may not be in teaching a useful job skill, but in getting the individual to exercise those skills later on, whenever asked. Even if the task itself may not be all that difficult for an autistic person to carry out, there needs to be a special structure in place to teach the skill initially, and later, a way of motivating the autistic individual to continue doing his task once he has learned it. Some individuals first need to acquire job skills in the context of a sheltered workshop, in the same way they may need a contained special education environment for instruction. Then, they can later take what they have learned and generalize it to work in a "mainstreamed" job.

Some autistic people who have a lower level of cognitive functioning remain indefinitely in sheltered workshops, which for them may be the "least restrictive" environment they can function in adaptively as a worker. In sheltered workshops, individuals do contract work that has been arranged by the workshop staff. I have visited workshops where seat belts are being assembled, maps folded, keys boxed, Twinkies shrink-wrapped, and medical equipment components sorted. Unlike a regular job site where the same kind of jobs may be done, there are many more supervisors, a higher level of prompts to stay on task, and immediate rewards for doing so. The level of output from a sheltered workshop is lower, but the pay is structured accordingly. Workshop workers are paid less (in order to pay their supervisors), and contractors tend to get a similar better deal on the work done than if they had hired non-handicapped workers. Most workshop programs that serve autistic people also serve others with comparable degrees of developmental disabilities, which may also help the autistic person to develop a peer network of friends at the same chronological and developmental level. In Chapter 13, alternatives for beyond the school years will be discussed in greater detail.

Day Treatment. A smaller number of autistic people are so severely handicapped that they really can't function in a sheltered workshop setting. These include autistic people who are severely to profoundly retarded, or who have severely maladaptive behaviors such as self-injurious behaviors that must be closely monitored, or who are medically fragile—such as those with poorly controlled seizure disorders. Mostly, such individuals are placed in residential facilities (see Chapter 13), or attend day treatment programs. Day treatment programs are also controlled by developmental services agencies. In day treatment, the goals include improvement of self-care and other adaptive behaviors, improving ability to function as part of a group, and leisure behaviors. Families that opt for day treatment may do so to give caregivers some respite during the day, or simply to provide a more varied environment for their autistic family member to practice his skills in.

Residential Placement. Perhaps the most difficult question that parents of autistic children ever have to ask themselves (and answer) is whether the child would be better served in some sort of residential placement. This issue was discussed in Chapter 7, and will be discussed somewhat more in Chapter 13. The point to be made here is that developmental services agencies, along with various other agencies, pay for part of the residential placement, and the autistic child or young adult's case manager usually orchestrates the process. Residential placement is virtually always at the discretion of parents. The only exception to voluntary placement is made when the parent can be shown to be psychologically unfit or physically unable to care for the child adequately, and cannot find a family member who will care for the child instead.

Case management is invaluable in planning residential placement: The maze of agencies and funding sources that may be involved given the child's legal status (such as being a minor, or a ward of the court, or a conserved or unconserved adult); as well as medical status (presence of concomitant physical handicaps), level of cognitive and adaptive functioning, and family finances is a bureaucratic morass of constantly changing rules and priorities that vary by locale and according to how overburdened the existing resources already are.

Where Developmental Service Agencies Leave Off. Developmental services agencies or regional centers provide one layer of support needed by parents with an autistic child. For many families, these agencies are most helpful before and after the child is school-aged. The main treatment milieu for most children between the ages of three and twenty-two who have autism or PDD is the educational system.

Eligibility for Special Education Services

Children are eligible for special education services if they have received a diagnosis of autism or mental retardation, or have significant delays in certain areas of development, particularly language development. Usually a child with a delay in one area of development that places him fifty percent behind peers, or delays in two areas of development of at least twenty-five percent each, is considered eligible for special education. So, for example, a thirty-six-month-old autistic child with an overall "communication" age of fourteen months is eligible for special education. Similarly, a four-year-old autistic child at a three-year level in expressive language, and adaptive functioning at that level too, would also be eligible for services. Different states implement these general guidelines somewhat differently. As a parent, it's important to find out what kind of criteria and cutoffs will be used to determine your child's access to services at different levels of intensity.

Federally Guaranteed Rights to Special Education

The first thing that all parents need to know about special education is that you are entitled to special education for your child *free of charge* no matter how young your child is. This includes infant stimulation programs discussed earlier in this chapter (and also covered in Chapter 9). Universal special education was mandated in the United States in 1977 by an act of Congress known as Public Law (PL) 94-142. Before PL 94-142, some handicapped children were simply not offered an education at all. More recently, PL 94-142 has been supplemented by PL 99-457, guaranteeing special education services to handicapped infants from birth to three years old. PL 94-142 has, in fact, been itself recently revised and supplanted by PL 101-476, known as IDEA (the Individuals with Disabilities Education Act). In addition, in 1990, the U.S. Congress approved the Americans with Disabilities Act, which guaranteed further rights to both developmentally and physically disabled persons.

Originally, PL 94-142 established the policy that every child was entitled to an education in the "least restrictive environment" ("LRE" in special education legalese) needed to remediate his or her disabilities yet provide opportunities for him or her to be a part of his or her larger community of peers. PL 94-142 also established that every child was entitled to an individually determined, *appropriate* program. "Appropriate" means that each child's program is individually tailored to provide remediation for that child's disabilities; goals and objectives for each child are formulated annually by teachers and assessment experts who review the child's level of achievement and set reasonable and specific goals for specific accomplishments the child can be expected to make by the time of next annual review.

As might be imagined, there are all sorts of ways of establishing what is "appropriate." It depends on whom you ask. Often, protracted battles over IEPs arise when parents obtain expert opinions saying their child needs one kind of education, and school system officials maintain that another (less intensive, less expensive) alternative is appropriate. While PL 94-142 does guarantee each special education child an *appropriate* education, it does not obligate the school to provide the *best* possible education for that child. As is the case with nonhandicapped students, parents are always free to seek a private school if they feel it will deliver a standard above the norm for the public schools, and that the extra quality is worth paying for. This whole situation presents several problems that will be discussed in the rest of this chapter.

Legal Issues and Rights Related to Obtaining Special Education

When a child becomes eligible for special education services, the parents basically enter into a contract with their school that assures both parties that there is agreement that an appropriate program will be delivered. This contract lists what the school intends to do to educate the child, and how it will be possible to determine later whether they have delivered the education they are promising. This contract is called an *Individual Education Plan,* or *IEP* as it is almost always called by school staff. The school is under certain obligations to make sure that parents understand what the IEP process is about, but many parents, at least at first, are so overwhelmed by having to put their child in special education that they just sit there, listen to the school district members of their child's IEP team, and at the conclusion of the IEP meeting, sign the IEP as requested. Probably because parents are accustomed to having no or few choices in determining what kind of public school education their non-handicapped children will receive, it does not occur to them that the rules are very different with a special education student. Most autistic children attend special day classes (SDC) which are provided in lieu of a regular education class, and in addition may receive other needed services separately (such as speech) or as part of the SDC program.

Costs of Special Education Programs

One of the dilemmas presented by the funding of special education is that it is an all-or-nothing game. Either you get what you want and the school district pays for all of it, or you can go off and choose a nonpublic school that you pay for entirely yourself. The fundamental problem is that special education costs a great deal more than education for a nonhandicapped student. Public school education for a nonhandicapped child costs between about $3,500 and $5,000 per pupil per year. Special education tends to cost at least double that, and special education that entails schooling in very small groups, significant amounts of one-to-one instruction, or a residential component can run upward of $60,000 per pupil per year. When a child is assigned to nonpublic special education because there is no public alternative, the public school must pay the full cost. So far, there is no system of vouchers or sliding scale fees wherein parents can apply to their districts for the average "per pupil expenditure" for special education, and then apply it to a certified nonpublic school, and pay the balance themselves if they so choose. Actually, the individual school district does not itself pay the full cost of special education either. It receives a substantial reimbursement for the costs for each special education student through a complex formula that brings in state and federal monies. Nevertheless, most school districts resist having any money outside their district.

Some parents try to help construct a more intensive special education program for their child by offering to provide (free to the school district) a qualified one-to-one aide or other special therapist for their child who would work with the child in his public school special education program. Some school districts who really want to do a good job, but have their hands tied, agree to such financial arrangements. Other districts, fearing they'll somehow be sued by advocates representing parents who cannot afford such extra help, shy away. Other districts reluctantly agree to such schemes after multiple reassurances that the parent is bringing in an individual who is as professionally qualified as someone the school district would hire (if they had the funds).

When parents go into an IEP meeting to ask for certain features in their child's educational program, they can find themselves in a tough spot. If their child's school does not give them what they want, there are only two choices: to pay for a program themselves or to negotiate. For many young families who cannot even begin to face having to pay for a special education program themselves, there is no choice but to negotiate with the school. Needless to say, such families are hardly negotiating from a position of strength. And, as in any negotiations, if the opposite party sees you have no leverage, it has very little motivation to make concessions to you. The only leverage parents have is to know their legal rights and insist upon them, and let the school know that you will not agree to your child's IEP until you feel you are getting what the law promises you.

Professional Advocacy

Sometimes parents negotiate their child's IEP with the assistance of their child's case manager from the developmental disabilities agency (as already discussed), or with the help of an advocate or attorney who specializes in special education rights. Case managers frequently accompany parents to IEPs and can be a great resource to parents of younger children who have the least experience with the special education system. Most often, parents who seek outside advocacy do not bring in advocates or attorneys unless initial attempts to agree on an IEP have failed. Once parents "up the ante" by bringing in legal consultants, the school may do the same.

There definitely are benefits to having the school district see that you are serious about your child's education and will fight for what you feel he or she needs. School districts, without doubt, categorize such parents differently, and on average, such parents *do* get more—but not necessarily without a fight.

Defining an Appropriate Educational Program

So far, this discussion about IEPs and getting the appropriate special education has been in the abstract. How do you determine the content of the IEP? There are basically two ways. First, the school will make its own assessment of the child's disability using developmental, intelligence, and achievement tests of various sorts. Each school has tests that its school psychologists feel are most informative; mostly tests with national norms are used, and the results are reported along with observations about the child's behavior, including information about the child's general school-readiness, ability to attend, and cooperate. Many school psychologists have relatively little experience testing autistic and PDD children, who generally hate new experiences (like visiting the school psychologist's office), and such children tend not to be motivated by the school psychologist cajoling them to act like a "big boy" or "big girl" or to do a "good job." Such children often are initially classified by school districts as "untestable." In better school systems, the psychologist may also make home observations, observations of the child in his infant stimulation program, or extensively interview the parents about what the child can and can't do. In other school districts such children are simply started in classes for the severely handicapped (SH) or multiply handicapped (MH) (where they may or may not belong), and if they do better, they get moved to another class.

Even though some school districts do a very thorough job of assessment, it can be very helpful to get an additional outside opinion. Although the analogy of "the fox minding the henhouse" is too extreme to describe most in-house school system assessments, there is often an (economic) imperative, either explicit or implicit, not to recommend too many intensive services. In my own experience, a good school psychologist has an excellent sense of what kinds of services a student will benefit from, but knows that she or he is first of all an employee of a school district (that inevitably has finite resources) and must walk the line between what the student should have ideally, and what it seems most cost-effective to offer given the existing resources of that district.

"Appropriate" versus "Best" Education

By law, each school district must provide each special education student with an "appropriate" education; "appropriate" for that child's disability. The school district is not obligated to provide each child with the "best" education possible. As is the case with regular education students, parents have the right to pay for it themselves if they want the "best." However, by obtaining an outside evaluation of your child, you increase the chance that you can shift the threshold of an "appropriate" educational plan closer to the threshold for the "best" educational plan. There is a great deal of subjectivity as to where the threshold for "appropriate" and "best" lies. There *are* rules of the game for arguing where the line should be drawn: First, there is very little chance at getting a school district to support an intervention method that has not been proven valid in educational or psychological research. In years past, I've watched parents futilely struggle to get (what I call) the "Autism Cure of the Year" written into IEPs to no avail. "Cures" that have been the subject of a book on one child's recovery from autism, and/or featured on the "Donahue Show" do not fall within the purview of what the school districts have any legal obligation to pay for.

More problematic to the definition of "appropriate" educational programs are new therapies for autism that show very promising results but are very expensive. A prime example of this is the intensive one-on-one behavioral-cognitive therapy based on the research of Dr. Ivar Lovaas at UCLA. (This treatment approach will be discussed more in Chapter 9.) While some data on the efficacy of his approach have been published, there are fewer data on who are the best candidates for treatment, and how long a child should be maintained in the program. At issue is how and when a new standard of "appropriate" can be defined. How much better does a new educational program have to be than an old one to justify a redefinition of an "appropriate" level of services? Treatments like the curriculum model developed by Lovaas and his group basically require thirty-five hours per week of one-to-one education. When this treatment is highly effective, children receive significantly higher test scores than children receiving more traditional special education. Thus, it has been successfully argued that a new standard of "appropriate" is established. On the face of it, the clinical improvements have to be clear-cut for a new treatment to be considered more "appropriate": Obviously, talking in sentences is better than talking in single words; high compliance is better than low compliance; knowing your numbers, letters, and shapes is better than not knowing them; and playing appropriately, albeit concretely, with a toy truck is better than always turning it over to spin the wheels.

When parents take the route of choosing to "prove" the efficacy of a new educational treatment so that their school district will pay for it, they choose the hard road. These parents are to be admired for their altruism. If they succeed (usually after high legal fees, which the school has to pay if they prevail), they help establish new precedents for treatment of autistic children that may be used in subsequent, similar cases. It's not something every family can practically, psychologically, or financially risk to undertake, however.

The Best Use of Outside Assessment for Educational Planning. In acting as advocates for their child's education, most families find themselves taking a position between just signing the IEP without protest, on one extreme; and holding out through various rounds of negotiating, on the other. On both extremes, parents may be acting out of a lack of knowledge about what can reasonably be expected. A reasonable, and usually effective approach is to obtain outside evaluation periodically. One time that it is very important to get outside advice is when the child is about to have his or her *first* IEP. This helps parents become oriented to the IEP negotiation process and establishes with the school district that this family understands their rights and has solidly backed-up clinical recommendations for the program components they ask for.

Schools seldom take the point of view that "Mother or Father Knows Best," no matter how well-informed. Instead, schools are much more likely to be convinced by recommendations that come from a well-respected center or agency for developmental disabilities that school personnel know well. This can be especially frustrating to the well-educated, well-read parent who feels that he or she knows as much about his or her child's educational needs as any "expert" who sees the child for only a couple of hours.

Triennial IEP Reviews. IEPs are subject to triennial reviews: every third year the school undertakes more extensive formal assessment of the child to reassess how well things are going. This is also a good time to have an outside reassessment. Whenever there is significant disagreement about what the child needs, it is a good idea to get an outside opinion. Often parents seek such opinions if it seems that one or more years are passing without significant improvement (that is, without realistic goals on the IEP being met). Concrete examples of this would be if a three-year-old has still developed no communicative means by age five, if a six-year-old has made no progress on schedule training or toilet training in the course of a year, or if a child has failed to show a significant reduction in an interfering self-stimulatory behavior like collecting and staring at sticks despite a behavioral program supposedly implemented to extinguish it. If progress is not made, either the program for changing itself is faulty, or the program is not being executed appropriately.

Setting Goals and Objectives on the IEP: Reliability and Validity. Of course, all autistic and PDD children acquire new skills at different rates, depending on how fixed a particular behavior is, and what the child's cognitive capacity is. As we will see in Chapters 9 through 13, a diagnosis of autism or PDD alone is not enough to develop a treatment plan. This brings us to the point of how realistic goals and objectives are set. As defined on an IEP, a "goal" is a change in behavior, or acquisition of a skill that is desired, and an "objective" is how the attainment of the goal will be defined. For example, a "goal" may be to "increase compliance in group instruction settings," and the "objective" may be that "Christina will go to her seat at circle time by the third request, 75% of the time without physical prompting." The same goal may have been present in Christina's IEP the previous year, but the objective may have been that "Christina will comply with verbal and physical guidance to go to her seat 100% of the time without exhibiting noncompliant behavior." As a person who reads IEPs by the gross, the objectives themselves sometimes seem picayune and trivial. However, they *do* quantify a standard, and provide an objective measure of an agreed-upon goal. Sometimes however, one feels that such goals and objectives are *reliable* without being *valid:* It is easy enough to observe Christina at three consecutive circle times and count how many times she is asked to return to her seat, and how many times she does return to her seat, on the first, second, or third request. That is, the *objective* can be reliably measured. But how *valid* is the measure? What if the teachers just work on teaching Christina to go to circle time appropriately, but fail at the overall goal—to increase her compliance in other instructional settings? Further, how do we determine whether it was reasonable to expect that in one year Christina can go from needing to be led to her seat, to mostly being able to get to her seat and stay there herself with only a verbal prompt from a teacher who is at a distance? Does this mean we can expect Christina to do other things she is asked to do seventy-five percent of the time? Who determines how much she can be expected to learn? What are such judgments based upon?

Calibrating a Reasonable Rate of Progress. The goals and objectives set by the school district may not be realistic, and in fact may be rather arbitrary. Outside evaluations may give parents a better understanding of how much progress a child can be expected to make in one year. The clinician doing a psycho-educational assessment bases her or his judgment on several things. One, a child who has never received intervention previously will probably learn at a faster rate in the first year of treatment than in the previous year of no treatment. The rate of learning is partly determined by the child's apparent underlying level of mental retardation. For example, a moderately retarded child may accomplish developmentally about half as much in a year as an average child. A maladaptive behavior that is more frequent will be harder to get rid of than one that is less frequent. Learning to produce spoken language for the first time is more difficult if you do not yet babble than if you babble a great deal. There are many such guidelines that clinicians are aware of, based on clinical experience and research literature specific to different areas of the autistic or PDD child's development. This is one of the reasons it is so important to obtain evaluation for an autistic child from someone who is very familiar with autism and PDD. A language specialist, for example, with no real experience in autism may overestimate the rate of progress, and underestimate the concomitant disabilities of social development that interact to make language acquisition characteristically problematic for autistic and PDD children. For school evaluators, autistic and PDD children are usually only a small proportion of all the children they are asked to assess. Therefore it may be difficult for them to predict rate of growth and set reasonable goals and objectives.

If the child's IEP objectives are set too high, the child will be seen as a failure when he is really making satisfactory progress. If the objectives are set too low, the child may receive relatively less attention than he should in class because he will be seen as doing so well. Sometimes, especially with initial IEPs, well-meaning school personnel who are trying to ameliorate a parent's feelings of grief at finding that their child needs special education will set unrealistically high goals and objectives as a way of saying to the parent that the child is really going to improve a great deal. While a parent may be reassured by this sort of approach initially, after a couple of years during which the child has not yet met initial goals and objectives, the parent may come to feel the school is not delivering what was promised, or that the child is more severely impaired than they were originally told—neither of which is a pleasant thought (and neither of which is probably true). Therefore it is important that IEP goals and objectives be realistic. If the goals and objectives are reasonable and valid, there is then value in making sure that goals can be reliably, objectively assessed so that all parties can agree on whether or not the planned progress has been made.

Legal Advocacy

In the course of trying to obtain both educational and developmental services, parents sometimes feel unfairly denied access to help. Sometimes parents feel that they simply don't understand the process well and therefore are vulnerable to being taken advantage of. Some parents feel that just having formal representation at an IEP or other meeting to negotiate services tips the scales in their favor. In these cases, parents may hire an advocate or attorney to represent them and their child. Some parents who are represented this way immediately become adversarial (and some special education attorneys encourage this), which may or may not be helpful. Other families see an advocate as a consumer expert who can point out things you might not notice yourself— like taking a friend who has read every issue of *Popular Photography* with you when you go to buy a new camera.

Advocates versus Attorneys

Representatives who can work with you on obtaining developmental services are of two types. The first are *advocates*. Advocates are not attorneys, but people who specialize in knowing the regulations, procedures, and laws governing the operation of the developmental disabilities and special education systems. Some are veterans of these systems themselves—former teachers, administrators, case supervisors, and so on. They have inside knowledge of how the system works, and usually a good network of contacts inside the school or department of developmental services. The second type of representation comes from attorneys who specialize in issues relating to developmental disabilities. In a given geographic area there are usually only a handful of these, and they all will know (and usually respect) each other. Advocates tend to charge less than attorneys, and provide similar services. Attorneys are probably best used when the appeals process goes beyond the local or county level and is to be heard in some sort of state-level administrative hearing that follows courtroom rules of evidence and testimony. Attorneys and advocates who specialize in developmental disabilities issues can be found through a county or state bar association or through the state's department of developmental services.

Advocates tend to cost less per hour than attorneys, and for many families this is a decisive factor. (However, you should be aware that if you prevail, the public agency that loses will be liable to cover your legal or advocacy costs.) There are a variety of publicly and privately funded nonprofit agencies that offer special education advocacy on a sliding-scale fee basis. Such agencies may use both advocates and attorneys, depending on the issues. Some of these public law groups specialize in clients with developmental disorders, and some also represent mentally and/or physically disabled clients as well. With an autistic child, you may be best off if you can be represented by someone specializing in developmental disabilities or special education. Such a representative is more likely to have existing knowledge of the special educational needs of autistic children. If you do hire an advocate or attorney, it is essential that he or she either know (or be willing to learn) about autism in particular. I have worked with many sharp attorneys who specialize in disabilities; once they learn a little of the specifics of a particular case, it doesn't take long before they ask the right questions and pick up on the key substantive issues behind an appeal for services. A first-rate attorney who has never worked in the area of developmental disabilities before is probably not going to be as useful as someone who knows the special education "ropes."

Mediation and Fair Hearing

In negotiating services, parents contract with the developmental disabilities system through IPPs (Individual Program Plans), and with the educational system through IEPs. If parents alone, or parents plus their child's advocate, are not able to reach agreement on services to be received after a few IEP or IPP meetings, there is usually a call for *mediation*. Mediation is a (usually) nonbinding arbitration process wherein a mediator from an outside agency is brought in to hear both sides of the appeal for services in a semiformal way. The mediator is an expert in the regulations and laws governing developmental disabilities services and usually fairly well-apprised of what the standards of education or other services are. If mediation fails after one or more tries, the family and the agency go on to a state-level administrative *fair hearing*. The mediator at the mediation meeting really has two jobs: The first, of course, is to get the family and the agency to agree on services that the child is entitled to receive. The second function is to make recommendations that reflect the regulations and laws. The mediator's recommendations basically say "If you don't agree now, and decide to go to fair hearing, this is what the fair hearing officer will probably decide anyway." Both parents and schools and other agencies have a strong incentive to avoid fair hearings because of the legal costs and the time such proceedings take. Therefore, a good mediator who can foresee the result of a fair hearing is someone important to listen to. A mediator will make it clear in plain language if the family is asking for something that is beyond what other families get, or something for which there appears to be no proof of efficacy. The mediation process is more efficient than the fair hearing process. Fair hearings, like other state-level civil matters involve each side gathering evidence, perhaps ordering evaluations, and subpoenas for documents and witnesses to give testimony; also, compiling exhibits and lengthy transcribed testimony in which witnesses on each side are examined and cross-examined by opposing attorneys.

There are certainly situations in which the threat of having to go to fair hearing is intimidating to a school, and it will cut its losses and concede what the parent wants, especially if what is requested is somewhere in that gray area between "appropriate" and "best." School districts will most often hold their ground and go to fair hearing if they feel either that what the parent wants is really nonmainstream, or, more often, that the parent is trying to set a precedent that will open the floodgates to other families with similarly disabled children wanting the same services.

Fair hearings must begin within ninety days of being requested. However, many are held over, and decisions may take months to come down. What must always be weighed before going to fair hearing is whether the process critically delays the child getting needed help. Sometimes parents go ahead and pay for additional (requested) services in the meantime, knowing they will be paid back by the agency if they prevail. As the adversarial process accelerates, it can sometimes be difficult for parents if they may begin to realize that a program for which they have fought so long and hard may not be working as well as hoped. On the other hand, sometimes having the child in the desired program for a while may demonstrate that the program really does work better than what the child had before. Such evidence may allow the parents to make a stronger case than they would have been able to before the intervention started.

When Do Parents Go to Fair Hearing? Most often, when parents contemplate going to fair hearing with a developmental disabilities agency, it is because the agency refuses to rule their child eligible for services. This is most common with older and/or higher functioning autistic children who have received many conflicting diagnoses. In particular, parents may find it hard to obtain developmental services for a higher functioning autistic child who has previously been erroneously labeled as "severely emotionally disturbed" or psychotic, because many developmental disabilities agencies try to steer these children in the direction of the mental health agencies.

Within the school system, parents of autistic and PDD children most often run into trouble negotiating IEPs when the need for a nonpublic school placement or one-to-one instruction comes up. (In Chapter 10 we will discuss criteria for deciding on a nonpublic school, and on amounts of one-to-one instruction.) A school is more likely to eventually agree to one-on-one instruction if the IEP team members feel it is for a finite period of time, or that the child is going to be very disruptive without it, *or* that the parents will take them to fair hearing if one-to-one instruction isn't agreed upon.

I remember one very cute little three-year-old boy with PDD, Marc (who collected any and all sticks of the right size), whom I first saw just as his parents, both attorneys, were about to negotiate his first IEP. Marc's dad, a litigator, spent much of the four-hour initial evaluation pacing our playroom in his three-piece suit. His eyes really lit up when I read him the riot act about how he must be tough with his school district (actually a very good school district), and that he should let his school district know that he would not sign his son's IEP until it was right. For days after Marc's assessment, I received Fed-Exs and faxes from Marc's parents (do lawyers know of other ways to communicate?) Before I knew it, much to my delight, Marc was headed into an excellent nonpublic school—funded by his district. Most conflicts over IEPs don't resolve this readily, but if parents show temerity, and a knowledge of their rights, it certainly helps.

Eligibility for Services through Medical Insurance

In addition to receiving services through the developmental services agencies and the schools, a child who is diagnosed with autism, PDD, mental retardation, or severe language disorder may be eligible for services provided by medical insurance carriers, such as speech therapy and even, in some cases, physical therapy. Unfortunately, medical insurance is usually subject to fairly strict limitations with respect to what therapies will be covered and for how long. In the United States, the current medical insurance picture for autistic children may change if and when universal coverage is introduced. At least, it will probably guarantee that autistic children cannot be excluded from their family's policy for a "pre-existing condition" if the family changes insurance carriers. However, it is still unknown whether a national health plan would cover any developmental services or whether it would simply provide for the non-developmental disability–related needs of an autistic child.

Currently, many medical insurance policies specifically exclude treatments for developmental disorders. In the past, some insurers would cover what they considered a *physical* disorder such as mental retardation or epilepsy, but would not pay for the same services (for example, speech therapy) for autistic children because they still considered autism an *emotional* disorder (without a medical cause). At least one case has been argued to the level of the U.S. Supreme Court on this matter; the Supreme Court ruled that autism *was* a physical, medical disorder and should be covered as such. The result of "proving" that autism is a neurophysiological disorder through litigation, sadly, has not been more medical coverage of services for autistic children, but rather new wording in insurance policies that specifically excludes autism as a qualifying condition for services. What this means is that autistic children are still eligible to be covered for medical problems that *all* children are subject to (for example, care for ear infections, pneumonia, and broken legs), but often are not covered for services they need because of their autism or mental retardation. The rationale is that autism and mental retardation are chronic conditions, and that the insurance only covers "curable" illnesses.

The one major exception to lack of medical insurance for the treatment of autism is that some carriers will fund initial evaluations to determine if the condition that exists *is* a chronic one—so they can stop covering help for it! Therefore carriers often will cover fairly extensive initial workups including full genetic, metabolic, and neurological studies to rule out that there is anything that can be "cured" surgically or pharmacologically. If developmental evaluations of your autistic or PDD child have been made and your insurance carrier has refused to pay for them because you saw a psychiatrist or psychologist for the diagnosis (that is, they think the child was being assessed for mental illness), you can ask your care provider to write a letter to the insurance company explaining that autism is a neuropsychiatric disorder with physical causes, and that the child was not being evaluated for an emotional disorder. In the best cases, medical insurance will cover weekly speech therapy, or sensorimotor integration therapy—but not the costs of services that might be more exclusively construed as special education.

Books about Autism

There are a variety of books written about autism, autistic children, and developmental disabilities. Some clinicians dispute the usefulness or dangers of "bibliotherapy"—that is, getting help with a problem through written material. My own point of view is that there really *is* a place for self-help books on developmental disorders and autism—both to get information and to explore one's own feelings and reactions to facing the stresses of raising a child with a disability. Books can be of incredible supportive value, especially at that stage where concerns and anxieties are formed, but specific questions are not.

Obviously, books on autism cannot take the place of an evaluation by a clinician who is really experienced with autistic children. The complaint I hear most often from parents about books they have read on autism is that some of what they learn fits their child to a tee, and some of the information is way off base. Because autism is a syndrome, not every affected individual has all the symptoms (as I explained at the beginning of this book). Severity varies, too. So, as parents read, they may encounter information that is untrue with respect to their child (for example, about a symptom that is more closely related to mental retardation than to autism), or not get the whole picture of how *their* child's autism is different from what is seen in most children.

General Information Books on Autism

With those caveats in mind, there certainly *are* things parents can profitably read about autism. Some books, like this one, are designed to help you understand what autism is, and what you can do about it. Some are written for the parent who wants a great deal of detail and explanation; other books are better for the parents who just want the basic facts in a plainspoken way, or for relatives or friends who want to learn more, but don't have the same driving interest as parents of autistic children to know all there is to know. Here is a list of some good general books on autism:

1. *Autism: A Guide for Parents and Professionals* (1972) by Lorna Wing. This is a clear, concise book by one of the real world experts on autism. It's a frontline book for parents grappling with autism. Dr. Wing is also the author of a shorter volume published by the Autism Society of America entitled *Children Apart* (1974), which provides a briefer overview of the same information.
2. *Autism: Understanding the Enigma* (1990) by Uta Frith. This is an interesting, erudite volume that includes historical speculation about how autism has been viewed in the past, as well as insight from modern-day experiments involving autistic children that are helping us understand how they think.
3. *Autism* (1988) by Laura Schriebman. This is a fairly detailed description of autism that is either for the very information-hungry parent, or for teachers and other professionals who already have some grounding in developmental disabilities.
4. *Children With Autism* (1989), edited by Michael Powers. This is a resource book with chapters by different authors on various topics including diagnosis, treatment, and special education services. It's a good book to pick and choose from because each chapter is self-contained.

Treatment-Oriented Books on Autism

Other books are more purely treatment-oriented, some dealing with specific behavior problems or stages of development in autistic children—from toilet-training to vocational training. There is related literature that deals with specific issues such as special education planning or setting up conservatorships or trusts for older children. In this category, the book that I recommend most often is

1. *The Me Book: Teaching Developmentally Disabled Children* by O. Ivar Lovaas. It's a hands-on behavioral guide to getting your autistic child to dress himself, eat properly, not scream whenever he wants something, toilet-training, and so on. For some parents, reading this book is the best place to start. As far as their child's bad behavior goes, some parents adopt the attitude that if they *can* fix it, they don't really need to know why it's broken.
    Also helpful are . . .
2. *How to Teach Autistic and Severely Handicapped Children* (1981) by Robert Koegel and Laura Schriebman. Like the Lovaas book, this explains techniques of behavioral training for autistic children. It's a bit more technical than the Lovaas book and, like Laura Schriebman's other book, is one that is probably most widely read by teachers and behavioral trainers.
3. *Negotiating the Special Education Maze* (1990) by Winifred Anderson, Stephen Chitwood, and Deidre Hayden. This is a good book for parents embroiled in special education disputes.

4. *Disability and the Family* (1989) by H. Rutherford and Ann Turnbull, G. J. Bronicki, Jean Ann Summers, and Constance Roeder-Gordon. This is a place to get up to speed on issues related to wills, trusts, and conservatorships. If you read this before seeing an attorney, you won't need to spend $150 to $250 an hour being educated about the baseline information in this book.

Special Interest Areas of Autism

Others books on autism describe a subset of autistic and PDD children, such as those dealing with a particular variant of autism like Asperger's syndrome, or the special issues of adolescence in autistic teenagers, or books on siblings of autistic children.

1. *Autism and Asperger's Syndrome* (1991), edited by Uta Frith. This book is the best source of information about Asperger's syndrome—even though the book is a bit more scientifically oriented than ones parents might usually read. Like other multi-author books, it's easy to pick and choose from among freestanding chapters—some are of more interest to parents, some to professionals.
2. *Autism in Adolescence and Young Adults* (1983), edited by Eric Schopler and Gary Mesibov. This is a technical but very good survey of the issues faced by autistic people as they grow up. It is primarily written by and for professionals, but also fills a gap in the available literature for parents and providers involved in day-to-day treatment of adults with autism.
3. *What About Me? Siblings of Developmentally Disabled Children* (1994) by Bryna Siegel and Stuart Silverstein. This book (to which I have to admit a certain partiality), is primarily directed to adult siblings and parents (and their therapists) and addresses the problems faced by families of autistic and PDD children, and characteristic ways that siblings learn to cope.
4. *Brothers and Sisters: A Special Part of Exceptional Families* (1985) by Thomas Powell and Peggy Arenhold Ogle. This book details research on siblings, the effects of having a disabled sibling, and reaffirms *their* role in their families. It is a thoughtful resource for both parents and professionals.

First-Person Accounts

This category of books on autism includes descriptions of particular treatments and the psychological growth and development of autistic individuals. I have mixed reactions to some of these books because some are testimonials to a "miracle" cure of some sort. To me, the worst travesty you can foist on parents of autistic children is to get them to believe that the only thing that stands in the way of their child being "normal" is their own willingness to lock themselves into a bathroom and imitate their child's every movement for 72 hours, or to hold the child immobilized and scream to them to come out because he is loved. These books, as far as I can tell, attempt to fulfill the wish that the incredibly bad odds that produced an autistic child in the first place can somehow be counterbalanced by equally unlikely odds that a complete cure will take place. Some of the books of this kind that have formed the philosophical basis for nonmainstream therapies for autism will be discussed more in Chapter 15.

Below are some of the books of this category that are the most informative and insightful without being promotional materials for miracle cures. The books that are first-person accounts can be quite insightful as to explanations of autistic symptoms particularly for higher functioning adults with PDD or Asperger's syndrome.

1. *The Siege* by Clara Claiborne Park (1982). This is the story of a mother learning how to cope and get through to her autistic daughter, as well as a look back on her experiences after her daughter's early years.
2. *Emergence: Labeled Autistic* (1986) by Temple Grandin (co-written by Margaret Scariano) is an autobiographical book about an intelligent person who continues to deal with her PDD "personality." Anyone who has met Temple Grandin is unlikely to question her diagnosis, but one does wonder how much of the book was put together by the co-writer (and therefore how accurate a view it really gives us into the autistic world).
3. *Nobody Nowhere* (1992) by Donna Williams is also an autobiography, one completely in the author's own voice. As I read this, I could not decide whether the author's main disability was actually autism or PDD, but some descriptions of experiencing autistic symptoms ring very true.
4. *Let Me Hear Your Voice* (1993) by Catherine Maurice is one parent's story of using the intensive type of intervention approach that will be described in Chapter 9. This mother tells how she successfully helped her first child deal with autism, and then found herself confronted with the same challenge again when her second child was diagnosed autistic.
5. *Family Pictures* (1990) by Sue Miller is a novel, but one that tells a very realistic story of a family with an autistic boy, and how his development affects every family member. (The book is a wonderful substitute for going to Autism Society support group meetings, since support groups are not everyone's cup of tea.)

Research on Autism

There is the whole body of research literature on autism, full of jargon and codes and innuendo that is difficult for even a well-educated professional to fully comprehend. Generally, I don't recommend that parents, even parents who are teachers, psychologists, or physicians, try to get into the research literature. It is a piece-by-piece accretion of knowledge that does not always directly or even vaguely relate to treatment, or even to understanding a puzzling or problem behavior that an autistic child shows. If as a parent you feel you *must* make a foray into this literature, you are probably best off to start with some of the major research compilations. These are books that would be found in a university or medical school library. Here are some suggestions:

1. *The Handbook of Autism and Pervasive Developmental Disorders* (2d edition) (1995) edited by Fred Volkmar and Donald Cohen.
2. *Autism: Nature, Diagnosis and Treatment* (1989), edited by Geraldine Dawson.
3. Any of the series on autism edited by Eric Schopler and Gary Mesibov including *The Effects of Autism on the Family, Communication Problems in Autism, Social Problems in Autism, Neurobiological Issues in Autism*, and *Diagnosis and Assessment in Autism.*

Most of these books, plus others, can be special-ordered through a local bookstore or ordered through the Autism Society of America, which distributes a mailing list for a "by mail" bookstore that is run by the Autism Society of North Carolina, 3300 Woman's Club Drive, Raleigh, NC 27612–4811, (919) 571-8555.

Books provide a kind of private support, something you can read and reread selectively at your own pace. Emotionally, there are always times when we are more able to hear some things and not others. Books on autism provide a resource that can be returned to as new issues or new understanding of issues arise or as an autistic child changes and matures. Another, more active form of support is through contact with other parents experiencing similar difficulties.

The Autism Society of America and Other Parent Support Groups

For many parents, belonging to an organization that understands what your experience with your autistic child is all about is essential. Other parents couldn't imagine anything they would like to do less. Having suggested parent support groups to many families and gotten reactions ranging from anticipation and relief to looks of horror, it's possible to begin to realize who benefits most from such activity.

Who Benefits from Support Groups?

Most American families respond well and feel they benefit from autism and developmental disabilities support groups. These families like the idea that they can go to a picnic with other families with autistic children and not have to be embarrassed if their autistic child doesn't respond to an adult who speaks to them, or if their child flaps his arms in delight after going down the slide, or if their sixteen-year-old son wants to ride the merry-go-round for twenty minutes without getting off. For parents of newly diagnosed younger autistic children, support groups help parents develop an understanding of how their autistic child is like other autistic children. Just to hear that someone else faces life with a child who wakes up every two hours for a half an hour twice a night, is helpful. One can feel a little less alone with the extraordinary stress of raising a handicapped child. It can be good to go to a support group function and learn that parents of other autistic children are not autistic too, but businessmen, professionals, or whatever—nice intelligent people like oneself.

As parents who attend support group functions informally network with one another they gain practical knowledge that is not available elsewhere. Parents learn about particular teachers in their school system, and how satisfied other parents of autistic children were with her teaching in previous years. They learn about doctors to avoid and doctors to seek out. Parents get tips from one another about where to buy child proof latches for their refrigerators and toilets. The learn about barbers, and babysitters who can handle autistic children. They learn about dentists who don't throw you out of their office when the autistic child bites.

The most educated or economically well-off families (probably those with the most personal experience with individual psychotherapy), on average, seem to participate less in parent support groups. For some parents, their child's autism may be, at least in part, a personal emotional event that they need to deal with in the context of one-to-one therapy before they feel they can really be effective in helping the child.

Support through Parent Pairing

As was mentioned in Chapter 7, we sometimes pair up families who come to our clinic with demographically similar couples. (We always obtain mutual consents before releasing anyone's name.) Usually we try to match parents of slightly older and younger children. It is hoped that the parent of the older child can gain a sense of altruistic helpfulness by what she or he passes on, and that the parents of the younger child learn the ropes of parenting an autistic child. Also, because autistic children can be so different from one another, it can be helpful to meet another parent whose child has similar symptoms (say, pairing a mother whose son is obsessed with fans with a mother whose son is obsessed with electrical extension cords). Every now and then I manage to pair parents who become fast friends, as well as mutual supports because of their autistic children.

The Autism Society of America

The main American support organization for families with autistic children is the Autism Society of America (ASA). (This group was formerly known as the National Society for Autistic Children, or NSAC.) It was founded in 1965 by Dr. Bernard Rimland, a pioneer in searching for the biological origins of autism, and himself the father of a (now adult) autistic son. The ASA has about 11,000 members of whom about eighty percent are parents, and twenty percent are professionals or agencies. Other families belong to, or participate in activities of, their local and state chapters but may not take part in activities related to national ASA membership. ASA has its national headquarters in Silver Springs, Maryland, from which it conducts policy and lobbying activities to legislate better services for autistic children and adults. They can be reached by mail or phone at 8601 Georgia Avenue, Suite 503, Silver Springs, Maryland 20910, 301-565-0433.

The national office of ASA coordinates several activities: One is the annual national ASA meeting, usually equally attended by parents and professionals working directly with autistic children—teachers, speech and language therapists, infant stimulators, and others. The meetings span a long weekend each summer and rotate across the country. Speakers cover a variety of topics, from parents who describe individual success stories, to panels of family members and high functioning autistics describing personal experiences, to teachers talking about particular methods to achieve specific skills, to researchers describing advances in understanding the behavior of autistic children, to molecular biologists giving summaries of studies on the cutting edge of the neuropathology of autism. Parents who attend these meetings tend to be very involved with their local ASA chapters and serve as reporters to those back at home who are interested to hear what is being learned.

The ASA also maintains a mail order bookstore (actually run by the North Carolina State Chapter—see above) that stocks many of the books described earlier, as well as abstracts from presentations at each year's national meeting. The national office of ASA also publishes a quarterly newsletter, *The Advocate*, which contains a similar mix of personal and research updates as found at the annual meetings. A subscription to *The Advocate* is included in national ASA membership.

All states have a statewide chapter of ASA, and within each state are regional and local groups. In many states there are separate annual meetings, usually for one day, with a similar mix of speakers as are at the national meetings. The statewide meetings tend to focus more on local resources, with some spice coming from purveyors of the most recent exciting scientific finding or grassroots story on autism making the rounds of the state meetings. These meetings provide more information on local resources to families than the national meetings, and so provide an opportunity for numerous families to learn firsthand about new ideas for working with autistic children. It can also be a way of learning about great autism treatment resources in your own locale that you simply hadn't heard about, or had wondered about, but had no firm knowledge of.

Local chapters of the ASA encompass families from more limited geographical areas, and are the smallest, most grassroots unit of support. Families may meet monthly at someone's home, a local restaurant, or at a church. Sometimes there is a set agenda, sometimes the gathering is more for social/networking purposes. Sometimes, local groups split into parents of younger and older children, or parents of children in a particular school or residential care facility, or parents from a particular language or cultural group. If you are interested in joining a chapter, a doctor who evaluates autistic children or a

DDS caseworker can probably provide a local contact person. The national ASA office requires ten people to start an official chapter; more information about this can be obtained from the national ASA office at the address above.

Autism Societies Outside the United States

England has a large and active autism society with local chapters in many counties. Their main office can be reached by writing to The National Autistic Society, 276 Willesden Lane, London NW2 5RB England, or telephoning 01-451-1114. There are also additional autism societies in Ireland and Scotland. Canada also has an active autism society (which sometimes has joint annual meetings with the ASA). The address and telephone number for the national office for the Autism Society of Canada is 129 Yorkville Ave., Suite 202, Toronto, Ontario M5R 1C4 Canada, telephone: 416-922-0302. The Autism Society of Canada has chapters in most provinces, even most of the vary sparsely populated ones. Other English-speaking countries with autism societies include Australia (with chapters in most states), New Zealand, and South Africa. Western European countries that have autism societies include Austria, Belgium, Finland, Denmark, France, Germany, Italy, Luxembourg, Portugal, Spain, Switzerland, Norway, Sweden, and the Netherlands. Eastern European countries that have autism societies include the Czech Republic, Estonia, and Hungary. Middle Eastern countries with autism societies include Israel and Turkey; Far Eastern countries with autism societies include Thailand, Hong Kong, Japan, and Taiwan. South American countries with autism societies include Argentina, Brazil, Chile, Mexico, Peru, Uraguay, and Venezuela; in the West Indies, Trinidad and Tobago. The ASA also has some Spanish-language materials available for parents. The addresses of autism societies in the countries named above can be obtained from the Autism Society of America, or from doctors and hospitals in those countries.

Other Parent Support Groups

In some areas, there are just not enough people or enough interest to get an ASA chapter going. In these locales there may be support groups for parents of developmentally disabled children run through Easter Seals, the local branch of the state developmental disabilities agency, or a special education program. There are also nonprofit organizations like Easter Seals, March of Dimes, and the Association for Retarded Citizens that operate on similar lines as the ASA but provide support to families with children with a wide range of disabilities. For parents of autistic children, these groups may or may not be as helpful as an ASA chapter. Obviously, if you are interested in participating in a support group and there's no ASA group around, joining a more general developmental disabilities support group makes sense. Such generic groups can be particularly helpful if they focus exclusively on children under three and your child is under three, or on children in residential placement and your child is in residential placement, and so on. The main drawback to being part of a group that serves families with children with a range of disabilities is that it is likely to contain parents who may mainly focus on the physical handicaps or medical fragility of their children, or who have children who are very social and mainly mentally retarded. It can be difficult (and maybe even frightening) for these other parents to relate to your main issues as the parent of an autistic child (and vice versa).

Support organizations help many people, and for a few, become a major organizing feature of their lives. But there are some families who will never be comfortable sharing their distress in public. For these families, support from within the extended family, and the parents' support for one another, may be key factors instead of support groups.

Chapter Summary

In this chapter, we've discussed what kind of help is out there for your child and for you. It is no easy matter to negotiate the developmental disabilities and special education system—especially at first, when you are just getting used to the idea that your child has a disability. Over time, as parents gain knowledge, and see what does and does not work for their individual child, they definitely become their child's most important resource. While you may need to enlist help from doctors, therapists, teachers, advocates, and lawyers to play the "getting services" game, *you*, as the parent, are the chief executive officer. Professionals can give you ideas, but you will be the one seeing the bigger picture of how all your child's services fit together—and know how much these services help in living with your child day-to-day. Unfortunately, services for disabled children are chronically underfunded, and unless you take an active role, you will almost certainly get less rather than more.

Autism is a fairly rare disorder, as we've discussed, and you'll encounter many people with plenty of misinformation, or complete lack of information, about autism. Your job will be to educate these people while finding a way of educating your child.

CHAPTER 9

◆ ◆ ◆

The Importance of
Very Early Intervention

"The Sooner the Better" Philosophy

Initiating Early Intervention

There are many reasons why early intervention—the sooner the better—is important for children with autism and PDD. Many of the reasons seem intuitively obvious to parents, but often parents encounter a "cart driving the horse" mentality from professionals unfamiliar with the treatment of young autistic and PDD children. For example, some parents are told that an early diagnosis doesn't matter because the child can't go to school until he's five, anyway (which is untrue)—or until he's three (which is also untrue). As we discussed in Chapter 8, there is now a federal law in the United States that mandates developmental services for any child identified as having a developmental disability from birth onward. While primary care providers offer somewhat less of this "wait and see" attitude these days, many remain unaware that there are treatment resources out there. Some who are aware of treatment resources for very young children may have only a partial knowledge of whom such services are for. Only a very few primary care providers have much of a sense of the efficacy of very early interventions for autistic and PDD children. Among these are pediatricians who have taken special training in dealing with children with developmental difficulties and are usually called "developmental" or "behavioral" pediatricians. Seeking out such a developmental or behavioral pediatrician is a good idea if you want regular pediatric care from someone who can also appreciate and help with the difficulties of raising a child who needs extra help.

Pediatricians as Gatekeepers to Early Intervention

The "if it doesn't go away on its own, then we'll think about fixing it" philosophy offerd by pediatricians who have not had training in developmental disor-

196

ders assumes that fixing something that has been "broken" for a while is just as easy as fixing something where problems have just started to appear. What we know about neurodevelopment, as we will see, just doesn't support that point of view. In fairness to pediatricians, the wait-and-see attitude stems from the difficulty in distinguishing the persistent complaints of anxious parents who have normally developing children from the persistent complaints of anxious parents who have atypically developing children. All pediatricians providing primary care see many more of the former. If the pediatrician's own sample of the child's behavior is limited to three minutes spent with a screaming, half-naked child who is sitting on an examining table with an otoscope in one ear, it is easy to see why all toddlers look pretty much the same despite what parents may say.

The Need for Early Intervention Research

The first thing that needs to be made clear when talking about early interventions for autistic and PDD children is that there is still far too little treatment research. What we know about the possible advantages of early treatment comes from child development theory, studies of adult recovery from brain injury, clinical experience, and a small number of scientific studies on young autistic children. There is a lack of hard facts about early treatment of autistic children for two reasons: First, the "big" research money goes to studies of the basic neurology and genetics of autism. This research is essential if we are ever going to *prevent* autism, but yields almost no implications for treatment with the exception of the occasional contribution to psychopharmacology. Second, it has been very difficult to study early intervention for autism because of the lack of well-defined, well-diagnosed groups of very young autistic children. It is generally recognized that autism does not look exactly the same in an eighteen-month-old as in a five-year-old, just as normal eighteen-month-olds and normal five-year-olds resemble one another very little! Early treatment research cannot begin until everyone agrees on who the subjects of such treatment would be. In some of the first studies of treatment for young autistic children, critics claimed that those who improved the most weren't autistic to begin with. So until there is an agreed-on standard for early diagnosis of autism, it will be hard for most professionals to believe the results of early intervention research done of "autistic" children.

Support for Early Intervention from Theories of Neuropsychology

What is currently understood about the treatment of young autistic children comes mainly from our general understanding of how autistic children differ from non-autistic children in the ways they are able (and unable) to learn. There is still not a great deal of research on exactly how early interventions work neurophysiologically, nor on the relative benefits of programs that more strongly emphasize different things like language, social skills development, or behavioral management. But from the wider literature on other developmentally disabled children who are not autistic, it *is* clearly established that earlier is better.

Our understanding of the benefits of early intervention, neuropsychologically, come from what is known from working with adult patients who have had a stroke or traumatic injury to a particular part of their brains. It is understood that in the adult brain, specific cognitions (specific kinds of information) can be localized (found) in certain physical regions. After a stroke or injury like a gunshot wound to a particular region, a specific ability or type of memory may be lost. Generally, the earlier and more intensively rehabilitation is begun, the less permanent loss there is. The brain has the capacity for "reduplication of function" or "transferability," allowing information or sensory ability to come from an area in the brain not usually used for that purpose.

The Neurological Basis of Developing Skills

We know that most brain growth and development occurs in the first five to six years of life. After that, major brain structures are in place, and they are, hypothetically, ready to begin to carry out their various functions. A newborn baby's brain is like a well-mapped geographic area but one that has no roads, or even pathways or dwellings. As specific kinds of information are stored, the landscape develops features of human habitation—"pathways," "storehouses," and things that are stored in the storehouses. Pathways to each storehouse open up as more and more information is fed in. In a very young autistic or PDD child there can be problems in the building of either the pathways or the storehouses. Through extra stimulation—*compensatory stimulation* in special education jargon—new storehouses and pathways can be built so that the pathways don't "erode," and so that the storehouses are constructed securely. Then, information can be stored in an organized way.

Another analogy for understanding early brain development and the effects of early intervention is to think of how a computer might function with a permanent "glitch." Around birth, the brain is like a computer with a big hard disk that has some software, but for which few files or applications have yet been written. If there is a problem with a particular software package—say a spreadsheet program that multiplies wrong fifty percent of the time, you might want to use the built-in calculator in your word processor to verify multiplication results. Of course, this would be awkward, and could take lots of extra time every time you had to multiply something. Assuming you were on a desert island with no mail delivery and couldn't get a new copy of the spreadsheet program, the next best thing would be to have the help of an expert computer programmer who could write a little program that modified your spreadsheet software and directed it to use the calculator on the word processor program whenever multiplication was needed. A real wizard programmer might be able to write an efficient little program that would make the rerouting almost invisible to you. A more average programmer also might be able to accomplish the same thing, but maybe the whole program would slow down for a few extra seconds each time it multiplied. If you had no programmer to help you reroute around the difficulty, you, as the computer user, would probably come to hate using the computer more and more over time because of the faulty results it so often produced, or because you had to go through many extra steps by hand just to get the answer to something that should have been simple to figure out.

Early intervention for developmental disabilities operates basically on the same pattern. The longer the wait until a "programmer" (early intervention specialist) shows up, the longer the "computer user" (the child) flounders with "flawed software" (the cognitive disability), and the more the child comes to dislike any activity that requires the use of a disabled function (in the example, the "multiplication"). Another problem that can occur is that the child may do some natural reprogramming of his own, and since he is no computer wizard (but just a little kid), he is likely to come up with an adaptation to his disability that only partly solves the problem (like echoing what has been said when the meaning isn't clear). So, the idea of early intervention is to reroute around non-working areas of the brain where specific functions are usually seated, and instead think of clever ways of getting other parts of the brain to function in lieu of the original structures. Good early intervention can do as good a job as a computer programming "wizard" given a clear understanding of what needs to be reprogrammed.

In neuropsychological terms, this capacity is called *transferability of function*. It also takes into account another neuropsychological concept—*redundancy,* the idea that there are multiple sites for functions to originate from. The caveat, however, is that "transferred" function often does not work as well as the real thing. A concrete example of this is if a right-handed person lost use of his right hand and needed to use his left. Some people would naturally adapt better than others; some would benefit significantly from hard, disciplined training to learn to use the left hand instead; and, ultimately, some people would just have the innate capacity to make the transition from right-handedness to left-handedness better than others. What we do know is that children who have early left-handed tendencies and are forced to use their right hand actually make the transition fairly well—at least compared with people who change hands after years of experience doing everything with their right. Early intervention is based on a similar idea: that training a new skill is easier to do than undoing an old skill and *then* training the new skill to replace it. Usually if there is an old "skill" to be undone, it is something the child has developed himself to cope as best he can with his inborn "hardware" error. Over time, if the child is not helped to cope better—by training designed to take the best advantage of what he can learn—the child is at risk of developing another set of signs of his disorder; those represent "system overflow"—an inability to tolerate the frustrations of his own disability. Figure 7 summarizes

A Computer Analogy for the Neuropsychology of Autism

"Hardware" Flaw	"Novice Programmer" Problems	"System Overflow"
Child has brain "disadvantage" from time of birth due to:	*Child innately tries to make up for brain "disadvantage" with partially helpful results, like:*	*"Computer"/ brain overflows or short circuits due to inability to process input fast enough, resulting in:*
Genetic Causes: -inherited genetic defect -random mutation	Ex) Immediate echolalia: only partial language understanding	Ex) Tantrums, low frustration threshold
Pregnancy Risks: -illnesses/infections -obstetric problems -toxics (drinking, drugs)	Ex) Advanced puzzle skills: good visual recognition, weaker abstraction	Ex) Increased 1:1 social withdrawal, avoidance of busy scenes
Delivery Risks: -asphyxia at birth -prematurity problems	Ex) Unusual interests: intellectual curiosity, no imagination	Ex) Oral apraxia, understand, but not speaking

Figure 7 Computer analogy of the neuropsychology of autism.

200

the "computer" model of the neuropsychology of autism—where it comes from and where it can go without appropriate intervention.

The Bottom Line to Learning

The fact that autistic children will learn differently because of their inborn neuropsychological differences implies three important things: (1) Learning will be harder work for the child. (2) Autistic children must be taught in a way that is tailored to what they can and can't naturally comprehend. This means that special education may consist of more stimulation than most children need, or stimulation in new ways. (3) If intervention is started earlier, the job will probably be easier, because the child will not have to unlearn poor ways of coping with his handicaps that he will have developed on his own—like throwing tantrums as a way of getting things.

How Much Early Intervention Is Appropriate?

Many parents instinctively try harder and do more and basically add more stimulation when their child does not respond normally. With autistic children however, just adding "more" is not enough. The special difficulties experienced by autistic children warrant a form of special education unique to their disorder. Clearly, the message is that early intervention is better than later intervention, but how much? Depending on the funding levels in a particular locale, families with a newly diagnosed autistic or PDD toddler may be offered just a weekly group session at the local Easter Seals Society with his mother; or, at the other end, up to four times per week, morning-long one-to-one class sessions, plus a home visitor, and speech therapy three times a week in the afternoons. Sometimes the most severely impaired children—those for whom even the most intensive services will not make a critical difference—tend to be offered more services than children who have fewer initial impairments or who may be more ready to tolerate intensive work. In fact, children with the mildest disabilities typically are offered fewer services than more moderately impaired children because it is felt they may improve eventually on their own. To the extent that there are any real data on who should get how much service, there is reason to believe that more intensive interventions for more mildly affected children may be particularly efficacious.

Evidence That Intensive Early Intervention is Better: the Lovaas Method

The work of Dr. Ivar Lovaas at UCLA provides the best direct scientific support that intense early interventions may be the most effective way of helping young autistic and PDD children. In 1987, he reported a study of autistic children who had received forty hours per week of one-to-one intervention for two years. The children who had received forty hours per week of one-to-one work did the best. These children received behavioral training that focused first on acquisition of compliance, then imitation, then receptive and expressive language, and finally integration with peers. Incorporated into "drills" to accomplish these goals were pre-academic concepts such as vocabulary, shapes, colors, numbers, and alphabet, as well as opportunities to use language functionally. The program, which is currently being expanded and replicated with even younger children, requires specific responses to very intensive one-to-one demands, in which the adult presents a very specific task, such as choosing "dog," given a picture of a dog and of a cat. At first, even small approximations of a successfully completed task are rewarded. (For example, letting the therapist put a block in the child's hand, and then releasing the hand so the block falls into a box.) The "intensity" of this approach, as you might imagine at this point, comes from the effort it takes to get a very young autistic or PDD child, who almost by definition is not too interested in complying to someone else's agenda, to put a block in a box. And, as soon as the block *is* in the box, (and a reward is given), a second trial is begun. Initial days of therapy using this method are not for the faint-hearted. There's a lot of screaming and struggling in most cases. However, high rates of compliance are typically obtained within the first few weeks because the child is given a chance to experience success by being given chances to do things he finds easy. Then, program intensity consists of repeated trials until a certain learning threshold is reached with a schedule of numerous tasks introduced in succession.

Not everyone likes the way the Lovaas sort of intensive approach "looks." There is, to some degree, a philosophical issue to be considered when deciding to implement something as intensive as the Lovaas program since parents differ in how permissive or strict they are with their typical children. In dealing with a disability, you are overcoming an unnatural barrier, as illustrated earlier by the computer analogy. No parents want to see their child struggle and scream and be unhappy. But, the therapy is a rehabilitation process and as such *may* "hurt," even if administered in a caring way by caring people. The analogy I often give parents in my clinic is that intensive work with a young autistic child is like recovering from a physical injury of your own: If you broke your leg skiing, you'd be given a series of painful exercises to do in the days and weeks after the cast was removed. As an adult, you would do these exercises with the knowledge that they were necessary to your longer-term goal of recovering full function in your leg. The child in intensive intervention undergoes the same experience, but is recovering from a brain injury—and most importantly, does not know that the pain he is being put through will ultimately benefit him.

In fact, the "trick" of much therapy with autistic children is to show the child benefits he cares about as quickly as possible, (for example, getting a desired food, toy, or activity) so that he finds his newly acquired skill (say, pointing at a picture of a cookie to get a cookie) to be a more efficient way of functioning than the behavior it replaced (say, standing in the kitchen screaming while

Mom frantically offers different things to eat). Later, this type of instructional strategy, which I'll refer to as *instrumental teaching*, will be discussed in more detail.

The Lovaas program involves quickly repeated trials and a very vigorous style of interacting with the child that definitely works but also (in my opinion) reflects the vigorous style of Dr. Lovaas himself and the young UCLA student-therapists whom he trains to carry out the work. It may be that similar program intensity can be accomplished by simply maintaining insistence that the task be completed though Dr. Lovaas feels this style serves to "amplify" positive reinforcement. Whether a vigorous or otherwise insistent style is used, it works well because the child is always rewarded for his successes, counterbalancing any initial aversion or resistance to the task. More importantly, while very intrusive methods definitely teach skills quickly, it is then necessary to wean the child to more normal levels of reinforcement so he can continue to learn new things on the same reinforcement schedule as others his age.

Dr. Lovaas has been involved in intervention with autistic children for close to thirty years. The behaviorally oriented methods (that is, behavior modification) that he pioneered with handicapped children influence much of what is done in schools for autistic and PDD children everywhere. What he and his team are doing now that has introduced improvements over his earlier programs is work on higher-level "pragmatic" use of language, and work on integration of the autistic child with peers. And, since the publication of his 1987 study, renewed attention has been paid to his approach because of its success. More importantly, his program contains a highly structured set of tasks and record-keeping procedures that makes it relatively straightforward for therapists to be trained well and to know what to do next. While Dr. Lovaas has found that closer to forty hours of one-to-one work per week works best, we have studied programs similar to his and found that in initially higher-functioning children, similar benefits may possibly be derived from about twenty-five hours per week if parents consistently apply the methods during nontreatment hours.

Perhaps the most pervasive negative myth about the Lovaas program, or about "behavior modification" in general, is that it means using physical aversives like electric shock or spanking the child. Many parents believe this. (In my clinic, fears that using behavior modification means using physical aversives far surpass queries about the "refrigerator mother" myth these days.) Yes, years ago, Lovaas did use mild electrical shock aversives on hospitalized severely mentally retarded children with intractable self-injurious behaviors. The current Lovaas program does not advocate the use of physical aversives. Though Lovaas does not advocate it, similar programs may use verbal aversives such as saying "No!" in a loud, flat tone of voice and grabbing away materials that the child has not used as instructed. That is about as rough as any good program should get to achieve positive results.

A final point worth making here is that the Lovaas program is a kind of package—it is not a patent medicine. There are many one-to-one behavioral programs across the country that are instituting similar curricula, such as the Eden Center in Northern New Jersey and the May Center in Cambridge, Massachusetts. It is important that parents and teachers consider the benefits of similar models rather than feeling that if it isn't a "Lovaas" program, the child isn't getting the best possible intervention.

Intrusive versus Insistent Methods of Early Intervention

While there is no study that specifically addresses whether intense interventions have to be intrusive in the way the Lovaas program can be, it is interesting to consider the methods used in some other well-known programs for autistic children. The Higashi School (of Tokyo and Lexington, Massachusetts) was massively favored by parents in the late 1980s. Dr. Kiyo Kitahara, its (late) founder, ran the program, and it was my impression from speaking with her, that she herself was an especially gifted special education teacher. Videotapes of the program (which is not one-to-one like the Lovaas program) show how teachers (many of whom were soft-spoken young Japanese women) would insist that a child complete a task, and even physically direct the task in a very mild way, but were not intrusive either physically or verbally. The speed of compliance was generally slower when this approach was used, but like the Lovaas teachers, Higashi teachers would persist until an acceptable approximation of the requested behavior was offered by the child. The children I have assessed who have attended the Higashi School seem to have learned less but are very good at the things that they have learned.

In my clinical experience, the one-to-one component is essential to early learning, especially when the child still has low levels of compliance and imitation. The intensity (that is, high number of hours per week) also seem critical, as Lovaas's data support. However, for parents who are uncomfortable with the more vigorous pace of a one-to-one program, it may be worth considering whether a program can be devised that is equally insistent (like the Higashi program) but also one-to-one like the Lovaas program. (It is also worth noting here that the Higashi School is not a panacea; in the past several years there have been serious concerns raised about the quality of the non-instructional care of children there, and more than one child has died, possibly due to lack of supervision.)

Determining Frequency and Intensity of an Early Intervention Program

Thus far, reasons why early intervention is needed, why intensive therapy seems effective, and why one-to-one is needed have been explained. How can it be determined how much instruction an individual child needs, or how much a given child can be expected to benefit from a very intensive program compared to a more traditional group-based infant stimulation program?

Family Functioning

One factor in determining the appropriateness of an intensive early intervention program is the family ecology. This means the whole family, and how it will be able to function given how much attention is paid to the autistic child's education. There is no point in throwing out the baby with the bath water. Causing emotional disturbance in siblings because they are neglected or dealt with in an overly punitive way by parents overburdened by the demands of an early intervention program is no good. Giving Mom a nervous breakdown because she is trying to put in four hours a day of one-to-one time with her autistic child while ignoring everything else is not good. Dad quitting his job to work half-time in order to do therapy, thereby endangering family economic stability, is probably no good for Dad, the marital relationship, or the family as a whole. Selection of an intervention strategy must be done in the context of a risks/benefits analysis for the whole family. Recently, the intensive early intervention approaches have been gaining momentum. While this is largely good, such programs are not going to benefit all children equally.

The Child's Capacity

The next issue is the child's innate capacity. More severely impaired, more mentally retarded children, sadly, do less well in any intervention they receive. A three-year-old with a mental age of six months *will* learn more slowly than a two-year-old who is only six months behind. Nobody wants the responsibility of playing God, but it does make sense to provide more limited learning opportunities to the child who can learn less, and more intensive learning opportunities to the child who can learn more—when resources are limited, which is almost always and everywhere. Exactly how to construct rules to allocate amounts of intervention is more difficult. In the Lovaas program at UCLA, for example, they cut back on the therapy hours for nonverbal children who do not begin to imitate speech sounds after three months of treatment. It is their experience that these children do not benefit as much from the twenty to forty hour a week programs as the children who *do* begin talking within that period of time.

A good diagnostician, looking carefully at the course of a child's prelinguistic milestones, can give a parent some idea of where a particular child falls in terms of spoken language readiness. If a child is doing some spontaneous babbling, appears not to have a significant degree of mental retardation, and shows interest in a variety of toys (although she does not play with them in an age-appropriate way), she is probably a good candidate for a fairly intensive intervention. Children who seem to not even notice toys for more than a few seconds each, and who are practically silent, are, in my experience, not particularly good candidates for intensive programs—and do nearly as well in more traditional, less intensive programs. If they are put in a more intensive program, their problem behaviors (during one-to-one sessions) may get better, but many typically tend to begin to develop "overflow" symptoms which will be described in the section on burnout, below.

Initiating Intensive Early Intervention

If a child *is* a good candidate for an intensive early intervention program, a conservative approach is to plan to gear up the number of one-to-one hours (for example starting with two- to thirty-minute sessions per day), and to get to perhaps three hours of one-to-one per day (for example, between home and school) after a month or so. If the child seems to be showing marked improvements and is on the less developmentally disabled end of the spectrum, moving ahead into a full-time one-to-one program may be beneficial. If achievements are more modest—increased compliance, but not much increased imitation, for example—it might be better to hold hours of therapy down to a lower, less intensive rate (say, some group and some individual instruction time). Many young autistic and PDD children can do well with twenty hours per week of one-to-one, especially if it is combined with some special education class hours, so that most hours of the day are spent in some structured activity, and there is relatively little time for the child to fall back on his own less difficult (and less adaptive) ways of doing things.

Burnout in Children Receiving Intensive Programs

There *does* seem to be some sort of threshold beyond which intense interventions themselves may create behavioral side effects. Again, this is something that is yet to be studied well, but some parents report that their children progress quite well in intensive programs for a year, eighteen months, two years—and then seem to burn out. They start to throw tantrums at easy tasks, or bite, hit, scream, or pull their shirt over their face to hide from the requirement of the task. They develop sleep problems, or begin to bed-wet again. These are probably signs that the child is emotionally stressed out (just like any other child at the same developmental level who would do such things in response to emotional stress). Such negative behaviors have to be examined closely. Parents should be especially concerned about signs of stress if the child's negative behaviors are not a direct result of being asked to do something new or difficult, but rather appear even when the child is presented with tasks he can easily accomplish.

These kinds of negative behaviors are another way that "overflow" (as we discussed earlier in terms of the computer analogy) can present itself. Children with a higher cognitive capacity can be expected to take longer to reach overflow than children with more mental retardation; but they do seem to have limits too. When parents come in and describe these symptoms to me, they expect I'll conduct a behavioral analysis and give them some behavior modification "tricks" to make the difficulties go away. Parents who have seen behavior modification methods used quite successfully are naturally going to reason this way. Often, they are surprised (and, I believe disappointed) when I talk about overflow reactions. I tend to liken the child's increasing refusal to be taught to what I feel would happen to me if someone decided to experiment with me and make me into a high-energy physicist. Even with the best tutors, I would go only so far. At some point I would be ready to run screaming from the room. Cognitively, I can't assimilate information at the level of mathematical abstraction that is important to a complete understanding of high-energy physics. It is the same with autistic and PDD children. You can help them compensate, but there are still underlying structural limitations to how much they can learn.

Life Is Not One-to-One

Up until this point, the virtues of one-to-one instruction have been extolled. One-on-one is particularly important to young autistic and PDD children because they are not socially motivated to be part of a group, they do not engage in what behaviorists call "social learning" until it's taught, they seldom do something to please an adult if they can be pleasing themselves instead, and they do not spontaneously learn well through imitation. These social factors, coupled with the fact that autistic children tend to prefer repetitive stimulation rather than novelty, tend to limit how well they learn without direct adult guidance. However, life is not one-to-one. All children eventually need to function as part of a larger system with rules to which they must at least partly adhere. (Criteria for using one-on-one instruction will be discussed more in Chapter 10.)

In a special education class, the young autistic child, for example, does not learn what other children learn from circle time. Circle time, for the still uninitiated, is the nearly universal preschool/early elementary level school activity in which children sit in a semicircle and conduct a fairly routinized series of introductions to the classroom day. During circle time, most non-autistic children will at least partly attend while each takes a turn at various routines—velcroing his name to a bulletin board, touching a sun if it's sunny out, or indicating the day of the week. The idea is that each child can learn by modeling others. The autistic or PDD child, who typically has little or no interest in peers, does not watch. Instead he spaces out, or maybe, if it's his particular interest, quietly recites the alphabet pasted on the wall above the teacher's head while the rest watch the circle time activities. What the autistic child learns in this situation is that she must hold still, stay in her seat, and find a way to entertain herself quietly while something she is not interested in goes on. It is not bad for a child to learn how to handle boredom, but that is not the point of circle time. So, being in a group may serve some purpose for the autistic or PDD child, but perhaps not exactly the purpose intended. Nevertheless, autistic and PDD children need to learn what it means to participate in and comply with group activities such as lining up to go outside, waiting one's turn for a snack, or putting things away in a cubby. Furthermore, it is good to know from habit or routine when these things should be done, or to be able to do them when someone reminds you from a distance or gives instructions to you as part of a group.

Until the autistic child can begin to imitate and learn from instruction not specifically addressed to him alone, the group setting is of more limited educational benefit, and one-to-one—or for some forms of learning, one-to-two—instruction is probably the most enriching instructional strategy, and indeed the only one that gives the child an opportunity to progress toward academic goals rather than just follow routines.

In subsequent chapters we'll discuss the educational *content* of early intervention and later intervention programs for autistic children. Chapters 11 and 12, in particular, give information and ideas for parents interested in doing significant amounts of one-to-one early intervention at home with their own child.

Chapter Summary

In this chapter, we have addressed some of the basic considerations in favor of very early intervention for young children with autism and PDD. In the next chapter, we will discuss what to look for as you begin to select potentially appropriate programs by assessing the skills of classroom staff, supplementary services, staffing ratios, and use of staff time. We'll discuss the pros and cons of mainstreaming, and the values and drawbacks associated with having autistic children placed in a class with other autistic and PDD children versus placing them in classrooms with children who have other disabilities.

CHAPTER 10

◆ ◆ ◆

Selecting a Classroom: Assessing Teachers, Aides, and Student Composition

Selecting a Classroom

In working with the school system to find an appropriate educational program for a child, parents and their consultants can have the opportunity to visit existing classrooms to determine whether the staff and the curriculum of a particular class will meet the educational needs of their child. In this chapter, we'll discuss what kind of classroom may be best for a particular child, what to look for as you observe staff, and the necessary preconditions there should be before agreeing to have a child placed in a particular class. The qualities of every class change with the addition of each new student. Therefore, observations need to focus on how the available resources could be applied to the specific needs of the child you are planning to place in a given classroom. As each new year of special education is planned, parents should take the opportunity to consider their child's educational alternatives before sitting down to the next (or first) IEP meeting where the agreement for the next year's education plan will be written down, agreed to, and signed.

Selecting a classroom always requires assessment of the particular classroom and its staff. Measures of quality such as staff-to-child ratio, the teacher's training, or the educational diagnoses of the other students are just "quick and dirty" measures of the appropriateness of a class for a particular student. Parents need to begin with a good understanding of what constitutes an appropriate program for their child, and then begin to piece together services that will meet those needs. As we discussed in Chapter 8, *entitlement to an appropriate program is the law*. Every child in special education is entitled to one. It is never appropriate for the school system to claim that "this is all that we can do for now." No matter how rural the place you live in, nor how financially impoverished your school system is, your child is still entitled to an appropriate education.

This chapter focuses on developing skills for assessing classrooms and relating program characteristics to specific educational needs common to many children with autism and PDD.

Designated Autistic Classes versus Classes Grouped by Educational Diagnosis

Educational Diagnoses. Are autistic and PDD children best served in classrooms that contain only other children with autism or PDD? Diagnosis-grouped classes is one educational strategy implemented by many school systems. Other schools group children by educational "diagnosis" irrespective of their clinical diagnosis. While some school systems recognize autism as a distinct educational diagnosis, others do not. An educational diagnosis is spoken in a different language from the "DSM-ese" used by clinicians. Educators use their own system of diagnoses to group children more broadly according to the intensity and focus needed in special education. Different schools divide up students slightly differently, and with slightly different nomenclature: Programs for many PDD and some cognitively higher functioning autistic children focus on remediation of language delays, and include classes designated as serving those with communication disorders (CD), communication handicaps (CH), language disorders (LD) or severe delays of language (SDL). Children with more generalized cognitive delays (such as those with verbal and performance IQs in the borderline to mildly mentally retarded range) are often placed in learning handicapped (LH) or learning diability(LD) classes. Autistic children with moderate to severe levels of cognitive impairment are often placed in severely handicapped (SH) classrooms, and some are placed in multihandicapped (MH) classes, especially if they will need work on development of motor skills as well.

One might ask, "What is the point of having a child diagnosed as autistic or PDD if his or her classroom is not going to be one especially for children with autism or PDD?" The answer is that the teacher needs to be aware of a child's autism, even if the class is not specifically for autistic children. Programs not specifically designated for autistic children *can* provide a good education for an autistic child, especially if the teacher is interested in, and better yet, also experienced in the particulars of educating an autistic child. There are both advantages and disadvantages of autistic versus educational diagnosis–grouped classes.

Designated Autistic Classes. There are several reasons why designated autistic classes can be a better placement. As we have already discussed, the specific problems that autistic children have in understanding things constitutes the basis for autism being considered a separate disorder from other disabilities like language disorders or mental retardation alone. As such, autistic children have specific problems that require specific remedies. A key factor among these is that autistic children often, at first, do not respond to social rewards very well. Getting to sit on the teacher's lap, being called "Such a big girl!" in an admiring tone of voice, or being reassured with a cuddly stuffed animal does not go that far in getting most autistic children to do things they find difficult or unappealing. Instead, an autistic class is often set up with primary and sensory rewards (for example, food, tickling); these rewards are then paired with more social rewards so that the social rewards will eventually take on reward value too. So, when an autistic child is very young, an all-autistic class may be the best place to find an instructional environment using this type of instrumental motivational system.

Another advantage of autistic classes for a very young child is that very small group (say, one-to-two) and one-to-one instruction is usually more available, and young autistic children need that to gain the initial imitation skills that can later be generalized to include things beyond the model that is right in front of them. As long as the autistic child is having major difficulties in imitating *proximal* things (that is, things *close* to him, like building three blocks into a pyramid after it is demonstrated), it is not likely that he is going to imitate other things much more *distal* (like circle time activities).

Some parents worry that in an all-autistic class, their child will pick up bad "habits" like hand-flapping in response to distress. Although there are reasons why behaviors that occur along with a higher state of excitement *are* more easily learned, it is unlikely that a behavior that is neurologically symptomatic of autism, such as flapping, will be learned. If a child has not yet acquired a simple motor imitation skill (such as being able to touch his nose when some one else does), it is unlikely that he will flap just because another child is doing it. It is also unlikely that an autistic child who does not yet show spontaneous imitation of actions that are demonstrated to him one-to-one will imitate more complex and social behavior like biting another child to get a toy. However, biting might occur to the autistic child on his own—especially in a busy, poorly supervised classroom where he is constantly frustrated in attempts to have his needs addressed.

Overall, all-autistic classes probably offer the best advantage when the autistic or PDD child is very young and does not yet respond well to social rewards and still engages in relatively little imitation. After one or two years of special education, perhaps fifty percent of autistic children, and virtually all PDD children, are ready to benefit from a class with other, more socially advanced role models. Criteria for deciding to move an autistic or PDD child into a class with other non-PDD children will be explained next.

Ability-Grouped Classes. Autistic or PDD children may be limited by an autistic class when they get to a point where their imitation is somewhat improved, substantial one-to-one is not needed for compliance, there is some responsiveness to social praise, and there is an emerging interest in appropriate play with toys. At the point when the autistic child begins to notice more distal (distant from her) activities and can still model them, she is probably more ready for a class with children who provide more developmental challenge in terms of how they play and interact. It is often a good choice to move an autistic or PDD child into a class with other children who may be socially advanced, but who have a similar level of disability with respect to language delay.

Classrooms for PDD Children. For many PDD children, an ability-grouped classroom (such as as CH, CD, or SDL class) is, from the start, the right choice. A classroom with other children who have similar levels of language disability, but better organized social and play abilities, may provide a level and type of stimulation that can especially benefit PDD children with less marked cognitive problems. Some PDD children, and young children with Asperger's syndrome, may actually have more language *production* than other language-handicapped peers, but have less ability to use the language meaningfully. Reciting long soliloquies from *Beauty and the Beast* may be an impressive feat of memory, but may reveal no more functional language understanding than that of the child with language disorder who is still expressing herself in single words and gestures at age five. Even though each child may have a different kind of language disability, both need to build slowly on language that is tied to full comprehension. Putting such children together in one class can be advantageous to both children. The PDD child is exposed to a child who probably will have more meaningful, less repetitive play, and the child who has a language disorder is exposed to a PDD child who may verbalize more readily than she does. The PDD or autistic child in such a class should be approximately matched on the developmental level of meaningful expressive language to the other children in her class.

Social Skills Development and Mixed-Disability Classes. It is difficult to foster social interactive skills in an all-autistic class. For example, in a one-to-two language lesson, trying to get two autistic children to ask each other what each had for breakfast can be a real challenge. However, if one child is at least willing to ask and persist at the communicative attempt (even if he has word-finding, articulation, or other language use difficulties), the autistic or PDD child is more likely to eventually respond to the social nature of the overture.

If autistic and PDD children who have achieved some rudimentary imitation skills benefit from being with non-autistic children with language disorders, will they similarly benefit from being with non–special education children their own age? This topic will be discussed later and in more detail, but the brief answer is probably not—at least for the very young autistic or PDD child. The average normally developing three- or four-year-old is pretty egocentric and doesn't hang around very long if a conversational partner doesn't answer back in the expected fashion and in the expected time frame. On the other hand, children with language disorders or mentally retarded children who have the desire to communicate, but have learned through their own experience that it may take several tries until they are understood, may persist more in talking to an autistic child.

Some developmentally disabled children, like children with Down syndrome tend to be on the *hyper*-social side, and may persist, boss, and run circles around an autistic child, trying to get a response. This is generally good for the autistic child. I have been to many classrooms where an autistic child's playground buddy is a child with Down syndrome. If told by the teacher "Now don't lose your buddy!" the Down child will grasp the autistic child's wrist firmly and resist attempts by the autistic child to pull away; sometimes both kids end up in a heap on the ground if the autistic child tries too hard to escape.

Teaching to the Middle

An ability-grouped classroom, where children are grouped by educational diagnosis, by definition is one where children are placed together because they have a similar level of functioning in terms of their major area(s) of impairment. A major objective in finding an appropriate ability-grouped classroom is to identify one where your child is neither the highest nor lowest functioning child. Special education classes are small because each child is different and needs something different. The whole idea behind an IEP is that it is an *individual* educational program. Nevertheless, even the most excellent special education teacher can't run eight parallel curricula if she has eight very different children. To some extent, the focus of her efforts will be to the middle. If all the children except one child have adequate single-word vocabularies, you don't want your child to be that only preverbal one. If your child can read and speak words and phrases, you don't want him in a class with other children who are all preverbal. The "different" child who is less developed than the rest will probably get ignored some of the time. The child who is more advanced will probably be underchallenged at least some of the time.

One worthy exception to the rule of trying to have a child in the "middle" of his class is when the child is remaining with a teacher who has already had one or two years of marked success with the child and feels she can do more. It is usually not easy to find a special education teacher who seems to have perfect chemistry with a particular child. When that does happen, take optimal advantage of this opportunity. However, it may not make sense to be "in the middle" developmentally when it would involve being in a class where the other students are chronologically or physically much larger or smaller. Also, as we will discuss below, in some cases where a child has a full-time, one-to-one aide, the ability level of the rest of the class may be relatively less important.

Teachers and Teacher Training

One question that many parents ask is "What should I look for in a teacher?" An all-autistic class should definitely have a teacher who has specialized training or previous experience working with autistic children. Most special education credentialing programs include some training about autism, but it is preferable to have a teacher who has had some practical experience with autistic children as an aide or an intern before having her own class.

Most states have no specific statewide teaching credential for autism, but there are some teachers who have made autism a focus of their training. Project TEACCH (Treatment and Education of Autistic and Related Communication Handicapped Children and Adults), which is based at the University of North Carolina in Chapel Hill, provides the most comprehensive and excellent teacher training for working with autistic children; it also has a compilation of educational assessment and curriculum materials that are integrated with their overall educational approach. (By writing to Project TEACCH, UNC, Chapel Hill, Chapel Hill, North Carolina 27599, teachers can learn more about their available materials.)

Interviewing a Potential Teacher

In talking to a teacher about her experience and qualifications for teaching autistic children, it should be clear that she understands that autism and PDD are related developmental disorders, that autistic children are *not* emotionally disturbed children, and that there are severe problems in social relatedness that affect the ability to learn language. This means that the teacher should be able to demonstrate that she knows that, in teaching an autistic child, it is important to focus on language in context, including receptive language, turn-taking, language tied to visual prompts, and so on, and that the primary problems are *not* articulation, resistance or negativism, or "acting out." The surest formula for disaster is when a teacher interprets autistic aloofness and lack of interest in compliance for malicious negativism.

Establishing the Parent-Teacher Relationship

A parent-teacher relationship is a very precious, fragile thing. A parent needs to be able to depend on the teacher to do the right things with the child. The teacher needs to feel that she has the parent's support and cooperation. Often this relationship begins the first time parents visit a class that may be an appropriate place for their child. While the parent needs to maintain a consumer-oriented "caveat emptor" attitude, it is also important that a potential teacher not be alienated by a parent who has an overly critical attitude at the first meeting. Most experienced teachers realize that an initially hostile attitude on the part of an interviewing parent is masking quite understandable anxiety about making an important decision on behalf of the child.

It is important to look for what the teacher seems to be doing right. It is important to talk to a teacher, observe her, and to describe your child and get her ideas. Generally, teachers are not very receptive to parents who pre-emptively announce that the parents are going to be the ones to tell the teacher how to instruct their child. Generally, however, teachers *are* receptive to parents who express an interest in discussing what they've read about autism, as long as the parents are also interested in seeing what the teacher thinks about implementing ideas that she has for the child.

The parent can and should be an expert on his child, but the teacher should be the expert on teaching. The two perspectives need to meld. Turning program planning into a power struggle stresses everyone and seldom benefits the child. Parents need to really listen to a teacher's rationale for accomplishing a particular educational objective. Teachers generally acknowledge that some parents want to be more involved than others in their child's programming, and should be able to offer you the opportunity to do that if that's your choice as a parent.

Making Classroom Observations

Checking Out the Options

When deciding on a special education placement, it is important to consider all the viable options. By looking at multiple classes you'll know what's available, and the school personnel will learn that you as a parent (or as a parent's consultant in selecting a classroom) are going to be a discriminating consumer. It is often the case that a school district will suggest a couple of different programs for a parent to visit, even if the school personnel feel that one of those placements is vastly preferable. Do not, however, waste your time visiting classes that are clearly going to be inappropriate. For example, I was recently consulted to assess some classrooms for an eight-year-old, profoundly retarded, nonveral autistic boy whose parents were petitioning the school district to pay for a nonpublic school. The director of special education for the school district took me into a CH class of eight-year-olds who were pasting construction paper turkeys and writing sentences about their upcoming Thanksgiving plans. I immaitely made it very clear to the director of special education that I was ready to leave and see another class. Most school systems can be expected to have at least a couple of viable choices.

Sometimes, in a very sparsely populated area, there is no choice among classrooms because there is only one special education class in the region. Even in these cases, it is important to visit the class to know what you will have to work with—meaning that the classroom may have to be just one piece of the total educational package the child will need in order to obtain an appropriate education. As we will discuss later in the chapter, the classroom setting is one component of educational services that also may include one-to-one instruction, speech and language therapy, occupational therapy, and so on.

Classroom visits serve many useful purposes; deciding which class to choose is only the first of a list of reasons to make classroom visits. Classroom observations calibrate parents as to how much of their child's total educational needs can be fulfilled by the special education system (and whether the services of other outside therapists may also be needed to put together an "appropriate" program). When it's possible, it can be good for parents to visit private or experimental treatment programs, as well as publicly funded programs, just to get a sense of what's out there, even if all the programs might not be appropriate for their child at the moment.

The Emotional Experience of Seeing Other Handicapped Children

Visiting classrooms may also help parents get used to seeing other developmentally disabled children and become aware of how their child fits in. When first visiting special education classes, many parents say that they focus on the physical characteristics of other developmentally disabled children, and that this makes them feel uncomfortable because these children "look different." A very natural reaction is to not want one's autistic or PDD child, who is usually without physical stigmata, to be near such "retarded"-looking children. But for most families, exposure to these other developmentally disabled children on a day-to-day basis, as well as getting to know their parents, tends to lessen those feelings of initial discomfort. It is important to remember that autistic children need to be placed with others who have similar educational needs, not necessarily just with children who happen to "look" normal. Some children who may look quite dysmorphic ("retarded-looking") are not necessarily as retarded as they appear. Many children with Down syndrome, fetal alcohol syndrome, or cerebral palsy may look more handicapped than they actually are. In fact, most parents of dysmorphic children have a hard time realizing how different their own child looks to someone else—because they are so used to them and love them.

Classroom Visits as an Opportunity to Learn about Instructional Alternatives

Making classroom visits is a good way to get ideas about educating a particular child if you don't have a clear picture of *how* your child will go about learning the things you want him to learn. It is reasonable for you (as either a parent or consulting professional) to suggest that appropriate methods or materials you have observed in use in one classroom be used with your child, but in a different class that may be better overall for other reasons. Teachers are generally open to learning from one another. In fact, most special education teachers I talk with feel that they lack opportunities to benefit from one another's experiences. Suggesting that teachers communicate with one another in the process of setting up a program for your child is completely fair and reasonable, if done tactfully.

Behavior-Focused Observation

There is nothing like seeing a teacher in action to enable one to judge her abilities. There are very good teachers (both of handicapped and nonhandicapped students) who are fairly awkward, nervous, and even inarticulate with parents. In making a classroom observation, it can help to try to pick out another student who seems at the same language level as your child and focus on how language is used with him. Then pick out another student who may have the same kind of tantrum problems as your child (for example, a child who doesn't like someone else to decide when he should stop an activity), and see what methods are used when one of the classroom staff has to get him to stop an activity.

Classroom Observation Etiquette

During a classroom observation, a visitor should make him- or herself inconspicuous. Sit down on the floor or on a little chair in a fairly empty part of the class, but one with a good view of most of the class. Try not to move around a lot. Don't follow or tower over children, or even try to interact with them. (If a student tries to interact with you, politely turn him or her away, suggesting that the child return to what the teacher wants the child to be doing.) The point is that the flow of classroom activity should be as unaffected by your presence as possible. Regular classroom hours are not the time to talk with a teacher about your observations, or to ask questions about why they are doing what they are doing. You'll disrupt what should be happening and then you may underestimate how good the class may really be. A teacher can't be expected to focus on a parent and answer questions when she should be doing her job with her students. Scheduling a separate time outside of school hours to talk to the teacher (such as coming at the beginning or end of the day) is usually a better idea. It is also better to make an initial visit *without* your child. An autistic or PDD child in a strange room full of other strange children is seldom happy or complacent, and his presence may be disruptive to other children's routines.

In any classroom things will go wrong. Sometimes outbursts are due to a particularly uncontrollable or new student. Sometimes a student is wandering around because he is having a free period. Sometimes there is an aggressive incident between two students and there is not enough staff that day because an aide is out sick. Sometimes more than one visit to a class might be necessary to really evaluate whether your initial impressions under- (or over-) estimated the quality of the program in a particular classroom. Since so many autistic, PDD, and other developmentally delayed children are highly sensitive to changes in routine and don't cope well with unexpected changes, an atypical day caused by a staff member's absence or a field trip may make everyone and everything seem dysfunctional.

Sometimes a subsequent visit to a promising classroom is a good idea: seeing the ways in which the program is the same from day to day gives a more balanced view of the routine and degree of structure in the program. At the time of a second visit, it may be all right to bring the prospective student along, especially if the teacher requests it. Sometimes, and this is usually the better alternative, the teacher may be able to visit the child in his current classroom placement or see him first at your home. Parents need to realize that choosing a classroom is not a matter of seeing if the child will have a good time when he is there. In fact, many an autistic child prefers a classroom where nobody will ever force him to do anything! However, the classroom will be a place to learn, and that will sometimes be hard, disagreeable work for the child. A child's behavior on his first visit to a classroom, therefore, usually cannot be considered representative of whether he will ultimately do well in that setting.

Building and Maintaining a Good Parent-Teacher Relationship

There is a wide range of intensity and quality in parent-teacher relationships. There are individual tutors who practically become part of the family, and the mother's best friend. There are teachers who reach out with home visits to each of their student's parents once a quarter (whether the parents seem eager for it at first or not). On the other hand, there are teachers who don't want to know their student's parents because they feel it contaminates their ability to form their own relationships with their students. There are even good teachers who can only be described as parent-haters, who constantly worry that their students are being abused or neglected at home, and that the parents are trying to deliberately thwart the school's progress.

Classroom Visitation Policy. A parent does have a right to be kept informed about her child's program. Parents even have a right to visit their child's classroom. But the school has rights to determine policy about prior notification of visits, duration of visits, and how the visits should be conducted and monitored. A school that will allow visits only at very specific times (like a parents' night or an "assembly") but won't let you see the regular program is not to be trusted. It's a good idea to make classroom visits at least occasionally. For very young children who are starting school for the first time, it may be really beneficial to have a parent at school regularly, if possible, so that routines and expectations set up in the classroom can be consistently maintained at home. For older children, a visit once a quarter or a couple of times a year for a few hours may help keep the parent informed about what is going on in school. A visit opens up an opportunity for dialogue and exchange of information between parents and teachers—for example, if the parent sees the child not doing something at school that he can readily do at home, or vice versa.

It is always important that a child be expected to function to the best of his ability in both the home and school settings. If a four-year-old autistic child has to say "More juice, please" at school, just whining to get juice at home is inappropriate. Autistic children often do not readily or spontaneously generalize skills from one setting to another, and tend to try to get away with the minimal communicative effort that the setting will tolerate. Therefore, it's vital that parents and teachers keep abreast of the child's highest levels of functioning in home and at school, and demand the child's most capable behaviors in both places.

Parent-Teacher Journals. In addition to visits between parents and teachers, another, less intensive means of parent-teacher contact is exchange of a daily journal. This can be as simple as a photocopied checklist that the teacher uses to show how many successful bathroom trips a four-year-old had, or how many time-outs a ten-year-old needed, or the daily score on a job readiness drill for a fifteen-year-old. Sometimes a daily journal is just one handwritten line. Sometimes teachers use a a more extensive weekly report that includes test scores as well as behavioral records. In one family I see in which the mother speaks only Vietnamese, the daily log is a list of frequently made comments—listed in English in one column, with the corresponding Vietnamese translation in the next column, The teacher checks off her part in English, and the mother then reads the corresponding checked message in Vietnamese. Even though the mother and teacher can't speak face to face unless they have an interpreter present, they actually "talk" every day.

There should be a way for parents to return regular communication to teachers, too. One way is to be able to comment on the daily journal and send it back. More common is for parents to simply know the times of day that a teacher can be reached by telephone in her class during non-instructional hours and arrange to call. Parents who show interest in and positive acknowledgment of what a teacher is doing with a student usually evoke more interest in their child by their child's teacher. This is especially true in the education of autistic and PDD children, since they tend to provide less positive social reinforcement of their own to the teachers.

Classroom Structure

In addition to the educational diagnosis of children served in an educational program, and the teacher and her qualifications, it is important to observe how much structure the program offers. A highly structured environment is without doubt the most tried and true model for educating an autistic child. A major learning problem experienced by children with autistic spectrum disorders is that, if left unstructured, autistic and PDD children will tend either to perseverate overly long on a small number of interests, or will regard things in an unfocused, undifferentiated way. Perseveration is a major trait demonstrated by higher functioning individuals with autism and Asperger's syndrome, and these narrow interests get in the way of further learning. It takes structure and externally imposed limits to broaden their horizons. Younger children with autism and PDD, on the other hand, more often suffer from being unfocused and uninterested in things around them, and a higher degree of structure imposes awareness of new things on them, so they can learn.

The tendency of autistic and PDD children is to *not* "go with the flow."

Typically, an activity does not seem inherently interesting to an autistic person just because everyone else is doing it. In fact, there is generally quite limited imitation of the activities of others unless the activity strikes an autistic chord, like swinging on a swing, or meets an instrumental need, like constructing peanut butter sandwiches. Autistic and PDD children need structure—rules that force them to do things—in order to ensure that they are exposed to a diversity of stimuli.

"Food for Thought"

One particular concern about young autistic and PDD children is that while other two-, three-, and four-year-olds are learning through copying others and then modifying what they've taken in with their own experiments, the autistic or PDD child is not spontaneously taking in information imitatively, and thus has much less "food for thought." This cycle of self-imposed understimulation can set a child farther behind, the longer he goes without intervention. (In the last chapter we discussed this in terms of a computer analogy, with the child as a "novice programmer" who really doesn't know how to fix what's broken and who therefore hobbles along with an information-processing system that is circuitous and inefficient.)

One remedy is to provide a highly structured environment that demands a certain level of varied behavior and forces attention to various types of stimulation that gives the child experiences he might not give himself. This doesn't mean that the child has to be completely regimented. Teachers can counteract the demands of high structure by giving choices. For example, a child may have to draw a circle, but can choose a red or green marker. Or the child can be given a marker and can then choose to trace a circle or a square. High structure helps the child become aware that there are rules to be followed, people who monitor them and who need to be checked with, and that there are negative consequences for not following rules. These are all lessons worth learning.

Capitalizing on the Autistic Child's Resistance to Change

At first, high structure is usually strongly resisted by autistic children because it interferes with their own agenda. However, the very resistance to change that characterizes so many autistic children, and can make adjustment to a new class difficult, may eventually flip over and serve them well. Typically, once an autistic child gets used to a new routine it becomes his. The once recalcitrant and tantrum-throwing little six-year-old who wouldn't hang up his coat, put away his lunch, or line up from recess when leaving the snack table becomes the model student at all of these activities. Woe to the teacher, however, on the day that the class needs to exit from the front door of the class for a field trip, instead of from the back door of the class for recess! One teacher told me about a small four-year-old autistic boy in her class who pushed a tall, heavy coat rack back into its "right" place on three successive days after she had rearranged her classroom.

The autistic child's tendency to prefer routines can be capitalized on in teaching adaptive behaviors (like dressing and table manners). Teachers must also introduce autistic students to the idea of being flexible with routines. They can do this by rehearsing changes in routine with students ahead of time— talking about a field trip, showing pictures of what will happen and where they will go, and repeating what new routine will be followed on the special occasion.

Working in a Low-Stimulation Environment

What should the physical environment of the classroom look like in order to provide a high degree of structure and an atmosphere conducive to obtaining and maintaining the child's attention? Typical pre-school and elementary classrooms tend to have all sorts of bulletin boards, papier-mâché planets hanging from the ceiling, and numerous examples of artwork based on the current season of the year or holiday. The autistic or PDD child is easily distracted by such extraneous stimuli around him, and will even find things to be distracted by that others don't really notice—like the sound of hot water in radiators, certain fluorescent lights, and buses driving by outside.

Some of the best-organized classrooms for autistic children I've seen have partitioned-off areas with small tables or beanbag chairs with just room enough for a teacher and one or two students. The partitions are free from decoration, and there is nowhere to go and nothing else to look at except the curriculum materials the teacher has on the table immediately in front of the child. In our clinic, where we give IQ tests to autistic and PDD children, we go one step further, with an adjustable-height trapezoidal table that pushes against one corner of a bland, empty room, confining the child to a small triangular area just big enough for him and his chair. The examiner sits directly across and takes out only one thing at a time. Confined environments such as these help the autistic (and hyperactive) child to focus and to disregard other stimuli that are not relevant to his current learning situation. Some children who are very hypersensitive to sounds and easily distracted can benefit from wearing heavy headphones that block out outside sound. At times, headphones can be wired or remotely connected to a microphone, which the teacher can use to give instructions. The fewer the sources of distraction, the more likely the autistic child will be to attend to the materials at hand.

Contained Classes versus Changing Classes

One issue related to the generally positive response that autistic and PDD children have to highly structured programs is how they may handle a school program that calls for multiple daily class changes versus remaining in a contained classroom. This usually does not become an issue until middle school/

junior high school age, when special education students may start changing classes along with other non–special education students. While the scheduling of a class change may be routine, what happens during a class change is generally quite chaotic: Often, class changes, especially on a non–special education site, involve hundreds of preteens making primitive noises that resound in the hallways, as they dart back and forth with an organizational flow that can only be characterized as an early pubertal mating dance. This level of energetic social interaction overwhelms a teen with autism or PDD and has no particular benefit. In fact, if the other students notice the autistic teen at all, the words sent his way are likely to be rather unkind.

Despite parents' and teachers' hopes for an enlightened attitude on the part of the typical preteen, it is virtually never there when adults are not around. The teasing that a young person with autism or Asperger's syndrome receives in this sort of setting is gross enough that despite his näive social skills, he can perceive he is being humiliated and it hurts. Sometimes teachers can set things up to help the autistic teen pass among his nonhandicapped peers more readily. William, an intellectually gifted spelling whiz with Asperger's syndrome, was able to enter the cafeteria without taunts after the teacher of his learning handicapped class sent him to lunch accompanied by two of his classmates—boys who were on the high school football team.

For most of the autistic or PDD teens in special education, at least some reduction in classroom changing is preferable, or a schedule modification, such that the partly mainstreamed teen can arrive at his next class just as others are leaving and so avoid most of the mass confusion. This type of program change needs to be carefully considered for any child. Later, when we discuss some of the special developmental concerns of teenagers with autism or PDD, the need for gradual mainstream exposure will become clearer.

Use of Classroom Paraprofessional Teacher's Aides

Another major factor in how well a classroom works is the presence of and utilization of paraprofessional teaching aides. These people are classroom assistants, usually with little to no formal training in special education, or only a little community college–level training in child development or early education. These assistants are usually referred to as aides, or in some school systems, "paras" (for paraprofessionals). Although teacher's aides generally have little formal training and are also poorly paid, some are very good. The largest category of really dependable, creative aides often is made up of women in their forties and older, whose own children are in high school or grown up, and who really like to be with children—and are naturally good at it. Some aides are young college graduates who want an altruistic job for a couple of years before they commit themselves to their "real" job. Some are young women filling in a few years between the end of their own education and starting their own families. There is a great deal that a talented teacher's aide can learn on the job from her teacher. Many are able to develop a relationship with a particular child that promotes learning even better than the relationship between the teacher and student. In most very high quality classrooms, teachers and aides cannot be distinguished from one another by *how* they teach. The teacher is the program innovator and program manager. It is her responsibility to see that aides carry out her instructional goals in the way she wants. In a well-run classroom, though, every instructor should appear equally competent and knowledgeable about his or her assigned task.

In the remainder of this chapter we'll discuss how judicious use of a teacher's aide's time (or the parent's herself—as a classroom helper) can have a multiplicative effect on accomplishing the goals set in the child's IEP. Mostly, we'll discuss the one-on-one use of aides. However, one-on-one is not *always* the best way to use an aide. Sometimes, an autistic or PDD child benefits more in terms of social skills development, and in terms of generalizing from learned material, by working with an aide along with one or two other students who interact together over a single activity that the aide or teacher directs.

Observing the Activities of Teacher's Aides. When you observe a classroom, what should an aide be doing? The use of aides was discussed briefly earlier, in terms of the one-to-one instruction that can be of great benefit to very young autistic children. When aides are used one-to-one with very young children, they are usually teaching early skills of basic compliance, imitation, and receptive language. Since imitation tends to remain a difficulty for many autistic children, a good use of classroom aides is for one-on-one instruction with a child when a new type of task is being introduced. The aide can provide hand-over-hand assistance or repeated trials to achieve a specific objective. For autistic children with very marked difficulties with imitation, one-on-one is needed to successively break down tasks into smaller and smaller components until the task is defined in a way that the child can begin to master, one component at a time. Non-autistic children with similar degrees of developmental disorder tend to be relatively better at imitation and can usually benefit without so much need for intensive one-on-one and task analysis.

Aides are also used during transitional periods. When a child starts a new program, an aide can guide the child through new and unfamiliar activities step by step, until he can participate with the same level of prompting and redirection as other students. Sometimes an IEP will specify a schedule of one-to-one time with an aide as a child adjusts to a new program. If the child is very young, an alternative strategy may be to have one of the parents act as a one-to-one aide during the initial transition period. If a parent does come into a classroom essentially to function as an aide, the parent must be willing to take direction from the teacher.

One-to-One and Transition Times. The presence of parents in a classroom as aides for their children raises the issue of when or whether parents should be present in class at all. Parents often ask if it's a good idea for them to be present as a young child gets used to a new school setting. This really depends on the nature of the parent *and* the child. A child who has the tendency to cling to a parent when there is something not to his liking is probably going to use his pattern of clinging to ignore what is going on in a new class. If the parent can serve as a secure base, and encourage the child to pay attention to the class activities and not to her (or to the child's own feelings), the parent *can* probably be of help in the transition period. However, if the parent feels that the child will take the mother or father's relatively cool attitude as rejection, and cannot behave toward the child in the way that the classroom structure demands, that parent is probably best off out of the classroom in the first place.

In reality, planning for a first day of school for an autistic child, in this respect, is no different than for other preschoolers. Parents and teachers should work out how or if there will be parent time in the classroom in the first few days of a new school. This should be agreed upon in advance. A particular teacher may have a strategy that works well for her. If the teacher insists on introducing the child to the class, say, without the parent there, the parent should respect the teacher's expertise by trying it her way for at least a couple of days. The first few days of leaving a child with someone else are at least as emotionally difficult for the parent as they are for the child. When the child is just beginning special education, the child may be seen as even more vulnerable, and the parent's feelings about the separation are likely to be even stronger than when a nonhandicapped child starts at a day care center or a preschool for the first time.

The Use of Privately Funded Teacher's Aides. Sometimes, parents want their child to derive the benefits of education in a group setting, but still feel strongly about one-to-one. As we discussed in Chapter 8, it *is* possible to get a school to agree to one-on-one time in an IEP, but it is not always easy. Increasingly, parents in some areas are hiring private aides to go into the public schools with their children. In this case, the parent has a great deal of control over who will be providing one-to-one instruction for her child (although schools usually insist that the person meet the educational qualifications of aides they would hire.) Parent-hired aides have become particularly useful in helping children make the transition from in-home one-to-one programs into more mainstreamed public school settings. Getting a school to agree to a parent-funded aide can be a cost-effective approach for a parent who may be willing to pay, say eight dollars an hour to an aide, four hours a day, five days a week, and cannot find a nonpublic school that would offer an equally individualized program; or can find one, but doesn't feel up to the fight of trying to get his or her school district to pay for it.

Using Teacher's Aides to Increase Exposure to Speech and Language Therapy Goals. Another important way in which aide time can be used is in providing backup for more expensive supplementary (ancillary) services that the school may not be willing or able to provide as frequently as the child may need. For example, a speech and language therapist may see the chld once per week on a "pull-out" basis (that is, taking the child out of his regular class and into her own office). If the aide goes along to the speech therapy session, the speech therapist can demonstrate to the aide how to work with the child, and the speech therapist can then focus on the role of diagnostician—setting new goals and trying out new material with the child—which then can be reinforced on a daily basis during one-to-one time with the aide. The technical, program development part of the speech and language therapy is still done by the more highly trained professional, but the practice drills, which require more time and patience (but relatively less expertise) are done by the aide.

Teacher's Aides for Behavior Control. There are times when ont-to-one aides are used because a child's behavior is out of control. Usually schools offer one-to-one aides for children who are considered a danger to themselves or others. This is probably the easiest way to get members of an IEP team to agree to a one-to-one aide, but playing cops and robbers is probably the least productive way for the aide and the child to spend their time together. When aides *are* assigned for behavioral control purposes, a school psychologist or behavior management specialist should be enlisted to devise a behavior management plan to reduce noncompliant and dangerous behaviors as quickly as possible so that the child can use some one-to-one time for learning. One-to-one behavioral control of autistic children is not the same as for other developmentally delayed children. (This will be discussed in detail in the next chapter.) For example, constant high intrusion (like the aide sitting in back of the child during circle time and keeping her legs wrapped around his) is likely to accelerate negative behaviors rather than provide some kind of effective containment and limit-setting as it might with another mentally retarded child. Instead, the aide needs to be helped to find situations where she can be with the child where the triggers for negative behaviors are absent, and the opportunity to display negative behaviors is controlled as much as possible by removing things the autistic child will find overstimulating or aversive (like too much physical contact). One-to-one time is a valuable resource, and, in a good classroom, it should be put to instructional rather than managerial use, if at all possible.

Mainstreaming and Full Inclusion

"Mainstreaming" and "full inclusion" have become the latest buzzwords in special education. *Mainstreaming* refers to putting a special education student into the mainstream, that is, into non–special education classes as a kind of a special education environment. If that sounds like a Catch-22, it is. The logic is that if you need special education you can benefit from mainstreaming. But mainstreaming means *not* being in special education; in which case, you are being educated like someone who *really* does not need special education. One type of mainstreaming is *full inclusion,* which means being fully main-streamed.

Mainstreaming and full inclusion are positive words. They sound much better than saying that the school district can save money by partly or fully depriving a child of the special help he or she needs to best overcome a learning disability. The term mainstreaming is a great example of Orwellian doublespeak—implying that something that is nothing *is* something. If I sound negative about mainstreaming—I am. There is relatively little research on the effects of mainstreaming autistic children, and even less on full inclusion. What little research there is does not support the ultility of mainstreaming for autistic and PDD children as it is most often carried out in public schools. Nevertheless, the PC (politically correct) revolution has launched main-streaming as a keystone of special education policy in many areas in the United States.

Is there a role for mainstreaming children with autism and PDD? Defi-nitely, yes. In this section, I'll qualify that "yes." There are several factors that need to be considered. First is the developmental level of the child in the area for which he is to be mainstreamed. The second is the child's social mental age. The third is the type of instructional support that will be available in the mainstreamed setting.

Limitations to Mainstreaming for Autistic and PDD Children

One of the chief limitations in using mainstreaming as an educational method for autistic and PDD children is the children's lack of spontaneous imitation, and more specifically their lack of social mimicry. As we discussed in Chapter 9, early intervention programs now often focus on teaching imitation so that the child with autism or PDD can learn more readily. Some children with PDD never have significant imitation problems to begin with, but just don't imitate spontaneously very often. Even after imitation skills are acquired through special instruction, imitation tends to occur only when requested ("Look at me!" "Do this!") rather than spontaneously, in response to some-thing the child sees someone else doing (and therefore wants to do himself). Not only do autistic children tend to imitate only on request, but they also tend to imitate only things that are happening quite close by, rather than things that are happening farther away. (The tendency to preferentially attend to things close by is probably a way of fending off a sense of being overstimu-lated by too many things.) This tendency to prefer closer (more proximal) stimulation further limits how an autistic or PDD child takes things in when in a classroom setting and makes it difficult to understand that if everyone in the class is doing one thing, it would be considered natural for him or her to do that one thing, too. I mentioned earlier that having a lot of routine and struc-ture helps children with autism and PDD in a classroom setting because they learn what to expect. A structured routine is also helpful because it helps circumvent the need to be constantly aware of what everyone else is doing and to begin doing it, too. If there is too much unpredictable change, most autistic and PDD children become overwhelmed and become more withdrawn or behaviorally difficult. This is because they have to work so much harder to imitate (follow what others are doing) compared to following pre-set "rules."

In addition to the difficulties that many autistic and PDD children have with imitation, almost all lack a desire to do things just because everyone else in the group is doing them. This can present a barrier to learning in preschool and the early elementary grades, as much instruction is predicated on following the leader (like doing an art project where everyone is pasting a brown tree trunk on a piece of paper, and then everyone is pasting a ball of green leaves on the paper, etc.). Most often, autistic and PDD children are not motivated to complete a task just to join in. Instead, they are motivated by their own internal system of rewards based on what pleases them, rather than what pleases others. This means that in a preschool art project the autistic child is just as likely to paste the trunk on sideways and to paste the leaves on himself, as he is to do it the way everyone else does. (This type of instrumental motivation will be discussed in detail in the next chapter.) The bottom line is that it most often takes extra help to integrate autistic children into a "mainstreamed" classroom because the others are more socially motivated whereas the autistic child is more instrumentally motivated. This is different from mainstreaming a non-autistic, developmentally disabled child who will tend to try what everyone else is doing, but may need more adult intervention to succeed.

Prerequisites to Mainstreaming Autistic and PDD Children

Proponents of mainstreaming tend to imply that it works like magic. Just put a child with a disability in a regular class and he'll learn to act "regular." Certainly there is considerable value in providing more normal role models for learning specific skills and for peer interaction. However, the autistic child needs to be *taught* how to join in these activities. It doesn't just happen to him naturally. Mainstreaming, done appropriately, is not just throwing the baby bird out of the nest to see if it will fly; it needs to be a gradual and supported procedure, with an adult helping the autistic child make the transition by stepping through activities with him and gradually pulling back as the child achieves mastery.

The first thing that needs to be considered is the purpose of the mainstreaming. There are two general goals: academic mainstreaming and social mainstreaming. Academic mainstreaming will be discussed further in Chapter 13. The purpose of academic mainstreaming is to assure that the child gets to learn at a rate that best stimulates his cognitive potential—especially if that child has a normal rate of learning in a particular area. Social mainstreaming is more often the goal with autistic children, especially young autistic children. The purpose of social mainstreaming is to give the child an opportunity to learn how children his or her own age play together and generally carry on in group situations.

Reverse Mainstreaming in the Special Education Class

Most often, mainstreaming consists of having the autistic child in a class with "typical" non–special education students. In such cases typical students are the majority, and the special education students being mainstreamed are the minority. Such classrooms focus on the typical children's emerging skills—not necessarily on the special education student's emerging skills. Therefore, if the special education student is not at or above the cognitive level of the typical children, he can be left in the dust, and that doesn't feel good to any child.

Reverse mainstreaming was developed as an alternative form of mainstreaming in which typical students are brought into the special education setting. Advantages of this approach include the fact that the instruction is still mainly geared to the developmental level of the special education students, that the special education students get to stay in a familiar environment, and that they are not as likely to be outnumbered by typical students who can form their own "critical mass" and exclude the special education students. There may also be advantages of destigmatizing special education for the typical children by letting them see and play with the materials in the special education class.

The Use of "Shadow" Aides in Early Education Mainstreaming

More often in the United States and quite routinely in Canada, autistic and PDD preschoolers are integrated into regular preschool education with the use of what is most aptly described as a shadow aide. Typically, the child is ready for such mainstreaming when she has the same cognitive skills as other preschoolers—such as knowing letters, numbers, the names of animals, and so on, even though language use may still be lagging. It also helps if the child has been taught some play "scripts," that is, age-appropriate activities and toys found in a preschool classroom. The shadow aide serves as a sort of Jiminy Cricket (to use a Pinocchio analogy), quietly assisting the child to do the right things. The "right things" can include paying attention to a group activity, following through on directions that have been given, or using play scripts to initiate or sustain play with other children.

Preschool mainstreaming is much less appropriate for the child who does not yet have any of the preschool level cognitive skills. If a three-year-old autistic child is still playing with toys in a primarily sensorimotor fashion (banging, sucking, feeling, looking), and doesn't know basic preschool pre-academic concepts, it's going to be very hard for that child to derive any meaning from the mainstreamed preschool environment. It would be like taking a mathematically bright five-year-old who can already add and subtract and putting him in a high school algebra class. Yes, with an aide, you could get the five-year-old to stay in his seat in the high school class. With an aide, the child could also use the time to learn multiplication and division—but nothing would be gained from the environment around the child. The five-year-old could not extract any more meaning from an algebra class than a mainstreamed three-year-old autistic child if he's cognitively at an eighteen-month level of development.

However, a three-year-old autistic child who is cognitively at the eighteen-month level of development *might* benefit from more socially appropriate role models who are at *his* developmental level—eighteen months. This may mean placing the child in a special education class with other children who also have fifty percent cognitive delays, but who are socially more gregarious than an autistic child. For example, children with Down syndrome or children with attention deficit disorder often are quite persistently social and may pair up well with autistic children who are in their class. In a sense, this is still a form of mainstreaming, because it is still predicated on the idea that the autistic child will learn social skills from someone whose social skills are better than his own. However, if the autistic child still markedly lacks imitation, no such tranfer of skills may occur. In this case, the child may still benefit from being in a class designated for autistic children where acquiring imitation is a major curriculum focus.

Peer Tutoring

For children who still have major difficulties with imitating, especially imitating more social activities such as reciprocal games and toy play, "peer tutoring" may be a more suitable approach. Peer tutoring occurs when a slightly older student is recruited as a special buddy or helper for a younger special education student. The idea is that an older child can be more persistent in getting the younger autistic child to do things, without being perceived by the autistic child in the same way an adult is—who is inherently less fun. Many elementary schools have formal or informal peer tutoring programs. For the older, non–special education student, the motivation to participate in peer tutoring is altruistic—wanting to help another child. Elementary teachers often like certain students to be involved in peer tutoring because it exposes them to students with disabilities and may help sensitize a child who otherwise has not spent much time thinking about other people. For more bossy children, peer tutoring can be a constructive outlet.

Typically the peer tutor does not need much training—in fact, significant amounts of training might defeat the purpose. Often, a peer tutor can just be guided with simple instructions like "Demonte really doesn't know how to play with trucks, why don't you show him," or "Kendra never plays with the dolls; why don't you go over there and show her how to feed them and put them to bed?" Sometimes a few tips to the peer tutor, such as "Demonte/Kendra might not want to play, but you try to get them to play with you anyway," authorizes the peer tutor to be a bit officious—which is likely to be necessary. As long as the peer tutor is not so young that he or she just goes off and plays with the toys him- or herself, this can be a useful approach.

Peer tutoring can be implemented at home by hiring a "junior" babysitter at a discounted rate to come over just to play with an autistic child. Usually I prefer same-sex peer tutors, because—to the extent that autistic children play with toys—they usually enjoy more gender-specific play. When I talk about peer tutoring with parents, some automatically point to their autistic child's older sibling. This is acceptable, but not wonderful. The sibling naturally has plenty of opportunities for interacting with his or her brother or sister. Peer tutoring should be cast as a "job." A sibling should not be put in the position of having to be "hired" or "fired" from the job, depending upon how well the job's goals are achieved. Neighborhood kids, friends of older siblings, cousins, and children the family might know from a Sunday school are good potential peer tutors.

Day Care and Social Mainstreaming

One nice way of achieving both kinds of mainstreaming we've discussed (with comparable mental-age peers, and with older peers) is to place the child in a mixed-age day care arrangement. Many parents need after school care for their autistic children anyway because they are working, or they could benefit from the respite time to take siblings to Little League or Girl Scouts. In my opinion, family day care (someone who cares for a small group of children in her own home) is often the best way to achieve this. If an autistic child is four, it is likely that the parallel play of two-year-olds will attract most of his spontaneous interest, but if a few six- and seven-year-olds include him too sometimes, this provides a form of peer tutoring. Having a small consistent group of peers makes it easier for the autistic or PDD child to form friendships; in a larger peer group, like a preschool, a typical four-year-old will quickly give up and try elsewhere if another four-year-old he approaches doesn't answer back fairly promptly. If there are a limited number of others to play with, a nonautistic child is likely to be a bit more persistent.

Most after-school day care is free-form play, nonacademic and unstructured, except perhaps for a snack or nap time. To me, school is for instruction—and on that account is a precious resource, to be used for learning, not peer socialization. After-school day care provides an excellent opportunity for socialization—*after* the part of the day when available instruction has taken place.

Chapter Summary

In this chapter we've discussed what you'll see when you visit different sorts of classrooms. In particular, we've focused on attributes of teachers and aides, and how they use their time, as well as the importance of taking into account the range of developmental disabilities being served in the classroom, and we've given some criteria for deciding whether mainstreaming might be appropriate for a particular child. In the next chapter, we will discuss hands-on behavioral and educational techniques specific to working with children with autism and PDD.

◆ ◆ ◆

CHAPTER 11

Behavior Management and Teaching Methods for Children with Autism and PDD

The central issue in the education of children with autism and PDD is the ways in which they learn differently. The Individual Education Program (IEP) as the name implies, is an individualized educational plan, based on the assumption that every special educational student has a somewhat different profile of problems that need specific remediation. The idea of special education is to provide an environment for learning in which the child can be taught at a slower pace, with more emphasis on particular subjects, and appropriate instructional techniques so as to help him compensate for his difficulties. In this chapter, we will focus on special methods of instruction that work particularly well with many autistic and PDD children. Thus far, we have discussed different types of classrooms. Which type of class a child is offered depends in part on how far behind he is when he starts school, and how specific his deficits are.

Once a child is assigned to a class, there is the matter of *how* to teach the child. In addition to knowing specific instructional methods and strategies, teachers of autistic children must have considerable expertise in the application of the principles of behavior management when working with autistic children. Therefore, the first part of this chapter will deal with applying principles of behavior management to autistic and PDD children in the classroom. The second part of the chapter will cover specific curriculum concepts and special education instructional methods as they apply to the special learning disabilities most often found in children with autism and PDD.

Since the first part of this chapter deals with approaches to behavior management, I'll clarify now what this term means. *Behavior management* largely refers to the application of principles of behavior modification, or what is also sometimes referred to as learning theory in experimental research. For some, the term "behavior modification" has negative connotations. These negative connotations may come from having watched too many TV news-docu-dramas—ones that show out-of-control, severely retarded teenagers being shocked with electrical devices, being exposed to loud, high-frequency sounds, or being tied down to chairs. These methods, collectively referred to as "physical aversives," are virtually outlawed by educational and residential care facilities today. While aversives of these sorts can be used as part of a behavior modification strategy, they seldom are, simply because they are considered inhumane. The types of behavior modification approaches that will be discussed here involve the use of "positive" teaching strategies. The main types of "physical aversives" that will be covered are a few things that autistic children find aversive, but that other children mainly view as rewards (such as being confined by a tight hug).

Primary and Social Rewards in the Classroom

A big issue is how best to reinforce positive behavior and positive attention to learning tasks so that the child will do more. There are several considerations here. The first concern is whether or not the child understands the concept of doing something desirable and then getting a reward for it. Children who have "social ages" below about the six-month level have usually not yet figured out that a particular behavior may bring them a desired consequence. Usually children who don't yet understand this type of cause-and-effect are very young or very developmentally delayed. Occasionally, there are also children who live in such chaotic, unpredictable environments that there has been no opportunity to figure out this basic principle of human interaction.

Instrumental Learning

Although autistic children have difficulty figuring out most principles of human interaction, they are usually pretty astute about cause-and-effect principles, especially in *instrumental* contexts. This means that the autistic child is usually quite good at understanding what he needs to do to get something he wants for himself. Parents usually first notice this with respect to a desired food. For example, the child may use his only verbalization to obtain a really desired food. The autistic child will try his hardest when the issue is obtaining something *he* wants (as opposed to something others want for him) like being a "big boy").

Constructing a Reward Hierarchy

The first thing to do in devising a reward system that will work for a particular autistic or PDD child is to ask "What does the child find rewarding?" A list may start with foods and also include particular activities like tickling or interactions with particular objects. Initially the list may not contain social rewards, like being called a "big boy" or being told "good job." It is important to think realistically about what the child in *his* view values the most. Next, a short list should be made of things the child can be given in small, metered amounts. If

Table 4 Reward Hierarchies

Mostly Primary Rewards (meets child's instrumental needs)	Mostly Social Rewards (acquired in association with primary rewards)
*Favorite foods *Favorite activities *Sensory stimulation (clapping, tickling, patting) *Termination of an undesirable activity	*Cheering *Verbal praise *Smiling *Token economies/ Delayed gratification

he like graham crackers, a graham cracker can be broken into ten pieces. A container of apple juice can be meted out in many, many separate sips. In general, food reinforcers are good ones because a food is something "appropriate." Sensory reinforcers—a toy that the child likes to look at, tap, or hold in a certain way may be just as reinforcing, or even more reinforcing than a food, but it should be used sparingly, because using it as a reward also reinforces the atypical behavior associated with its use. However, for children to whom food reinforcers mean little, a sensory reinforcer may be one of the only alternatives. Table 4 summarizes some of the concepts behind reward hierarchies we will discuss.

Initially, social rewards may mean little. The child may ignore verbal praise and even find physical reinforcers such as a pat on the cheek to be aversive. Through "paired-association" learning, however, the child can be trained to respond positively to the reinforcers that other non-autistic children respond to. This means that when the child is reinforced with a sip of apple juice, an enthusiastic "Good girl!" should be given as well. Some autistic and PDD children really like vestibular (movement) stimulation and so a tickle, a squeeze, or a bounce may be a more "normal" sensory reinforcer that can accompany foods used as a reward. Over time, the pairing of food or sensory (primary) rewards with more social rewards will cause the positive effects of the primary rewards to rub off onto the social rewards. (This is what is meant by "paired-association" learning.) Gradually, the food rewards can be taken away, or "faded" and social rewards can become the main mode of reinforcing appropriate behavior and responses in a teaching situation. As the child becomes more responsive to social rewards, it is easier for him to function in a group instructional setting where the teacher does not have to be within arm's reach to give the reward, but can verbalize "Good job!" from a distance.

Reinforcement Schedules

How often should primary rewards be used? When should they be faded? How do you know when to change reinforcers? These are all questions pertaining to the construction of a reinforcement schedule. A general principle is that the more unfamiliar the task, the more undesirable the task is likely to be for the autistic child. Thus, more frequent rewards will be needed. Some autistic and PDD children who stay on-task well after getting social rewards for familiar tasks will need a return to primary reinforcers when beginning a new, more difficult, or intrinsically less interesting task. Reinforcers should preferably be given for successful task completions. However, if a new task is very difficult for a child, she may need to be reinforced periodically for just maintaining an attempt to do the work, or for steps in the completion of the work. As the child becomes more proficient at an activity, the successful completion of the task itself will likely be, to some degree, rewarding. Then the reinforcement schedule can be cut down to one reward at the completion of every few tasks instead of one reward at the end of every task. As long as a child seems interested in doing more work, there is no reason to keep popping food in his mouth, or interrupting his concentration with clapping for successful completions. For example, on a familiar four-piece puzzle, a child may be eager to do more puzzles just by being verbally praised when the puzzle is complete. If that child is given an eight-piece puzzle she has never seen, she may need food reinforcers every thirty seconds or every minute—as long as she continues moving pieces around trying to find a solution (or watching as she is being shown the solution).

A child should never be given any reinforcer as a "bribe" to become interested in the task while the child is actively off-task. The bribe strategy will only reinforce off-task behavior. Similarly, a child should not be given a reinforcer to soothe crying or quiet tantrums or other protest. The effect will be to reinforce the undesirable behavior. A reinforcer can be given as a protesting child pauses in his shrieking for few seconds as a way of reinforcing the deceleration of the undesirable behavior. (As soon as the deceleration is reinforced, the child should be quickly re-directed back to the task he was doing, or to an easier form of the task so as to sustain the focused attention that the child has probably directed to the reinforcer.)

When using reinforcers of any type, it is important to vary them so that the child does not become satiated. As wonderful as the first M&M may be, after five, ten, or fifteen (or for some children, fifty), they will become less wonderful. Having a variety of primary reinforcers on hand, and well as a variety of sensory, play, and verbal reinforcers that can be used is important in the reward's quality. Rewards can be varied as task difficulty varies—for example, with food rewards used toward the beginning of a new task, and verbal rewards toward the end of a task, when the child can see he is almost done, and the reenforcing qualities of the task completion itself becomes more apparent to the child.

Sometimes when beginning to introduce an autistic child to functioning in a group setting, it is helpful if the group is doing work that is relatively easy for him. That way, he can stay with what is going on without needing frequent or primary reinforcers. When an autistic or PDD child is initially instructed in a group (especially after having been acclimated to significant amounts of one-to-one instruction), the group setting itself may be perceived as aversive. Therefore, a task that is easy for him to do one-to-one (for example, recognizing a card with his name printed on it), may seem "harder" in the group setting and should be reinforced as such. This is because autistic children often perceive the group situation as negative; which is in contrast to other, non-autistic children who may find it *more* rewarding to show what they know in a group setting. For the teacher who has had little or no previous experience teaching autistic or PDD children, this is an important point. Group situations are basically non-reinforcing, and this is one main way that autistic and PDD children are different from other special education students. They do not want to show off for peers or be admired by them, and at first, will mainly work to maintain their isolation (such as by staring at their hands or "spacing out") when placed in a group cooperative learning setting.

Token Economies

As children get older, they begin to be able to tolerate more delay of gratification and will work longer for a reward that comes at the end of the task. Most special education classes, and many regular elementary classrooms, have some sort of a *token economy* system. In a token economy, a child accumulates "points" over some period of time that can be later traded in for a reward. Usually, the longer the wait, the bigger the reward. A token economy can be considered a more natural reward system, a little like getting a paycheck once a week or once a month. It is also easier for a teacher to manage than giving M&M's every fifteen seconds.

Sometimes, though, autistic and PDD children have a hard time changing over from a primary or sensory immediate reward system to a token system. The tokens tend to be too abstract a concept to comprehend—as a promise of goods-in-the-future is really a social contract. A gradual transition between immediate rewards and a token system can, however, be designed for an autistic or PDD child if the principles of the system are introduced gradually and visually. For example: Step 1—Reinforce on the same schedule, but deposit the reinforcers into a cup with a small hole on top using the word "later." At the end of the activity period, let the child have all his reinforcers at once. Step 2—Increase the period of time that the reinforcers accumulate. Step 3—Deposit surrogate reinforcers (paper chips that look like M&M's, Fruit Loops, or whatever). At the end of the activity, count out the tokens and exchange them for their equivalent in real M&M's (or whatever). Step 4—At exchange time, give the child a choice between the several small reinforcers he's earned, or one big reinforcer (for example, twenty raisins for one fig bar). Step 5—Switch to a picture of the reinforcer cup and make marks with a pencil to represent points that are exchanged for rewards at the end of the day or at the end of the week. Not all children may need to be taken through all steps. But, if a child is in a class where other students function on a token economy (as is often the case in many elementary school classes that PDD children find themselves in), it is reasonable to plan to help the PDD child become better integrated into this aspect of his classroom milieu.

Reducing Interfering Negative Behavior

One of the great challenges in working with autistic children is in how to reduce negative behavior to the point where they can be easily instructed. Probably the greatest cause of burnout among really talented teachers of autistic children is having to deal with so much negative behavior. Negative behavior is behavior that is disruptive to, or incompatible with learning, or incompatible with what the child is supposed to be doing. This includes screaming, lying on the floor and refusing to get up, running out of the classroom, knocking over furniture and toys, and other things that no one really wants to deal with. There are a variety of methods that may be useful in the control of negative behavior, and which technique is used depends on how disruptive and hard-to-eliminate the child's negative behavior is. The methods we will discuss here (which are summarized in Table 5) are *ignoring, mild aversives, time-outs,* and *physical aversives.*

Ignoring. Many negative behaviors can be extinguished by ignoring them. This is particularly true in a one-to-one instructional setting when the child begins to act silly or decides to test a teacher's limits. Ignoring a child's negative behavior takes away one aspect of the child's reinforcement—your attention and aggravation. Autistic and PDD children often seem to perceive emotional response in others in "absolute value"—irrespective of the positive or negative valence others might attach. Many will work as hard to get a negative response from an adult as a positive response. It is as if they are reinforced by the excitation value of the interaction. In addition, the child's negative behaviors are often easier to produce (for example, climbing on a desk top) than are the behaviors that produce positive responses (for example, finishing the puzzle on top of the desk). By ignoring the child, at least some of the reinforcement value (fun) goes out of the negative behavior. Then, if the adult pays positive attention to any renewed attention to the task at hand, the child's positive behavior is being more strongly reinforced. Ignoring, done correctly, can work fairly well some of the time, especially if it is instituted before the child gets really wound up. However, if the child becomes self-

Table 5 Eliminating Negative Behaviors

Ignoring. "Short-circuiting" the emotional charge from negative behavior

Mild Aversives. Examples: Negative or slightly loud voice; unsolicited physical holding

Time-out. Time to defuse, "clear buffers," separate from antecedent (cause) of negative behavior

Physical Aversives. Spanking or grabbing (for endangering behavior); more forceful physical restraint

stimulated enough by his own negative behavior, it will be hard to cancel out the negative behavior simply by ignoring it.

How do you ignore an autistic child? Don't autistic children like being ignored? Using an ignore strategy with them *is* more difficult than with other children. The ignoring must include a withdrawal of social attention and also a withdrawal of as much stimulation as possible. For example, if a child has gone off-task by flapping a piece of paper he should be writing on, holding the paper flat on the table while ignoring him should help. If the child grabs at the paper and tears it up, grabbing his hands firmly and holding them together on the surface of the desk (while still looking away and ignoring the child visually and verbally) would be the next step. Most of the time, ignoring is a good behavior modification strategy when the child is simply faltering in completing a task. A simple "ignore" would be looking away for a few seconds while withdrawing expression from your face. As soon as the child returns some attention to task, you should look back, give some verbal praise, and smile. The preceding "ignore" will tend to have an amplifying effect on the praise that follows it.

Ignoring can also be used to interrupt more aversive behaviors. Say, for example, a child is sorting cards with animals, buildings, and vehicles into different piles and begins to bite each card before placing it. A loud "No!" in a neutral tone of voice, followed by taking back the card abruptly, and making a solemn face and looking down for a few seconds will probably result in the child correctly placing the card when you hand it back a few seconds later. If the child accelerates instead and reaches to spread all the cards all over the table, another loud "No!" plus quickly retrieving the piles of cards so that the child cannot proceed further (and ignoring cards on the floor) comes next. A more prolonged solemn look, plus a sharp turn away from the child with arms folded, can further emphasize the withdrawal of attention. As soon as you hear the child settle down a little, turn back, smile, give an encouraging "Good!" and proceed. Some children continue to accelerate further, and other mild aversives may have to be added.

There are times when a child will try to get you to do the ignoring "game" five or six times in a row. If he consistently gets the same (unrewarding) consequences from the game, his negative behavior will simply become extinguished. Ignoring can work best when the child is in a fairly structured or contained setting, like a high chair or in a small cubicle, where the opportunities for accelerating negative behavior are more easily controlled by the teacher.

Mild Aversives. A lot of people will say that they don't like the idea of using any aversives. Actually, we all use aversives of various degrees in all our social interactions. Aversives do not have to be physical, and they don't have to hurt the child. In fact, there are some things that children with autism or PDD find aversive that other children find pleasurable. These constitute some of the most mild aversives and can be quite effective. For example, in getting the attention of an autistic child, reaching for his face and orienting it toward yours as you speak may be perceived as aversive by the autistic child. If you release his face as soon as he begins to respond, you are reinforcing the responding. If the child knows he must speak to have his face released, he will try to say something. (A few very clever little autistic children discover they can close their eyes and avoid much of the unpleasantness of having their face held directly toward another person's face—this method doesn't work well for them.) If the child knows that his face will be held if he does not attend when spoken to, he will attend better to avoid having his face held. Most non-autistic children, however, like being touched gently on the face, and enjoy direct eye contact with a teacher or parent; for them, the procedure is not aversive at all.

Some other mild aversives are designed to counterbalance negative behaviors that are accompanied by over-excitation. My personal favorite is to gently but firmly hold an autistic child's hands down in front of him on a table while saying "No" in either a soft or loud tone of voice, depending on how difficult I feel it will be to extinguish the negative behavior. Other methods of gentle physical restriction, like holding a child in his seat by resting your hands on his shoulders, may accomplish the same thing. Another way of breaking into overexcited off-task behavior (like flicking a block that should be getting stacked) is to abruptly pull the material away from the child. This "clears the field" and gives you an opportunity to start over again after the child has had a few seconds to get calmer. Also, at that point, he is no longer engaged in the negative behavior because the stimulus for it has been removed.

Autistic children often fill the void of having nothing to do by starting a new, negative behavior. Therefore, in using ignoring or mild aversives to stop a behavior, there must be great sensitivity to the pace of the interaction. You can't expect a three-, four-, or five-year-old autistic child to sit perfectly still for ten-seconds as "punishment" for off-task behavior. Without a doubt, the child, in the absence of other, more positive stimulation will think up another negative behavior before the ten seconds is up (like staring at his fingers, flapping, or humming). Therefore, positive redirections onto a more appropriate activity should be initiated as soon as the negative behavior is decelerating. This means that if an autistic child is waving his crayon around (rather than coloring with it), it should be taken away, but handed back almost immediately—but with initial hand-over-hand guidance to keep the crayon on the paper.

Accompanied Time-Outs. A very powerful method for controlling behavior is time-outs. Time-outs work very differently for children with autism and PDD than they do for other children, however. The purpose of a time-out period is to punish a child for misbehavior by isolating him, giving him time to calm down, and giving him time to reflect on his misdeeds. Usually time-outs are used for specific, predefined violations like hitting another child on the playground, stealing someone else's toy after a warning not to, or overturning a chair or desk. With children who are not autistic, the child is usually sat in the back of the room facing a wall, or out in the hallway by himself. This type of time-out works poorly for autistic and PDD children because, by and large, they do not find isolation to be aversive.

Parents come see me and say "Time-outs don't work for my child." I say, "Tell me how the teacher does them." The parent says, "Well, they sit Jose out in the hall—but in five minutes when the teacher comes back, Jose has run over to the playground and is swinging and having a great time." So I say, "If you didn't like math, and every time you had to do math you could go have a free cappuccino instead, just by turning over your desk, do you think you would be trashing your desk more or less over time?" The isolation of time-outs is generally very reinforcing to autistic children. At home, parents can make the same mistake by sending a child to his room alone for a time-out. In fact, parents have often observed that when they return to their autistic child's room after a half-hour "time-out," the child is playing contentedly or has gone to sleep. If time-outs are used the same way for autistic and PDD children as for other children, the negative behavior will be reinforced.

So how do you make the time-outs aversive? Most importantly, the time-out needs to be *accompanied*. An accompanied time-out *is* more work for the teacher, aide, or parent, but it will be much more effective. When the bad behavior occurs, the child is removed from the "scene of the crime" and taken to a designated spot in the classroom (or home) for time-outs. This should be a place where the child has little to look at and nothing in his reach to do. Some classrooms have an adjacent walk-in supply closet they can use. Some teachers even use a big cardboard box (like from a washing machine) with a flap of fabric over the front. One point of the time-out is to give the child a chance to empty his overflowed "buffers." However, someone must stay with the child to make sure he does not try to leave, and also does not experience positive effects of isolation. A good way for the adult to make his presence known is to count. With two- and three-year-olds, I usually suggest a count of ten or twenty; thirty to fifty for older children. (Some children learn the sequence of the alphabet before counting. For these children, extending a time-out for the duration of a recitation of the alphabet may be a better way to mark time.) If the child is still resisting the time-out at the end of the count, the adult starts the counting over. This goes on as long as necessary. Initially, time-outs can be very long. Then, the child may get himself another time-out as soon as he is finished with the first by testing the parent by returning to the forbidden activity. The parent must be prepared to immediately give another time-out. While this is time-consuming, it shows the child that no matter how hard he tries, his negative behavior will always be timed-out. It is typical for children to initially respond to the use of time-outs by trying even harder to do the wrong thing to see if the punishment *still* happens. (The technical description for this type of behavior is an "extinction burst.") After an extinction burst, the rate of the undesirable behavior tends to go way down.

Eventually, a child will learn to sit and calm himself fairly quickly in order to end the time-out (if the time-out is being done in a way he really finds aversive). The time-out is not the moment to explain to the child what he did wrong or to negotiate future behavior. It is not a time for a soothing tone of voice or for a parent or teacher to tell the child she's sorry he's so upset. The adult should not directly interact with the child during the time-out, but stay there more as a form of human restraint. If there is concern that the child may attempt to leave the time-out, having the adult stand in back of the child with his hands on the child's shoulders may be sufficient. As children get bigger, it can be difficult to keep a really agitated child seated for a time-out. In these cases, there are two alternative positions that some teachers use. The first is to have the child sit cross-legged on the floor with arms crossed. The child's arms can be restrained from behind if necessary with a big bear hug. Another position is the "turtle" position, in which the child crouches on his knees and elbows with head down. This can be particularly helpful for an over-excited autistic child who needs to calm down, as the turtle position limits movement and visual stimulation.

When the time-out is over, it is important that the child immediately be positively redirected back into an acceptable activity. This may be the activity he was involved in before the time-out, or something else. If it is possible to remove antecedents of the behavior that caused the time-out, that's helpful too. If the child hit another child with a truck, it would be better to return him to a different area of the classroom away from the other student, and to give him another toy.

Physical Aversives. Physical aversives are perhaps the most controversial topic in the treatment of autistic children. Most maligned is electric shock, a method that is no longer used except in very rare cases of severe, intractable, serious, self-injurious behaviors (sometimes called SIBS) that do not respond to behavioral or psychopharmacological interventions. I have recommended electric shock only twice in the last 1,500 children I've seen (intractable SIBS in autistic children are *very* rare). One was Jenny, a fourteen-year-old severely retarded autistic girl who was hitting her head so hard that, even with a helmet on, she had caused intracranial bleeding and had almost detached an optic nerve (which would cause permanent blindness). The other, Brady, was a moderately retarded seven-year-old autistic boy who was hitting the side of his head so hard that he had recurrent bleeding into the ear; he had lost part of his hearing and part of his external ear on one side. For both Jenny and Brady, intensive behavioral interventions in their schools had failed, as had a number of medication trials. The type of electrical shock that is recommended for children like Brady and Jenny is usually conveyed by a helmet that has a motion detector and a small electrode attached to the child's thigh. When the motion of head-banging or head-hitting is detected, it is followed by a mild shock to the thigh. The immediacy of the response, and the unpleasantness of the shock (which is not a dangerous dose), tends to stop the child cold. Usually, the interval to the next SIB is longer, and in a brief period of time (sometimes a couple of hours), the behavior disappears altogether. However, the child may later realize that when the helmet is off, he can't be shocked, and the helmet (or *a* helmet) may have to remain in place for some time.

American parents do not need to worry about schools using serious physical aversives, and certainly not electrical shock. It is against the law in U.S. schools. Nevertheless it is worth discussing physical aversives here, and learning more about what they can and can't do to change behavior. One concern about physical aversives that is raised by learning theorists is that when behaviors learned through aversive conditioning are withdrawn, the behavior fades more quickly than if it is learned through positive forms of reinforcement (as the example with the SIBS helmet suggests). Another problem with using physical aversives on some autistic children is that many have a diminished pain response (a high pain threshold or tolerance). For example, some parents of autistic children will notice that their children don't respond negatively when they are spanked, and so spanking does not deter the behavior for which the child is being punished.

There are times when limited physical aversives may have a natural role: Arlo, an autistic three-year-old was a major hair-puller—particularly his six-year-old sister's. At first, Arlo's parents, solid upper middle class liberals, preached endless forbearance to the six-year-old. Late one afternoon when everyone was irritable, Arlo pulled his sister's hair again, and this time, Arlo's mother gave his sister permission to pull Arlo's blond ringlets in return. She did. After that, Arlo didn't pull his sister's hair anymore. (Psychologists call this one-trial learning.)

Spanking. Although spanking children isn't allowed in school, it is a form of discipline that some families choose to use on all their children. Parents who use spanking as a judicious punishment will have set clear limits as to what kinds of bad behaviors incur spanking. When I am asked about spanking an autistic child, I give parents the following guidelines: If other children in the family get spanked, then the autistic child should, too. (The other children should not feel their autistic sibling is exempt from the family's rules.) However, if the child has a diminished pain response, spanking probably isn't going to be very effective, anyway. The child should only be punished for those things that it is reasonable for a child of his mental age to understand and control. Finally, spanking should be limited to behaviors of the child that endanger himself or others, like running out into the street, pushing a toddler from a moving swing, or heaving heavy objects into an occupied bassinet.

Restraint. Another form of physical aversive is forcible restraint. Sometimes, in the process of a time-out procedure, the restraint needed to maintain the time-out can get fairly forceful. Forcible restraint is best carried out in as nonintrusive a way as possible. As long as the restraint doesn't turn into a wrestling match, the child shouldn't get hurt. The adult providing the restraint is always in the role of monitoring how soon the restraint can be minimized or released.

Another type of physical restraint is obtained from mechanical devices. Restraining a child mechanically with straps and bars is unacceptable. Occasionally I visit infant or preschool classes with special chairs that are intended to restrain/support the legs and arms of children with severe cerebral palsy. These chairs can be fine for children who have little or no muscle strength and need the support to stay upright. Sometimes, however, these chairs get used to force autistic children to stay put. Occasionally, autistic children will break or strain a wrist, ankle, or forearm struggling to get out of such devices. At school and at home, an autistic child should not be physically restrained by anything more confining than a high chair or a stroller.

Autistic children and adults tend to panic when physically restrained, especially if they are not able to understand enough language to know why the restraint is being used. I've seen a number of young autistic children who have injured themselves when being put in "papooses" in hospital emergency rooms. Papooses are meant to be used to physically immobilize a small child in emergencies during which the child might need a local anesthetic to get stitches or where his own movement might create more severe injury. When an autistic child is injured, it might be safer to consider a general anesthetic rather than a papoose. On occasion I've even learned of physical restraints being used to immobilize an autistic child for an EEG (brain test) or a BSER (hearing test). This is particularly horrifying, as the child is being put in physical danger for what should be a noninvasive procedure. Similarly, the occasional adult autistic person who becomes violent can injure himself if put in full body restraints by paramedics who don't know that autistic people can hate confinement enough to break their own thumb or wrist trying to escape from it.

So far in this chapter, we have discussed the application of behavior management principles to working with autistic children in classrooms, and to some extent at home too. The rest of this chapter deals with specific curriculum concepts in special education and early education and how they can be applied to designing day-to-day educational activities for autistic and PDD children.

Methods of Instruction

Cross-Modal and Multi-Modal Information Processing

A main idea in special education that has specific applications to the instruction of children with autism and PDD is the idea of *cross-modal* transfer of information. Basically, the idea is that if a child has difficulty perceiving information on one sensory channel, then the child should be helped to use another channel to compensate for that difficulty.

Visual to Auditory Transfer of Information. With autistic and PDD children in particular, the "language channel" is often the weakest. This is often the case with children who seem able to tune out much of the language addressed to them, and do not easily learn new words just by hearing other people use them. These children do not learn language "incidentally," meaning just by hearing other people talk (as opposed to language directed especially at them). There are a variety of reasons why autistic and PDD children seem to be "word-deaf" (or at least "word-hard-of-hearing"); this was discussed in Chapter 3. One idea for educating such a child is to supplement the weak signal on the language channel with a channel that gets better reception. For many autistic and PDD children, a stronger channel is the visual one. Therefore, pairing auditory stimuli with visual stimuli helps information be received and stored differently. In a little while, we'll discuss how this idea can be applied to language instruction through the use of communication boards and sign language. The main idea, however, is to think of ways of tying language to a visual representation.

In particular, using attention-getting visual representations (things the child *likes* to look at) is a good place to start. This might be favorite foods, a favorite toy, or a picture of some place he likes to go. A teacher can put together exercises that accomplish this type of information transfer with a series of flashcards, and physical objects like plastic foods or plastic farm animals. The child can be given *receptive* language work (choosing between two objects to show which is the banana and which is the apple), or *expressive* language work, like simply naming an object to ask for it, or by using a full sentence to ask for it. At a higher language level, visual stimuli can be used to foster more complex use of language—like describing the context of activity, for example, "The cow is riding *on* the truck" to label a plastic cow in a toy pick-up truck. Exactly what task is appropriate for a particular child depends on that child's receptive and expressive language level. When children are at the earliest levels of language learning, three-dimensional objects may be the most attention-getting vusual stimuli. Photographs are the next most abstract. Color pictures, and then line drawings can be subsequently used to increase abstraction. For some PDD children in particular, the alphabet is particularly attractive early on, and sight-reading words is a good way to provide a visual mnemonic for auditory comprehension.

Tactile to Verbal Transfer of Information. Some children with autism or PDD have heightened awareness of tactile sensations. At an extreme, this can be considered one of the symptoms of autism, in which the child touches certain textures repetitively, often with close visual attention as well. Heightened tactile awareness can be capitalized on in an instructional setting. Information that comes in on a tactile channel can be transferred to a verbal channel in the same way as visual to verbal information is transferred. For example, a teacher can take a box, and fill it with things that are hard, soft, smooth, bumpy, and so on. Students can stick their hands in the box without looking and "Get smooth" or "Get bumpy," and so on.

If a child likes things that are textured, letters of the alphabet or numbers cut out from sandpaper might be a good curriculum material. Objects with magnets attached to the back may appeal to autistic children who like interesting touch sensations. Another toy that can be used with tactilely oriented children is a "Light-Bright," little pegs that light up when plugged into a pegboard. A Light-Bright or something of that sort can be used to teach labels for colors, and shapes, or to improve imitation by having the child copy a pattern. In each activity, the tactile qualities should be used to call attention to a verbal label, or to a command, statement, or question about the object.

Whenever a teacher works with an autistic or PDD child, it always helps to call attention to as many channels of information simultaneously as possible—with the idea that the verbal (comprehension) channel is probably the weakest. This means repeating words, using accentuated intonation for a new word, using descriptive gestures, helping the child to touch or look at the corresponding tactile or visual quality of the object, and so on.

The Use of Computers in the Instruction of Autistic Children

Another method of instruction that is coming into classrooms everywhere is computer-assisted instruction (CAI). What are the pros and cons of CAI for autistic and PDD students? Computers, by their nature, are non-social interactants. There is a back-and-forth exchange, but only one of the interactants is human. For some higher functioning autistic children and many PDD children, this seems like a match made in heaven. I remember the first time, about ten years ago, when I first saw an autistic child using CAI in a Silicon Valley school for autistic children. Michael, age seven, was a high-functioning autistic boy who already read fairly well. Each time he would respond to the computer with the right answer, a series of bells and chimes would ring. This caused Michael to flap his hands excitedly. His teacher would prompt, "No flapping!" and remove the keyboard until the flapping subsided. Soon, Michael began to sit on his hands as soon as he would type the correct answer. This way, he wasted no time with flapping and waiting to get the keyboard back before he could begin another exercise. The task itself was instructional, but the computerized nature of the presentation was itself a powerful reinforcer—powerful enough for the student to devise his own strategy for eliminating an inappropriate behavior.

The content of almost any computer program is easier for an autistic child to learn than the same material taught by a person. As far as I'm aware, there is no computer software specifically designed for autistic children, nor could I imagine what it would be like. But most educational software, depending on the instructional level, can be beneficial in the teaching of autistic children. One of the prime advantages of CAI is that it substitutes in certain ways for the need for one-to-one by providing individually paced instruction and reinforcement that is immediate and completely contingent on the child's appropriate, on-task behavior. Higher functioning PDD and Asperer's syndrome children tend to have a great deal of intellectual curiosity, although it is not always expressed across a broad array of topics. Computers allow them to pursue a topic they are interested in without interference from others. Generally, this is fine, unless too much time is spent on the computer, or to the exclusion of all else.

One problem with computers, compared to a live instructor, is that they tend to have less ability to recognize the student's errors and re-present material in a too simple form to help get across a concept that may be particularly difficult. Presently, most CAI programs tend to emphasize rote skills. This can include programs in which you match a word to a picture, draw lines between things that go together (like a bird and a bird cage), or touch a picture on a special keypad to indicate recognition of a particular animal sound.

How early can CAI be used as an instructional strategy for autistic children? A child can't just be plugged into a computer like some sort of peripheral device. Initially a child needs a well-established sense of cause and effect so he can relate his own actions on the keyboard or keypad to the actions on the screen. This can be taught on the computer, but may initially need a good deal of one-to-one modeling. My own impression is that autistic and PDD children show relatively little self-initiated interest in the computer until their nonverbal mental age is at about the four-year-level. Earlier than that, the child must be specifically guided and prompted for most activities and it's not clear that doing the activity on the computer is in some way inherently better.

In terms of technical adaptations that computers can provide, many young children can do well initially with a power-pad rather than a regular keyboard. A power-pad is generally a flat surface with sensitive areas that allow it to be programmed as eight or sixteen cells, or sometimes as large squares representing letters of the alphabet and numbers. Power-pads require less coordination than a keyboard and the power-pads with cells can be used with overlays that guide the child to make one-to-one matches of power-pad icons with a corresponding action on the screen (for example, if a dog icon is pushed, a barking dog appears on the screen). Touch-screen technology can also be used for teaching early cause-and-effect reasoning via the computer.

Computers can also be thought of as offering a possibility for learning more interpersonal skills, such as those related to imagination and the capacity to engage in fantasy. For example, for autistic children who can read well, various mystery programs in which a story unfolds and the player chooses alternative courses of action may be a good way to develop understanding of a narrative plot. (Understanding narration is a relatively difficult task for autistic children because of their difficulties in taking the point of view of others.) Computer games can be used in conjunction with more child-initiated activity, like writing down the story plot that the computer developed. Pairing the more passive learning that comes about with the computer with the more active, expressive learning that derives from the child's own activities is a positive complement to the use of CAI in the classroom.

Most children with PDD prefer to play a game like hangman or ticktacktoe or checkers with a computer than with another child. The computer can be a fine modality for the child to learn the rules of these games. Once the rules of a game are learned, a teacher (or parent) is presented with a perfect teaching opportunity to help the student generalize his playing skills into a more social situation that involves turn-taking with another student. This can be in the form of two-joystick Nintendo or, if possible, away from the computer altogether. For example, a child who can play Tetris well could be encouraged to play a turn-taking, score-keeping game of three-dimensional Tetris using Leggos.

Computer Games. There are many little boys with autism and PDD I've met who were able to play Tetris on a Gameboy before they could really talk. There are many more who can't really play an electronic game properly, but are endlessly fascinated with operating the joystick (probably thinking they are playing). For these children the game itself is reinforcing. Some parents are concerned that their autistic child spends too much time with computer games, and wonder whether to limit access. Earlier, a six-year-old boy with PDD was described who would play Super-Mario Brothers on his Nintendo, forgoing meals and even wetting his pants if his mother did not turn it off. One day, after a long session at the Nintendo, his mother noticed he had developed a blister on his joystick hand. She asked whether she should take the Nintendo away from him altogether. The commonsense answer is that anything in moderation is better than anything in excess: If the child spends so much time at a computer game that the chance for other learning opportunities becomes more limited, then the computer game is being used too much. (Obviously, not making it to the toilet and developing blisters fall in the excessive use category as well.) Getting new computer games from time to time so that new skills and a new awareness of things can develop is a good compromise, as is limiting the time of day and duration of video game sessions. Video game playing can also be held out as a reward; for example, following a half-hour of appropriate dinner time behavior.

Gestalt Processing Difficulties, Task Modeling, and Task Complexity

Task Modeling. The autistic or PDD child tends to do what might be best described as *spontaneous problem-solving*. By this, it is meant that the autistic child will look at a pile of blocks on this desk, and then build with them whichever way he wants. A non-autistic child, given those same blocks and a model of an interesting-looking truck made out of the same assortment of blocks, is probably more likely than the autistic child to try to copy the model in front of him. The autistic child has a tendency *not* to imitate something or someone else, while the non-autistic child has more of a tendency to imitate. The ability and interest in imitation varies among individual children with autism and PDD. Some children with the diagnosis of PDD have little difficulty imitating things that are not social in nature (like building with blocks), but do have difficulty imitating the way other children act—since children begin to imitate one another mainly to impress one another and to fit in with a group.

When teaching a task that is built on imitation, it often helps the autistic child to break the task down into as many rote parts as possible instead of just letting him look at a model: Imagine a pyramid with four large yellow blocks of the bottom, three medium blue blocks on the next level, two small green blocks on the next, and a tiny, single red block on top. If you give an autistic child a box of blocks of all sizes and colors, it is likely he'll have significant difficulty replicating the design. Many autistic children tend to perceive such a complex design as a *gestalt* or whole, and have relatively more difficulty analyzing the components of the gestalt as they relate to one another. A teacher could show the child how to sort his blocks first by color and then by size within the color groups (or vice versa). Then showing just the bottom row of the pyramid, the child could be helped to select four of the largest blocks from among the yellow blocks, and so on. This strategy of breaking wholes into parts using rote sequences allows the autistic child to develop strategies to compensate for his ability to perceive overly large "wholes" by relying on his interest in rote and more obsessive interests like sorting.

Visual Gestalt Processing. "Gestalts" or literally "wholes" are cognitive units of information that are processed as one meaningful thing. Autistic children often seem to have gestalt processing difficulties: They fail to break things into small components when they should (such as echoing whole phrases). Autistic children can get stuck on processing visual gestalts as well, and a classic example of this is in how autistic children often solve jigsaw puzzles. Rather than finding two pieces that look as if they should be adjacent (for example, two puzzle pieces that each have an eye, and are part of a five-piece puzzle that makes a boy), autistic children tend to manipulate the pieces by fitting shapes together, irrespective of whether the contents of the pieces correspond. (In a study we did, we found that autistic children did equally well with the same jigsaw puzzle no matter if the front was blank, had an abstract design, or had a picture on it. Non-autistic preschoolers greatly preferred puzzles with pictures on them, and did better with such puzzles.) This unusual way of approaching puzzle completion—focusing on shape, not content—may explain why, as some parents of autistic children know, their child will readily put a puzzle together, even if it's turned over backward with no picture showing.

This over-attention to visual gestalts may be why some very young autistic children insist on certain routines, like always having apple juice from a certain bottle. This may be because they can't separate the characteristics of the apple juice from the characteristics of the bottle—and don't realize that the apple juice will still taste like apple juice, no matter which bottle it's given in.

Language Gestalts. A second gestalt-processing cognitive disability that many autistic children have is their tendency to perceive language in overly large chunks. Delayed echolalia can be an example of this. A whole segment of language gets used idiosyncratically to refer to a particular type of event, request, or activity. In these cases, the parts of the whole—individual words— are not being perceived with individual meaning. In a learning situation this implies that the autistic child may not readily see multiple aspects of an object simultaneously. For example, to an autistic child a "blue square" may corre- spond to all squares, which he will call "b-l-u-e-s-q-u-a-r-e-s," creating a new unitary concept as far as he is concerned. The teacher has to be aware of the tendency of autistic children to see things this way, and break down aspects of classification, such as demonstrating how color can vary regardless of shape, and vice versa.

Task Complexity. When a child fails to perform a task it may be because he isn't motivated, or because he doesn't understand. It is, needless to say, important for a teacher to be able to distinguish between these. If a child fails at a task but is eager to obtain the reinforcer, the task is probably too difficult. The challenge for a teacher in this situation is to think of ways the task can be broken down into smaller components, each of which can be separately taught (and reinforced), with addition components being added as earlier ones are mastered, until finally the child can perform the whole task.

This idea of *successive approximations* is common to all teaching in special education, but has a particular twist with autistic and PDD children. Autistic children tend to do as little as they can to hold up their end of the communica- tive turn: If for example, Daniel wants juice, and his teacher holds up juice, if Daniel can get the juice by reaching for it, that's all he'll do. If Daniel clearly knows how to reach to indicate a want, the teacher should request that he say "J-J" as well. If Daniel can say "J-J" fairly easily, she should require that he say "Juice." If Daniel can say "Juice," she should require that he say "I want juice," and so on. The autistic child does not do well if his only three-word phrase is "I want juice," and he is therefore expected to also be able to say "I want sandwich," "I want chips," etc. "I want juice" may have become his holistic phrase for obtaining juice, a single concept that he classifies as "I- w-a-n-t-j-u-i-c-e" with no separate meaning assigned to the "I" and "want" parts of the syntax. Therefore, using the "I want" in combination with other objects may not make sense to him at first.

Task Approximations and Record Keeping. In working with autistic children, it is important to keep a tally of how many times they have been presented a particular task, and how often they are able to get it right. This makes clear to the teacher—and other helpers in a class who may work with the child over the course of the day—what the child knows, what he is still learning, and what he may be simply refusing to do. Some sort of scoring sheet with individual tasks and assignments should be available in a notebook, posted on a wall or taped to the child's desk for this purpose.

Individual Differences in Response to Modeling. In getting to know an autistic child, it is quite worthwhile for a teacher to become familiar with what types of modeling the child can respond best to. Some children respond best to very unintrusive models. For example, in our clinic, as part of our standardized assessment, we conduct a play session during which, part of the time, an adult plays alone with toys in front of the child. We see many children who actively flee from attempts to engage in the hand-over-hand modeling of a task watch the adult obliquely and surreptitiously from a distance. As the adult puts the toy down (say a toy vacuum cleaner), the child approaches the vacuum and begins to operate the switch and push it around. For this type of autistic child, the hand-over-hand modeling of an activity (the adult holding the child's hand over the vacuum's switch) is so overwhelming that the child tunes out from the opportunity to learn from the situation, although he may be able to learn when intrusion is low, and the activity or object is something he finds inherently attractive.

There are other autistic children, however, who are so self-absorbed in their own activities that they seldom observe a model at a distance. Such a child, although he may also resist hand-over-hand modeling, may need this type of intrusion to be made aware of the possibilities of new toys and how to play with them.

Some autistic children need both intrusion and opportunities to be free of intrusion. In order to maintain attention, some children might need a fairly high level of intrusion followed by a cool-down period during which they might be talked to in a whisper. The whispering is probably more of a reward to most autistic children than is more intrusive (louder) instruction, and so should be used to reward compliance and sustained on-task behavior rather than to initially establish it.

Helping the Autistic and PDD Child Get the Most from Instruction

Follow-Through on Commands. From time to time I visit a new classroom that serves autistic children and see a really out-of-control child. Sometimes I am asked to consult on a particular problem student who has developed really uncontrollable behavior. The problem that is most common in such situations is a lack of consistency and follow-through. Once a teacher makes a demand of a child, she or an aide must have the time to follow through and make certain the child does as requested. For example, if a child is asked to line up to go out to the playground and he sprints out the door instead, it will only make things worse to call after him once or twice and then go back to helping the other students line up. The best solution is structure (such as keeping the door latched in some way that students can't easily open it) if there is not sufficient staff. If the autistic child can get away with bad behavior, the only thing the student is learning is that misbehavior has rewards. A classroom that cannot provide sufficient structure either through staff and/or the physical setup is an inappropriate placement for a child with negative behaviors that need to be re-channeled.

The same concerns about not letting a student succeed in acting inappropriately during routine activities like lining up, naturally prevail in work on instructional tasks. If the teacher requests that the student "Put the ball in the box" (and she knows from other occasions that he understands this), she should not let the trial be over until the student succeeds. A learning episode should always conclude with something the student has just done right (even if it was something easy for him to do) so failure or lack of completion does not become associated with the (desired) end of the lesson.

Positive Redirection. In some classrooms it seems that all the teacher can do is to keep students out of trouble. When you first see a class like this, you may feel that the teacher is really doing her best, but that the students are so difficult behaviorally that there is no opportunity for real teaching. In such a situation it is important to look for the use of *positive redirection*. Positive redirection is a technique that involves giving children something positive to do after they are deflected from, or punished for, doing something bad. Take, as an example, Samuel: Every time he has a chance, he rushes to the teacher's desk and grabs all her pencils and throws them in the air, giggling giddily. The aide rushes up and shouts "No," and then tries to teach him a lesson by taking him from pencil to pencil on the floor and guiding his hand while he picks each one up. So far so good. Then she returns Samuel (still slightly giddy) to his desk and tells him to sit. He sits at his desk, not really looking at the mimeographed sheet spelling "S-A-M" that he is supposed to be tracing. Forty-five seconds later, when the aide has turned her back, he goes for the pencils a second time. In this kind of situation, several additional things might have been done to make things better. First, the aide might have used an accompanied time-out at Sam's desk to calm him down before leaving him again. She might have removed the stimulus (the pencil jar) from where he could get to it. Redirection, however, might have been the most effective technique for not just getting rid of the bad behavior, but moving on to a good behavior. First of all, in addition to putting away the pencils, the aide might have moved Sam someplace where he couldn't look directly at the teacher's desk or get to the teacher's desk without going past an adult. More importantly, she should have chosen a new task for him that would hold his attention. Does he already know how to trace his name? If so, maybe he should have a more challenging worksheet to match words to pictures. If Sam has never traced his name before independently, he needs an aide to help him do it, or he needs another task (like sorting beads onto pegs) that he enjoys doing independently. Without a satisfactory task which the child can succeed at to replace the misbehavior, the errant behavior, because it is stimulating to the child, is likely to reoccur.

Getting and Holding the Child's Attention. A prerequisite to teaching effectively is to have your student pay attention to you. The autistic child is not merely distractible, like a child with attention deficit hyperactivity disorder (ADHD); he is often actively seeking ways to avoid interaction. Using multiple cues to get the child's attention before beginning to speak helps. This can include calling the child's name and saying "Look!" or "Listen!" holding curriculum materials up to your mouth so the child can observe more directly what is being said, speaking slowly and repetitively (depending on the child's language level), using exaggerated gestures, and, if possible, having the child repeat directions or explanations he's been given. Another helpful technique is repeating what the child has said, and then correcting usage as necessary. Repeating the child's words before answering or elaborating also helps to keep the focus of a child who has receptive language difficulties. Having the child focus and look your way while speaking to him provides an opportunity for the child to get to know facial expressions and emotions that go along with different kinds of statements.

Autistic children's tendency to not attend to speech appears to be part of their aversion to social contact. In avoiding language stimulation, autistic children may also be creating deficits in their ability to use language as an internalized guide in the way most children do by age two or three. Normally, two- to three-year-olds will have begun to use significant amounts of "private" speech to guide their behavior, saying things to themselves like "Snow White go nite-nite"; or "R-r-r-o-m, pow, pow" while throwing trucks in the air and letting them fall. The autistic or PDD child of a comparable language age more often plays fairly silently. In working with autistic children, private speech (talk children usually direct to themselves while playing) can be modeled through an adult narrating the child's play activity ("No, no! Don't eat me Mr. Lion!"). Hopefully, the adult's language will be interesting enough so the child will begin to use similar narration independently. For example, if a child is putting together a wood puzzle with various geometric shapes, the teacher might say "It's a *square*," "That one's a *square*," "It goes *there*," and so on as the child proceeds with his activity. Over time, the child internalizes the kind of thing the teacher says, and begins to label his own actions. This is a very important cognitive step, because internalized language is what allows us to develop the capacity, later on, to reason more abstractly.

Use of Physical Exercise as a Method of Focusing Attention

Some teachers feel they have definitely observed a relationship between physical exercise and an autistic child's ability to focus in class. There are many possible explanations that run from the simple, "They need to let off some steam," to more complex theories about endorphins, which are brain neurotransmitting chemicals. Whatever the reason, for many children, physical exercise before a work period does seem to promote an ability to hold still and pay attention. My favorite example of this comes from videos I once saw of the Higashi School in Lexington, Massachusetts. Part of the philosophy of this residential treatment program for autistic children was to "run" the children every morning. All the students (many quite young) would wear red caps, presumably to keep them from getting mixed up with non-students in public places. The teachers would amass all the children at one end of a large field, and then chase them down field. At the end of the field, they were regrouped and chased the other way. After several traverses, it was time to go inside. The teachers also got an early morning workout. While a structured part of the class day like early morning exercise may not be equally beneficial for every-one, it probably is good for any able-bodied child and is something a teacher can arrange to do with all or part of her class to determine its effects on individual students.

Chapter Summary

In this chapter, we have covered methods of behavioral management, and various ideas about curriculum that have been helpful in working with autistic children. The single most important content area of teaching for all young autistic and PDD children is communication. Building on the techniques of instruction that have been discussed in this chapter, the next chapter focuses exclusively on the teaching of communication skills.

CHAPTER 12

Teaching Communication Skills to Children with Autism and PDD

Autisitic versus Typical Language Development

Thus far we have discussed when education should be started, what to look for in a classroom and in a teacher, and how an autistic child should be taught. In this chapter, we discuss the specifics of teaching communication skills to children with autism and PDD who are at different levels of language development. To begin with, the same principles that apply for teaching an autistic child anything apply to teaching language: The child needs to be instrumentally motivated. This means that an autistic child is most interested in communicating when there are things he wants for himself and cannot get for himself. The first step in learning how to teach communication skills to autistic children is recognizing that the moment that the child wants something is the moment that the window of accessibility to language learning is open widest.

Talking to a Child at His Language Age

One difficulty that is encountered by all children with language delays, including autistic and PDD children, is exposure to language that is too difficult to comprehend. With little babies, we naturally adjust our speech to a simplified level that linguists call *motherese*. Motherese typically consists of small numbers of simplified words that are repeated frequently, and with exaggerated intonation. There are good reasons why motherese is helpful to a baby's ability to learn language: By saying a word several times, the baby gets a chance to pick up the pattern of sound. The baby's hearing apparatus is not yet as mature and experienced as an adult's and so the baby may experience *processing delays*. Processing delays occur when we really don't absorb the first sound or sounds that are spoken. The best way for an adult to understand what it feels like to experience a language processing delay is to consider how it feels when someone starts to talk to you in a different language, or in a language you understand only partly. If you miss the first part of what is said, it makes it all the more difficult to catch on to the rest. We all understand that babies need to learn language, and so we slow down input, and give them plenty of chances to catch on. In fact, in motherese, much of what the adult repeats is modulated by how the baby reciprocally responds by doing things like fixing her gaze, smiling, or waving her limbs at a familiar word.

This usual model of language learning through motherese presents some difficulties when the autistic child learns language. For some autistic children, the language learning problems started very early on. This subset of autistic children never acquire any early language. In these cases, the babies may not have been giving back signals to the motherese (like reciprocal gazing, smiling, etc.). Eventually, the baby's lack of response may lead to the parent talking to the child more in a way that she talks to other adults, or simply talking as if thinking out loud (that is, not really expecting a response). This further cuts down the child's language learning opportunities. When the autistic or PDD child has older siblings, the parents have already been pre-programmed to use a certain level of language complexity appropriate to the child's chronological age. If the autistic child's language age is not keeping up with the chronological age, the autistic child will get farther and farther behind until he has some special help to "crack the code."

What kind of special help is needed? The first, fairly intuitive answer is to speak to the child at his language age rather than his chronological age. Therefore, the first step is to determine the language age the child is at. One of the really useful aspects of formally assessing a child's level of intellectual functioning is to gain information about language age and how it relates to the child's overall level of development. Usually, the language portion of intellectual functioning is reported in two ways: *receptive language age* and *expressive language age*. Some parents and teachers are fairly accurate at deducing language age without any tests by comparing the autistic child to their normally developing children. Once it is established that a three-year-old's receptive language is at the eighteen-month level (he recognizes many labels of objects, follows common one-step commands—if interested), then it is beneficial to adjust the language input to that child back down to the eighteen-month level. The same child's expressive language age may be lower still, and so very early ways of stimulating expressive language—like putting the child's hand on your mouth as you make certain sounds, making funny noises, and repeating sounds over and over, can be helpful.

Using Natural Gestures to Enhance the Communication "Signal"

Another way that we communicate to babies is with natural gesture. Natural gestures include waving our hands around to indicate the dimensions of an object; direction, speed, or pattern of movement; pointing; and facial expression to connote associated emotion. Use of gesture to communicate is equivalent to using a second, visual language side-by-side with oral language. Autistic and PDD children have early problems with reference—that is, under- standing what a gesture might refer to. Absence of pointing and failure to follow pointing are early signs of autism that appear in the vast majority of autistic children and in most children with PDD as well. If we could assign an "age" to comprehension and use of gestural communication the way we do to receptive and expressive language, most toddlers with autism and PDD would be considered delayed. Therefore it is important that communication include a lot of exaggerated gesture in order to call the child's attention to its communi- cation value. Because an autistic child does not follow a point readily, at first, it is good to actually touch objects you are referring to (rather than just point in their direction), at least until the child's comprehension is developed enough so that he can demonstrate a concept of pointing by using it himself. Con- versely, an autistic or PDD child can be taught to point, by pointing his or her hand and leading it to a desired object, demonstrating the connection between referring to the object from farther away and from nearer to it.

Some autistic children appear to be basically word-deaf when they are very young. Often deafness is the first suggested diagnosis. For children such as these, using a lot of gesture in speech may be potentially as helpful as gesture is to a deaf child or to a person traveling in a foreign country and trying to communicate without a shared language.

Some children who receive the diagnosis of PDD rather than autism have relatively less marked impairments in social relatedness than children diag- nosed as autistic, but have their relatively most severe specific deficits in language reception and expression. In PDD children whose imitation and nonverbal communication skills are fairly good, the use of natural gestural communication may be especially important in helping the child to learn to compensate for what she has difficulty comprehending verbally.

Methods for Teaching Language to Nonverbal Children

Perhaps the greatest challenge in the special education of autistic children is teaching them to talk. For many teachers it is difficult to know where to start. Often the communication program that an autistic child receives is more a function of the classroom milieu than of his particular developmental needs. Over a long period of time in our clinic, we have worked out some guidelines for recommending communication programs for young autistic children. De- pending on developmental level, degree of imitative ability, and milestones in nonverbal communication, we start either on oral language development, sign language development, the use of communication boards, or some combina- tion of these. The advantages of each of these approaches for children with different developmental profiles will be described.

Communication Boards

Two-Dimensional Communication Boards. Communication boards, or pic- ture boards as they are sometimes called, are the most basic way of beginning communication skills. A communication board is simply pictures of everyday objects that the child encounters and sometimes wants. Many children benefit most from communication boards constructed out of color photographs of the specific things in their experiences. This means that if the child drinks juice in a green Gerber training cup, there should be a picture of the child's own green Gerber training cup, and not a tan Tupperware training cup cut from a catalog. Other pictures in a "starter set" might include two or three pictures of favorite snack items, or a photo of the outside cover of a particularly cherished video-tape. Pictures of foods can be placed on the refrigerator (if the food is refriger-ated), on kitchen cabinets, or wherever the child is likely to be when he makes a particular association to the things he wants.

The purpose of a communication board is to get the child to indicate what he wants by touching a picture of the object. In this way, the child begins to have the idea that there are symbols for objects. The difference is that he is starting with an object that is different from the real thing only insofar as it is reduced to two dimensions and appears smaller. A word is a much more arbitrary and abstract symbol and therefore, for some children, is more difficult to retain and associate with the corresponding physical object.

Three-Dimensional Boards. For some autistic children, particularly young ones with moderate to severe mental retardation, an even more concrete representation may be needed for the communication board concept to catch on. For these children, we use actual three-dimensional representations of the object they are requesting—like a plastic banana attached to a cardboard stand (with a bowl of sliced bananas hidden behind). Empty juice boxes and cookie boxes can be used in the same way. When first introducing communication boards to children, it is important to start with only one or two pictures or objects until they have mastered the procedure.

Communication Boards for Expressive Communication. Communication boards can also be used expressively. A teacher can keep pictures in class that show different activities like lining up to go outside, being on the playground, or sitting down at snack time. When it is time for a particular activity, she can show the picture as well as announce the activity. Some teachers keep a sequence of pictures that correspond to the daily schedule, or make arranging the pictures part of a circle time activity, first thing in the morning. A particu-lar child might benefit from pictures taped to his desk that include photos of himself on a swing, eating his favorite snack, and so on. The teacher can use these to help communicate to the child the upcoming activities and the need to begin the transition from one activity to the next.

When to Use a Communication Board. Which children benfit most readily from the communication board approach? A communication board requires less fine motor precision and less imitation to master than sign language. Therefore the communication board approach may be particularly helpful to the very young child who still has limited fine motor development and limited imitation skills. One of the problems that young autistic children have is that development of their visual recognition abilities tend to outstrip their receptive language development. This means that there are many objects the child recognizes and understands the functions of, but for which he has no verbal label. Therefore, when the child wants something, he may cry and have a tantrum because he pictures what he wants and doesn't have it, but doesn't know how to use any sort of communicative strategy to get help for himself in getting what he is picturing. Parents of autistic children know they've hit this stage when they find that they are rushing around showing their child one thing after another while the child continues to throw a tantrum until he sees what he wants. Introduction of a communication board is a very powerful tool at this point. The child soon learns that he can get what he wants more expeditiously by pointing at a picture, and the parents are relieved that needs can be met without prolonged exposure to their child's tantrums.

It is also worth noting that the behavioral methods, such as time-out, that were discussed in Chapter 11 for reducing tantrum-throwing behavior don't work nearly as well if the child is hungry and throws a tantrum because he is (in his mind) trying to indicate what he wants. It is therefore essential that behavioral methods and communication training be used in conjunction with one another to obtain the best improvements in the child's ability to communicate and stay in behavioral control.

Children who benefit from the introduction of communication boards the most are those who do not yet hand-lead. These children need to be taught the basic cause-and-effect paradigm of touching a picture and getting a desired result so that they learn that there is an important link between a picture and its corresponding object. The best way to teach this is to start with a food the child really likes (let's say Fruit Loops) and to put out a photo of the Fruit Loops box. The teacher or parent can touch the child's hand to the picture, and say "Fruit Loops! Want Fruit Loops?" and then give the child a Fruit Loop, praising him verbally. This should be made into a game, with as many turns as possible. Initially, getting the concept across with one picture keeps things simple. Even if the child is angry and frustrated that he can't just have the whole bowl of Fruit Loops at once, and eat as many as he wants, the teaching drill needs to continue. After a fixed number of trials (like ten), the drill can be ended. However, if the child is going to get unlimited Fruit Loops, juice, or whatever at that point, it is a good idea to move him away from the area where the drill was taking place before giving it to him, so he begins to feel that at least in one setting getting Fruit Loops is contingent upon being communicative. In fact, it would be even better if the child could be made to accept a different food altogether at that point so that Fruit Loops can be moved into the category of an "ask for it" food. As the child improves at this kind of game, the prompt (putting the child's hand on the picture) should be *faded* by letting the child move his hand toward the picture himself—at first, the last half-inch; then, the last inch; then two-inches, and so on, until he moves his hand toward the picture with complete independence.

Choice of Two. Initially, communication boards are introduced for the child to ask for one particular object that is pictured. When that has been mastered, the communication board can be used to make a choice between two things, such as two choices of snack or two choices of activity. Initially, the child will only want to use the communication board when asked, but if a communication symbol is consistently used, the child should begin to use it spontaneously on his own. One necessary technique for achieving spontaneous use of the communication board is that the child must not be arbitrarily asked to use the board some times and not at other times. If, for example, there is a photo of Tropicana orange juice on the refrigerator, it should be required that the child get juice directly from the refrigerator only by using the board. (This doesn't mean that if everyone is sitting down for breakfast, the child needs to be brought to the refrigerator before his juice can be served at the table.) There should be context-specific demands for communication at first, with later opportunities to generalize that knowledge in other settings (like having another copy of the picture of juice which can be brought to the table.) Once the child has been requested to indicate a picture before getting what is pictured, the parent or teacher needs to be careful to follow through consistently on her request or the child will learn that "holding out" may be as affective a strategy as communicating.

One indicator of readiness to use a communication board is whether or not the child naturally hand-leads to objects he wants. For the child who already hand-leads, the communication board may be relatively easy to get accustomed to. This child should need relatively little help in being shown how to touch the picture in order to get what he wants. For this kind of child, the communication board can be used to encourage more sophisticated communication skills, such as looking at the adult after you touch the picture to make sure that the adult sees your action. The adult can teach a more socially communicative use of the communication board by withholding the object the child has signaled that he wants until the child has looked or been guided to look at the adult, and the child's action has been acknowledged by the adult's words and facial expression.

How Far to Take Communication Boards. Some parents initially don't like the idea of communication boards because they don't see how it is helping the child learn to speak. It is. A communication board is teaching the child what the function of communication is, and that objects have separate and discrete symbols. Further, by pairing language with the use of the communication board, the child is able to adopt a visual mnemonic (the picture) to aid in retention of the word, thus improving receptive vocabulary. For most autistic children, use of the communication board can be considered a stage of language learning. As the child's frustration in having needs met diminishes by virtue of being able to use the communication board successfully, the child's receptivity to producing language increases. At the moment when a child is throwing a tantrum and crying because he cannot successfully communicate what it is that he wants, he is not very accessible to being taught anything. By being able to be calm while communicating, the child is more receptive to learning words, gestures, and other information related to communicating.

As the child's capacity to speak develops through these measures, the communication board will simply fall away. Saying "juice" is more efficient than having to go to the picture of "juice" on the refrigerator and touching it. Because the autistic child is interested in having his instrumental needs met as easily as possible (and usually without prolonged interaction, if he has his way), he will adopt the more efficient verbal means of communication as soon as he is able to figure out how to use it. On average, autistic children who take to the use of communication boards begin to use spoken language within a year and simply stop using the pictures.

Some children, however, have greater difficulty than others in comprehending language. Most of these are autistic children who also have moderate to severe mental retardation. For these children, communication boards are a more prolonged phase. Some of these children do well with a communication booklet or wallet. A communication booklet is a small series of laminated pictures on a key ring that the child can carry with him. When the child wants something, he can take out the picture and show it. Parents and teachers can also use communication booklets to show the child what is about to happen or what he needs to go and do.

A small percentage of autistic children have intact nonverbal intelligence but marked and severe expressive language deficits. These children fail to develop spoken language even though they can discriminate many, many pictures. Some of these are children who also qualify for a diagnosis of an expressive language disorder, as well as autism or PDD. For these children, a more complex form of a communication board can be devised. These boards can simulate grammar by having one column (or page) of pictures for subjects (such as the child, parents, teacher, siblings), one for actions (such as being in school, being in bed, going in the car), and one column for modifiers (such as things to eat, videos to watch, or toys to have along). The child can be drilled to use the board to indicate more complex ideas such as having himself, Mommy, and Daddy in the car and going to McDonald's to eat french fries. Most children do not have the unusual profile of skill strengths and skill deficits that call for this sort of an approach, but this is a useful way of expanding the communicative repertoire of those who do. This approach can also be useful for children with very severe articulation problems, who speak but are generally not understood, or children with severe fine motor problems who do not develop enough fine motor coordination to learn to use sign language well, but can point to target pictures.

Bells and Whistles. Running a clinic as I do, in the midst of Silicon Valley, I am sometimes asked about electronic communication devices such as portable communicators that a child can use to type letters that appear as words on a small built-in screen. Some communicators have special alphabetic, non-QWERTY keyboards; some have programmable keyboards designed to accommodate icons or pictures rather than letters of the alphabet. Some communicators or computers provide mute children with an electronic "voice" for what they have typed.

These devices are fine . . . Are they "better" educationally than laminated pictures glued to cardboard? I doubt it. Cardboard pictures don't need batteries, and can fall in the toilet without a $1,200 investment going down the tubes. Most children who are nonverbal can't spell, and if they can spell, it is usually a more arduous process for making their needs known than pointing to a picture. Some of the electronic devices aren't so portable. Michelle, a severely retarded ten-year-old autistic girl with cerebral palsy had a communicator with a keyboard and icons—all of which she could use. The problem was that the device (with battery pack installed) weighed about ten pounds. Michelle had only learned to walk at age six, was still not steady on her feet, and couldn't hold onto a ball or other small object for extended periods. Needless to say, picking up and carrying her communicator around with her was a significant challenge (and one she had not yet mastered). Her parents discovered she'd use the same icons on a cardboard (when the batteries went dead on her communicator, which they frequently did). I encouraged them to keep up the spelling and keyboard skills electronically in moving Michelle toward sight-reading, but as an instructional task—not as an everyday way to get basic needs met. A cardboard communicator can be less obtrusive than an electronic device, and pointing is less obtrusive that having an electronic voice speak for you.

Sign Language

Many infant programs include sign language as part of their program for developing communication skills. For many young children with developmental disabilities, sign language is a more visual, more sensorimotor, more concrete approach to communication than spoken language and can be acquired at an earlier developmental level. In fact, parents often report that baby siblings of developmentally disabled children who sign usually spontaneously begin signing around nine months of age. One advantage of sign language is that it is more portable than a communication board. The type of sign language that is used with developmentally disabled children is usually a simplified form sometimes referred to as see signing. See signing is based on American sign language (ASL), which includes gestures that indicate nouns, verbs, and various modifiers. ASL also has a system of finger-spelling, but this is virtually never used with very young or developmentally disabled children since you need to be able to read and spell to use it.

When to Introduce Sign Language. There are two main reasons why sign language learning can be an especial problem for children with autism and

PDD, although in many cases there are advantages as well. Sign language is gestural language. Children who fail to develop natural gestures such as pointing, or looking to see whether someone else is looking where they are looking (social referencing) are naturally going to have a harder time with a formal set of gestures for communication. My rule of thumb is that if an autistic child has marked enough deficits in nonverbal communication such that he is not yet pointing, then I start the child on a communication board. If he uses a point, or even follows a point readily, then sign language may be appropriate instead of, or in addition to, a communication board.

When I say this to parents, suggesting the use of a communication board instead of sign language, a parent often says, "But he's already learned one sign." Then I guess: "Is it the sign for 'More' or 'Please'?" Quite often, it is—or some equivalent. What happens with autistic children is that they can learn one sign that functions more as a behavioral regulator than as a commuinicative symbol. For example, a child will learn the sign for "More" (pursed fingers coming repeatedly together at mid-line, mid-body). Autistic children tend to overgeneralize this sign to mean "More juice," "More cracker," "More outside," "More bath time," and so on. Basically, the single sign comes to convey the fact that the child has something he wishes to have more of, or that there is something he wishes to continue. Granted, using the sign for "more" in this fashion *is* a whole lot better then having a child lie on the floor and throw a tantrum. However, such "communication" is not object specific. The teacher or parent is still bearing most of the communicative effort trying to guess *what* the child wants "more" of. If sign *is* going to be used, it is very important to avoid overgeneralization of "More," "Please," and so on, and to work on specific signs for specific wants so that the child learns that communication is a matter of using specific symbols. Overall, it is my experience that the instrumental nature of the autistic child's desire to communicate in as brief and abbreviated a manner as possible makes prevention of overgeneralization of early sign language an uphill battle. With the communication boards, overgeneralization is seldom a problem—children will not point to apple when they want cracker (especially if both pictures are presented as choices).

When children are initially learning sign language, they will need to have the sign demonstrated to them. However, since imitation is not a strong point for most young autistic children, a hand-over-hand, gradual approximations approach to learning a new sign is usually more effective. In initially learning a new sign, this means taking the child's hand and forming the sign, and then giving some of what is requested by the sign. In gradual degrees, the child needs to be encouraged to do at least parts of the sign independently, before getting what he is requesting. At first all children who are taught signing use kind of a "baby talk" sign, and so the signing tends to be less precise than in adults.

Some parents worry that they themselves will not know the signs the child learns in school and fail to recognize them when the child tries to use them at home. Fortunately, most adults learn faster than young autistic children. A good teacher can easily keep a parent abreast of new signs being taught and acquired.

Going with an "Oral Only" Language Approach

Some educational programs (and some parents) shy away from communication boards and signs because these are not used by typically developing children as stages in their development of communication. Fair enough. Some children with autism or PDD just need stimulation and direct modeling of verbalizations to begin language. Some just need to have language set into an instrumental context ("You won't get it unless you ask for it") to start using single words or word approximations.

The decision to try a nonverbal communication such as a communication board or sign language has, in my opinion, virtually no downside risk. It cannot hurt the child to be introduced to these methods as long as oral language is constantly paired with the nonverbal symbols, so that the child always has the opportunity to respond partly or fully with words, too. The upside risk is that if oral communication is promoted as the *only* modality for communication, the child who is not cognitively ready to master oral communication is likely to become increasingly frustrated, and therefore less open to interaction—since it is so unrewarding to him. As a general principle, once a young preverbal autistic child begins a fairly well-organized special education program, but does not begin to use some form of verbalization for instrumental requests within three months, it is reasonable to add a nonverbal form of communication to his educational plan as well.

Social Stigma and Nonverbal Methods of Communication

Some parents don't like the use of sign language because it seems stigmatizing. Sometimes the communication boards are more easily accepted as some sort of a game or as an educational exercise, but sign language is sometimes more closely associated with the lifetime patterns of the profoundly deaf. My response to parental concerns about the child "looking funny" if he is signing or using a communication board is that you must do what is most likely to work. With sign language, as with the communication board, the child will drop signing as soon as he is able to make his needs clear through verbalizing. As with the communication board, language usually begins to emerge within the first year of sign language training, usually when the child has acquired twenty single-word signs or less.

Signing as the Sole Mode of Communication

A very small proportion of autistic children with particularly severe language deficits continue to acquire signs and even begin to sign in sentences without ever acquiring accompanying development of oral language. These autistic children tend to show the same sort of problems with echolalia and pronoun reversals in sign language as other autistic children show in their spoken language. Another difficulty such autistic children may encounter as they gain enough sign to use it spontaneously, is problems in the language pragmatics of their sign communication. Just as with oral communication, the signing autistic child does not do much in the way of looking toward, or making eye contact with the person she is addressing before beginning to sign. At least with spoken language, the parent or teacher hears the child speaking and attends. The signing can be harder to catch, and when unobserved, can lead to frustration. I have seen some signing autistic children standing with their back turned to their parents signing things like "Go potty" or "Eat sandwich."

Among the few signing *deaf* autistic children I've known, there is a particularly odd phenomenon to be observed: They tend to prompt a comversational response from an adult by molding the adult's hands into the desired response, instead of the child himself signing, and then looking at the adult for a response. One boy I've been off and on ever a number of years, Frankie, is fairly bright, autistic, and deaf. On his last visit (at age thirteen) he repeatedly approached his father and tried to form "Go home" with his father's hands. He did not make eye contact with his father before or after he signed. This seemed to be Frankie's way of making sure he got his message across without having to make eye contact in the process.

A small number of autistic children remain mute thoughout their lives. I define mute as those children with no words, or with less than three or four words, or perhaps as many as ten words—but with such limited intelligibility that they can be understood only by people who are very familiar with them. The numbers of autistic children who remain mute was once estimated to be around forty percent; however, in my clinical experience, because autistic children have benefitted from the better quality earlier interventions that have been available in the past ten to fifteen years, the current figure seems more like thirty percent. Research has shown that when a child has received good quality early language intervention up to age six and still isn't talking, the chances of that child remaining mute are exceedingly high. Perhaps seventy-five percent of mute autistic people have nonverbal IQs in the moderate to severely retarded range. For these individuals, sign language may be a good longer term adaptation. As adults, mute individuals with signigicant degrees of retardation live in sheltered group homes or other residential facilities, or stay protected in their own extended families where caregivers can easily learn the signs that the autistic person knows. Given that living arrangements and staff change, sign language is the most universal way for such an individual to have a portable communication means that will be recognized wherever he goes. So, for children over six years old who have no language (and little or no babbling), a more intensive focus on sign language is justified to help longer term adaptation.

Mainstreaming Autistic and PDD Children with Hearing-Impaired Children

Some autistic children who take well to sign language and have fairly good intellectual functioning but seem unable to learn to use spoken language may benefit from "mainstreaming" with hearing-impaired children. Severely hearing-impaired children who have few or no cognitive delays tend to be very strong in the use of both natural gesture and sign when communicating with one another. This type of amplified quality to social interaction among deaf children has been helpful for some autistic and PDD children we've followed—getting them to develop better peer interactional skills. If an autistic child's only form of communication is sign, it is very difficult for him to benefit from a more socially normal peer milieu unless the peers also sign. Therefore, "mainstreaming" signing autistic children with signing deaf children can be used to provide such an experience.

Early Oral Language in Children with Autism and PDD

There is an old expression: "Before you walk, you must crawl." Similarly, before you can talk, you must babble. Prognostically, I pay a great deal of attention to the amount and quality of spontaneous vocal production a young autistic child has at the time of initial diagnosis. The level of language or pre-language the child acquires before beginning special education often is informative about how easily the child is likely to begin using language. Normally, first words are preceded by a variety of earlier language stages that must be passed through by autistic children, (and by all children). At the earliest stage of vocal development, the infant normally produces a whole variety of sounds—virtually a lexicon of sounds the human vocal cords can produce. Many autistic children begin to do this at the usual time (around four months until about nine months). However, by nine to ten months, children usually begin to selectively reproduce the sounds that go with their own language much more frequently. This is when we typically hear "ba-ba-ba," "ma-ma-ma," and so on. Often autistic children who go on to develop the most severe language problems don't get to this stage, or pass through it only briefly and then grow more silent. Quite possibly, the absence of this type of very early babbling is an early sign of the difficulties that the child will have later on with other types of spontaneous imitation.

Bilingual Homes and Early Language Development

A significant proportion of the families we see in our clinic speak a language other than English at home. Typically, such families use their mother tongue with young children, who then gradually are exposed to English through children's television and, later, pre-school. Using this approach, the normally developing child is usually fully bilingual by kindergarten. If both languages are used at home, the child may start talking a little later (for example, not speaking in phrases until two-and-a-half years, instead of at two), and they may also go through a prolonged period of mixing words of the two languages together, until, around age four, the languages become distinct and separate. It almost goes without saying that this process is not what happens to the language-delayed child with autism or PDD who is growing up in a bilingual home. If a child is having trouble attaching meanings to words, it does not help to have two completely different words with identical meaning. We generally recommend simplifying things for the child by using just one language—usually English, since that will be the language of instruction in school. This recommendation is usually fine with parents unless the parents don't speak English either. In these cases, we try to recommend a small target vocabulary of words to use in English (say, the labels of pictures for the child's communication board) and teach the English equivalents of those words to both the parent and child. While parents generally appreciate the benefits of simplifying things for a child who is having difficulty learning, it *is* also difficult to change. A number of years ago, I had a patient who was Pakistani, but where parents spoke English quite fluently; they assured me that they used only English with their eight-year-old autistic son, Omar. On one visit, Mrs. Khan was eager to show me that Omar had learned the names of all his colors, and so I watched from behind a one-way mirror while she completed a coloring lesson with him. What Mrs. Khan did not know was that I had a young Pakistani research assistant behind the mirror with me. When Omar began to make errors at choosing crayons, my assistant told me that Mrs. Khan was imploring him in their native language to "Give me the yellow one, not the red one!" Realistically, single-language consistency is desirable, but not always 100% possible.

Language Loss

Some autistic children go on to develop language to the one word stage, but after getting a small single-word vocabulary, language begins to plateau. For some children, this takes the form of losing old words when they get new ones, as if there were "room" for only a small number of words. In other children, the words just drop away one by one until there are no more words spoken. In one study we did, we found that among the one-quarter to one-third of autistic children who do lose language this way, most start talking again within a year. After more than a year with no return of language, the chances that the child will remain mute begin to increase. Of course, what kind of intervention the child receives and how soon it is received can make a significant difference. However, there is no special or separate language therapy approach for autistic children who have lost language versus those who have simply been slow to develop language.

We do not know why such a large percentage of children who develop autism or PDD go through a stage of language plateau or language loss. It may have to do with the early language acquisition being a fundamentally cognitively different type of process than later language skills. It may have to do with internal changes in connections in the brain. We do know that with language loss there are no specific brain abnormalities that can viewed by MRI or other methods. In children we have studied, language loss seems fairly specifically a phenomenon associated with autism and PDD, but *is* occasionally seen in children with other forms of mental retardation and language disorders.

Encouraging Early Vocal Production. It is important to observe when the young autistic child makes his sounds. Is it when he is uninvolved with other things? Playing intently with one particular toy? Only when really pushed to "say" something to get what he wants? At these naturally occurring times, it can be helpful to provide feedback to his language production in the way we normally do with babies—making the child's own sounds back to him, or helping to modify the sounds if it seems like the sounds are an attempt at a particular word. When possible, encouraging speech sounds (phonemes) over non-speech sounds is useful. Some autistic children are more attracted to non-speech sounds, however, and will selectively imitate them. I've seen young autistic children who don't talk but who could do very nice imitations of vacuum cleaners, fire engines, and garbage disposals, as well as various animals. If you have a child who seems receptive to nonverbal sound imitation, do encourage it. The earliest goal is really to increase overall amount of vocal production, and then to bring it under imitative control.

Increasing Oral-Motor Awareness. Some autistic children need help developing better oral-motor awareness. This means that the child may not be that aware of how well he can control his mouth muscles to make different sounds. Sometimes parents make this observation themselves because they notice that the child stuffs too much food into his mouth at once, or tries to fit things in his mouth that are too big, or that the sounds that he makes are indistinct.

Most speech pathologists are very familiar with oral-motor awareness exercises, which actually are more often needed with other language-delayed children than with autistic children. Activities to increase oral-motor awareness can include blowing bubbles, blowing out candles, making raspberry sounds, sticking out the tongue certain ways, having the child watch his own mouth in a mirror, and biting into hard things. These activities can and should be worked on at home by parents too, and should not be limited just to speech therapy sessions.

Videotape Viewing and Language Development. Parents, naturally, are concerned about whether it is bad for their children to watch videotaped movies as much as the child may seem to want to watch them. There are retionales to support both yes and no answers to that question. First, there probably *is* benefit to language development in terms of stimulating listening to language, and stimulating attempts to repeat language. There also are real benefits to letting an autistic child watch videos and giving parents some peace, and time for other things, too.

In Chapter 3, we discussed speech intonation (prosody) processing and prosody use problems in autistic children. In that chapter, it was mentioned that videos and records—especially the same ones over and over—are often preferred sources of language stimulation because prosody is fixed, and what you hear, sounds exactly the same every time. So, for children at the earlier stages of acquiring language comprehension skills, videos are probably at least somewhat helpful. However, when the language development of the autistic or PDD child progresses further—to the stage where the child can use sentences or multiword phrases—then constant video watching may be *maintaining* the use of holistic, delayed echolalia type speech and become counterproductive to other language development goals.

Once again, the example of an adult learning a foreign language can be applied to how autistic children may be helped in learning language from videotapes. For adults learning a new language, it can initially be helpful to learn songs, or to just read aloud in the language. It gives the learner a sense of the sounds, the rhythms, and a growing sense of where words begin and end. But after a while what is needed is slower speech, with more emphasis on specific words and often-used phrases, so that meaning can be better extracted. Similarly, for the preverbal or just-verbal autistic child, videos (and any delayed echolalia produced) are probably okay. Then, when his or her language capacity improves, encouraging the child to experience a greater diversity of language stimuli and less repetition is probably better.

Language Pragmatics Interventions

Early language development consists of speech, and it also consists of the nonverbal message sending and message receiving that goes along with all acts of communication. The nonverbal part of communication, which encompasses skills like eye contact to punctuate meaning, turn-taking, topic maintenance, and topic elaboration, is part of what is referred to as the *language pragmatics* of language development. Language pragmatics requires certain social as well as linguistic skills. As such, it is at the core of what autistic people have the most difficulty with. Typically, language pragmatic skills are acquired at the same time as spoken language, but are learned mainly from the example set by those who talk to the child, rather than being something specifically taught. Since autistic children have difficulty learning by example (modeling), this makes the acquisition of language pragmatic skills all the more difficult for them. For autistic children, language pragmatics skills need to be specifically taught. It should be noted that poor language pragmatics tends to be characteristic of even the most high functioning autistic adults and even those diagnosed with mild PDD. Depending on how you interpret that observation, it means either that language pragmatics deficits are very much a part of autism, or that it is particularly hard to remediate difficulties in language pragmatics totally because they are difficult skills to learn by rote.

Eye Contact. The most easily addressed difficulty in the development of better language pragmatics skills is in the use of more appropriate eye contact. Training a child to give better eye contact is not just cosmetic. It is not just a way of making his conversation "look" more typical. There is a great deal of information that we get from looking at the face of a speaker, or the face of someone listening to us. Going back to our example of speaking to babies in "motherese," one of the features that it includes is exaggerated facial gesture. In the early stages of communication development, exaggerated gestures help draw and fix the baby's attention, and get the message of the facial expression (for example, surprise, happiness, naughty behavior) across very clearly. To begin improving eye contact in autistic and PDD children, it is important to provide them with equally clear signals that draw them in. At first, autistic and PDD children often need to have their face turned toward the speaker because they do not know the information embedded in facial expression and eye contact is there until you show them that it is.

Before beginning to force eye contact from an autistic child, one must understand why they avoid it. For the autistic or PDD child, eye contact appears to be aversive in the same way as it is in a child who is being looked at by a parent who has caught him being naughty. In those situations, even the non-autistic child tends to look away because the eye contact is somehow psychologically intimidating. Therefore, the adult has to surmount this by insisting on the eye contact, but must also be aware that being too intrusive for too long may be counterproductive to maintaining the eye contact. Starting with a demand for a little eye contact and working up to demands to prolong it for normal durations is the most sensible approach. With young children the best way, initially, to get eye contact is to call the child's name and say "Look!" while turning his face gently toward yours. Talking in a quiet, gentle, nondemanding tone (the way you would to a baby) is the best way to start. Keep the interaction brief, and try to punctuate it with facial expression that matches the words. Some children are more resistant to passively being co-opted into making eye contact. A more vigorous, intrusive demand for eye contact that matches the child's own level of resistance may work better with such a child. Always verbally praise the child's ability to make eye contact, no matter how brief at first.

Some educators who are very behaviorally oriented feel strongly about praising a specific behavior (such as saying "Good looking!" when the child looks). I tend to just use a "Good!" "Good boy!" or "Thank you!" By using praise, one is probably reinforcing the immediately preceding event, even if it isn't specifically labeled. I prefer the latter formulation because it seems more conversationally natural than a phrase like "Good looking!" which one would not use in praising a non-autistic child for responding to having his name called.

Getting eye contact is important, because it is you best assurance that the child has heard what you have to say. Gradually fading the prompts for eye contact (a prompt may be moving the child's face in the direction of yours), can begin once the child begins to respond to having his name called. Like other aspects of teaching autistic children, you will initially do better at getting eye contact if you try it when communication pertains to instrumental topics like food the child wants or a toy he particularly prefers. One way of maintaining initial eye contact is to hold a desirable topic of the conversation close to your eyes as you speak. For example, if you have a Matchbox car, and you want the child to tell you "What color?" and "How many wheels?" and "Is it a car or a truck?" the car can be held up to your eyes so the child will inadvertently get some facial cues as well as attending to the inanimate object he finds interesting.

Making better eye contact seems to be a sort of desensitization process for most autistic and PDD children. As they become more accustomed to doing it, it is less assiduously avoided. However, even teenagers with autism and PDD who have long ago learned to make fairly good eye contact need occasional reminding, as they tend to backslide into what is more comfortable for them.

Turn-Taking. The next major skill area in the development of language pragmatics is in turn-taking. Another basic aspect of language and social interaction consists of the fact that the listener and speaker constantly shift roles. Since language is a difficulty all its own for children with autism and PDD, the best way to begin some inculcation of turn-taking skills can be in the nonverbal domain. This can include all sorts of simple one-to-one activities like rolling a truck or a ball back and forth, or taking turns putting blocks into a box. The idea is that the child learns to observe and wait for the other, taking his cue for *his* turn from the completion of the complementary activity by the other participant. Early turn-taking activities can be embedded in rote activities the child likes. For example, a parent or teacher's aide might try swinging a child on a swing from in front, counting one number with every push of the child's feet. If the child likes to swing, he learns to get ready for his "turn" (sticking his feet out to be pushed), and stays tuned in as the counting, alphabet, or nursery rhyme progresses. (The swing activity is also a good one for eye contact.) As the child becomes better at turn-taking, the goals should be to (1) increase the length of each turn, (2) increase the overall duration that the turn-taking activity can be maintained, and (3) elaborate the content of the turns. If a game starts out with adult and child taking turns putting shapes in a shape sorter, a more elaborate turn could be naming a shape first, then finding that particular shape, and then putting it in. Next, sorting and labeling could take place before the shapes are put in, and so on, thus making the turns longer and more elaborate.

Turn-taking can and should also be encouraged on a verbal level once the child can turn-take on a nonverbal level. Again, rote activities are a good place to start. For example, a teacher might have a basket full of plastic jungle animals, and say "Bring me the lion." After the child brings the lion, the teacher would proceed with each of the other animals in turn. On a more complex level, the teacher and child could then switch roles, and have the child say "Bring me the lion," which the teacher would then have to find and bring to the child. Games like these can be mastered step by step and made more complex so that they successively encompass further language and cognitive skills in addition to turn-taking. For example, the teacher might try hiding four or five animals while the child watches, and then asking the child "Is there a lion hiding?" thereby testing the child's memory as well as the ability to maintain an activity. The only "trick" to teaching this type of turn-taking with autistic children is that the "rules" of each simpler game must be well mastered before changing the rules to something more complex. Children with autism and PDD tend to lack a great deal of flexibility and spontaneity, so the kind of arbitrary, changing, make-it-up-as-we-go type of play that other children the same age do so much of, needs to be eased into slowly through these types of more structured activities.

Topic Maintenance and Topic Elaboration. For many autistic and especially PDD children, topic maintenance is not so much a problem as is topic elaboration. In broad strokes, these two concepts refer to the individual's ability to identify a topic to talk about, and then to talk about it in a way that is of interest to both parties, and to include new information that the speaker is able to discern that the listener does not already have about the topic. Both of these skills are universally difficult for the child with autism or PDD to acquire. Often the verbal autistic child *does* have a topic that interests him, but in a very rote way. At a very early level of development, this can include a nearly endless fascination with lining up the magnetic letters on the refrigerator, verbally labeling each as it is included in the line. At a higher level, some autistic children will develop a fondness for a children's dictionary, and expect you to sit while they go from front to back labeling each object. The "topic" of conversation in these cases tends to be one-sided (the child reciting what he has learned), and the information included in the topic is a well-defined set that is not modified by the fact that the listener is already familiar with the information being given. Typically, adult attempts to expand the conversational topic do not go all that well.

What is behind the topic maintenance and topic elaboration difficulties that autistic and PDD children have? One major component is the child's lack of imagination. Usually, lack of topicality in language pragmatics is not a function of vocabulary size. Even an infant can have a "conversation" with you, cooing and changing the cooing in successive turns. Autistic children seem permanently stuck in a very egocentric phase of development where the topic revolves around "me" with little or no ability to be aware that other people can grow weary of the child's topic. This can be a little more tolerable with nonautistic, egocentric three-year-olds who have plenty of imagination. One very bright (not autistic) three-year-old, Jason, was endlessly fascinated by firemen, fires, and fire trucks (as is common in little boys that age). He would tell elaborate imaginative tales of how the buildings were plastic and a million degrees, and melting, and the people and the firemen would melt too . . . and so on. Given the same fascination with fires, but without imagination, the autistic child will label parts of fire trucks, line up fire trucks, memorize stories on cassettes about firemen, etc. After parents have heard a recitation of the same fireman story for the fiftieth time, they are usually wondering how else the child can be taught to use his abilities.

Improvement of topic maintenance and topic elaboration skills can come from stimulating the child's imagination. Repeating the same story endlessly falls under the heading of perseveration, a repetitive behavior the autistic person probably enjoys, but which blocks his ability to learn anything new about the topic at hand. As mentioned earlier, this is a behavior worthy of extinguishing in and of itself, because time spent perseverating is time *not* spent learning something new. However, the drive to perseverate can be very strong and thus can be capitalized on as a reinforcer. Therefore, appropriate topic maintenance may be best taught, initially, on a topic the child tends to perseverate upon. Permission to go speaking on with the topic will provide reinforcement for the continuation of the conversation, but the adult/teacher must force the child to acknowledge or introduce new information into the topic. For example, if a child is lining up trucks, then finding something that is a suitable "garage" and parking the trucks, washing the trucks, putting the firemen in the trucks, deciding what's on fire, and so on can be logical extensions of the conversation and the activity. Similarly, if a child verbally perseverates on a story, it would be a useful topic elaboration activity to stop the story in mid-recitation, before another page is turned, and require that the child answer (at least brief) questions before proceeding. Thus, strongly encouraging topic elaboration serves to jump-start imagination, which feeds back into future conversational possibilities.

Some parents are afraid if they don't allow the child to talk about his perseverative topic, he won't talk to them at all. This is not true. The perseveration needs to be reduced and confined as a maladaptive behavior. For example, Gregory, age eleven, who was diagnosed with Asperger's syndrome, enjoyed reading the Encyclopaedia Britannica to family members. He stated that his goal was to start at the beginning and read the whole set of volumes. His parents told him that he could read out loud to them each night after dinner, but he would have to choose what he wanted to read for each night, and then stop after fifteen minutes.

Brendan, a 10-year-old autistic boy, was, at the time I met him, perseverating about particularly high elevations on maps of Pakistan and India. At one point, he came out of his house and ran down the driveway after his mother and me as we were driving away, trying to start a "conversation" about altitudes. His mother handled it just right: She told him they would spend some time that evening looking at the maps together and discussing them. She reinforced his conversational attempt but also showed that his perseverative interest had to have bounds.

An autistic person needs to be actively shown what is an appropriate length of conversation about a topic. There is nothing wrong with saying that "We've talked about elevations on this map of Pakistan long enough," and then offering a conversationally adjacent choice like "Do you know the name of the highest peak in the Himalayas?" or "Let's see how deep the deepest seas are around India." Sometimes an autistic person needs to be asked if he has anything *new* to say about his topic, and if he does not, it is time to tell him to stop talking about his topic.

Multiword Language Development and Reading Skills

Representing More Abstract Language

One big leap in language development occurs when the child must begin to comprehend words for which there is no fixed physical, visual analogue. The first words acquired by autistic children are usually nouns—things the child wants, usually followed by classifications of things like numbers and letters. Using pictures, gestures, signs, and actions, you can also teach most verbs—like walking, running, and eating. You can even teach relational words like big and small, and first and last. Prepositions can be taught with physical models too, like showing "on" and "under," or "in" and "out."

Children with autism and PDD tend to have more persistent problems with "wh" words like "what," "where," "which," and so on. Sometimes the child makes pretty good guesses from context, especially if the "wh" question is asked about a familiar situation like "Where's the kitty?" or "What do you want to eat?" Sometimes, teachers (or parents) have to devise systematic tests to see if their child *really* is fully comprehending—like asking a question out of context or at an unexpected time. Teachers can devise practice materials for "wh" question drills by using complex pictures where several "wh" questions can be asked. For example, "Which one is Bert?" "Which one is Ernie?" "Who has the cookie?" "What is Bert doing?" Using stories that are already familiar to the child helps in these types of activities so that the progression of the plot is already understood.

Other Higher Level Language Skills

Other kinds of exercises can be used to improve higher level language skills, such as knowing when to say "I don't know," or to detect "silly" nonsense words. These kinds of activities further fine-tune comprehension. Higher level skills such as these can be embedded in other classroom tasks. An example could be a lesson on telling time: As the teacher moves the hands of the clock she can ask "Is it twelve?" "Is it six?" getting yes or no answers. Then she could ask "Is it twenty-five?" To which the child can be taught the response "No, that's silly." The same sort of response can be taught to questions like "Do cows bark?" and so on. Teaching a "that's silly" response is important in the development of self-reflective thinking and judgment, and moves the child away from the tendency for minimal rote responses that terminate the language interchange as quickly as possible. Similarly, giving the child opportunities to reflect on the *difference* between simply saying "No" in response to a question versus "I don't know" when that is a more accurate response also minimizes rote responding.

Chapter Summary

Once a child's language has proceeded to the multi-word stage and he is using various parts of speech, language can continue to develop in the more academic contexts of reading, writing, and verbal reasoning. In the next chapter, we will cover the things children need to learn in elementary school and beyond. We'll discuss educational models for both the higher functioning, more academically oriented child with autism or PDD, as well as the more practical skills that become an increasing focus of the curriculum for those students whose mental retardation is as much a disability as their autism.

♦ ♦ ♦

CHAPTER 13

Forks in the Road: The Elementary School Years and Beyond

Mental Retardation and Prognosis

Language instruction is usually the primary focus of the first few years of an autistic child's educational program. As we've seen in the preceding chapter, all of the various language activities that can be done in school can also be done at home—and in fact *should* be done at home. There are other skills that some autistic children learn mostly at school; these include learning to read, do math, and other regular academic tasks. For some other autistic children though, those with the more marked cognitive impairments, schooling consists of a focus on learning to be more independent in the functions of everyday living. In this chapter, we'll discuss how both these sets of skills are taught to children with autism and PDD.

Level of Mental Retardation and Determining Curriculum Focus

In educational planning for autistic children, the first few years of school are the same for many of the children, although children will progress at very different rates. Some three-year-olds will go from being mute at the beginning of their first year of school to speaking in two- and three-word phrases a year later. Others still have no words after a year of equally intensive efforts. Other factors being equal, for the most part these differences are due to the child's overall degree of mental retardation.

In my years of working with families with autistic children, it is clear that the hardest thing for all parents to hear is that their child has some degree of mental retardation. Aside from our society's stigmatizing attitudes toward the mentally retarded, parents fear this diagnosis because they know that mental retardation will limit the child's potential as an adult. Some parents therefore take the position that they do not want to be told that their child is mentally retarded. Some prefer to believe that it is not possible to know if a three-year-old is mentally retarded. Parents are understandably afraid of the day when, they imagine, their child cannot learn anything more. There are two main problems with adopting this position. First, it is wrong—even very retarded children continue to learn all their lives, although slowly. However, the degree of abstraction in the child's thinking and the child's ability to generalize knowledge become limited by the degree of mental retardation. Second, it is important to know a child's degree of mental retardation because it gives us some indication of how fast or slowly the child can learn, and thereby a metric for determining whether an educational program is doing as much for a child as can be reasonably expected.

It *is* possible to tell from tests and observations, if a child is mentally retarded and approximately how mentally retarded the child is. In fact, this can be determined at a fairly early age. The more severely retarded the child is, the younger the age at which mental retardation can be detected. Profound mental retardation—which is rare among children with autism and PDD—is usually apparent in the first year. Severe retardation is usually detectable by an experienced clinician in the second year. Moderate mental retardation can be detected fairly accurately by the third year of life; mild mental retardation between ages three and four. Depending on how much intervention the child has received, how he has responded to it, the special skills of a clinician in testing young delayed children, and other factors, the degree of mental retardation may be detected at even earlier ages.

Information about a child's degree of mental retardation is very important to curriculum planning because it gives us some ability to know what we can expect a particular child to be able to learn. Because there are enough individual differences in the progress some children will make, only broad judgments about severity of mental retardation are usually made—but these judgments very much *need* to be made so that a child is not unduly frustrated by endless attempts to learn things that he does not have the capacity to learn. One reassuring point that I make to parents in this regard is that *everybody*, not just autistic children, has a ceiling to what he or she can learn. If someone persisted in teaching me beyond my capacities, I would feel like a stupid failure and not want to interact with the people who were constantly making me aware of my deficits—and this happens to children, too. Determining degree of mental retardation in a child with autism or PDD is a way of estimating where the child's ceiling is. The tactic is to strategically plan the child's instruction so that she learns all about the things she *is* capable of absorbing, and that things above the ceiling are not hammered at, in order to avoid creating an unhappy, learning-averse child.

The reason for making the above points is the following: There are a few major forks in the road to learning for autistic and PDD children that relate to their degree of mental retardation and which predict the general direction they will head in life. Initially, most are placed in similar infant stimulation programs, and/or instructed with the language-learning strategies we've discussed. Depending on the rate of progress in the first few years, children diagnosed with autism, PDD, or Asperger's syndrome can follow very different paths after that.

The Communicatively Handicapped Educational Track

Children who are speaking (albeit more or less autistically by age three or four) are generally placed with other children with communicative handicaps (CH). These children tend to either have specific language disorders or are functioning in the borderline mentally retarded range. Classes for CH children typically are continued up until fourth, fifth, or sixth grade. Children in such classes are taught to read, write, add, and subtract. In later grades, some of these same children are placed in classes for the learning disabled (LD) or learning handicapped (LH); these classes deal with a variety of learning disabilities in addition to language handicaps, often including many children with mild mental retardation but with relatively few behavioral or adaptive problems. These children acquire similar academic skills, and as such children get older, they also learn multiplication and division, and may study history and science. In the past, children at this level educationally were sometimes referred to as educably mentally retarded, or EMR.

The Severely Handicapped Educational Track

The next tier below CH, LH, and LD classes are for more severely handicapped (SH) students who are functioning in the moderate to severely mentally retarded range. As preschoolers, these children start out with the same language goals, but may be eight or nine years old before they have as much language as a CH class student had at five years. These children may learn some reading, but it is usually what is described as "sight" or "survival" reading (recognizing the "look" of words, rather than reading phonetically), and learn basic concepts of quantitation through the use of physical manipulatives (like blocks or coins that can be counted one by one). In the past, students with this level of disability were sometimes referred to as trainably mentally retarded, or TMR.

By fifth grade or so, in the better programs, children in SH classes are learning everyday skills like cooking, cleaning, and how to act in public. Some schools for such children, however, still have twelve-year-old SH students tracing eight-inch models of the first letter of their names for the fifth year in a row. In my opinion, these schools are anachronistic abominations. How can any child be interested or happy in his work if he has been given the same task year after year? Teachers in these classes often report many more severe behavior problems and spend more time in behavior management. It is understandable that children will protest being forced to do tasks that have no meaning for them. These children do not need to be treated with drugs, or "better" behavior modification (as is often concluded), but with different educational goals that give them something they find meaningful to do.

There is definitely a point at which parents and the school, working together must decide that a student is ready for a more "everyday skills" curriculum, and that it is time to mostly leave academics behind. This can be a really hard decision for parents because for some it feels like locking the child into some sort of prison cell that will always separate him from mainstream society in some way. It is perhaps more helpful to think of making the "mainstream" more diverse, with roles for people with limited cognitive ability, but who can be helped to feel useful doing a small, well-defined vocational job. If it takes a child ten years to learn to talk, and then can only use his language to answer in one- and two-word phrases, then age ten is not too soon to start teaching the child the skills he needs to function as independently as possible at age twenty.

With that said, the rest of the chapter will deal with specific instructional issues beyond the early language learning years. First we will cover some topics that pertain to the children who do acquire formal academic skills. Second, we'll focus on the children who follow the everyday living skills track.

Academic Skills for Higher Functioning Autistic and PDD Children

How Do Autistic and PDD Children Learn to Read?

Many PDD and some autistic children learn to read on their own. Even more teach themselves the alphabet unbeknownst to parents. I remember the mother of Damon, age 6, who told me that she had realized that her son could read one day when they were in the living room with the game show *Wheel of Fortune* on the television. Damon had said "Michael Jackson" for no apparent reason. In a few minutes, it became apparent that "Michael Jackson" was the phrase being uncovered from the tiles on the game board as they were turned over one by one. Tyler, at age four, had selectively begun to read overhead freeway signs out loud as he rode in the car with his family. Michael, also age four, read street signs and signs that regulated traffic. I have met a number of children who first read the word "Toyota" off the back of a pick-up truck, and then began to recognize the word everywhere—on TV commercials, in parking lots, and on billboards. The youngest reader was William, an intellectually gifted boy with Asperger's syndrome who at age fourteen competed in the national spelling bee. His mother recalls his fascination at ten months with an alphabet quilt. At fourteen months, he pointed to the words "cat" and "dog" and said them. To test whether he was reading or memorizing, his mother showed him the word "elephant," and William read "elephant."

Autistic children seem to find letters naturally interesting because they can be endlessly rearranged and are concrete and finite. There are plenty of opportunities to observe words paired with pictures of words—in books, on TV, on the menu at McDonald's, and on every car that passes by. Some autistic children seem to learn to recognize words as complex patterns rather than as separate phonic elements. By the time they can sight-recognize several words, it is usually fairly easy to introduce the concept of phonics. Autistic children who read generally do so for their own satisfaction, on topics that interest them. Early books usually include ones that focus on classifications (such as types of whales) or labels of objects (such as colors and shapes), rhymes, or children's dictionaries, rather than books with story lines.

In teaching young autistic children to read, their propensity for labeling and classification should be kept in mind and turned to the advantage of the teacher. Books with one-word vocabulary items are usually the easiest to begin with. Pointing to the individual letters as you say the words helps the child see the phonic relationships. At the next stage of reading, some autistic children can do well with rhyming, Dr. Seuss–type books because the visual element is strong, and the plot is not very important.

Autism and Hyperlexia. One oddity that often occurs with autistic children as they begin to read is that they develop a special form of learning disability known as *hyperlexia*. Children who are hyperlexic can read better than they can comprehend. I have seen children who read a book by starting on the first page and reading the title, the publisher, the publication date and place, the copyright infringement warnings, etc. Then they read the story. Usually, children who are doing this are not comprehending all that they are reading. In certain ways, hyperlexia is the written word's equivalent for echolalia in speech, when the autistic child speaks but does not understand all the component parts of what he says. Hyperlexia is like an English-speaker reading but not understanding Spanish—a language with similar phonics, but completely different vocabulary.

Working with Hyperlexia. The autistic child's ability to read can be used to improve comprehension of written and oral material and to improve his overall ability to analyze social situations. There are several ways of going about this. For children who can read, teachers can photocopy pages of simple children's cartoons like Garfield or Snoopy. The child can be shown the page and asked to read it. For example: Frame 1—Garfield sees a lasagna (caption: "Oh boy, my favorite—Lasagna!!"); Frame 2—Garfield jumps into the lasagna (caption: "Slurp, slurp, slurp"); Frame 3—Garfield is found by his owner in an empty lasagna dish, licking his face (caption: "Glad I got here in time!"). After showing the child the three frames, the teacher can make a few sets of materials: (1) the series of pictures plus separate captions for the student to attach to each one; (2) the series of captions with separate pictures to attach to each one; and (3) separae pictures *and* captions so that both visual and written materials have to be sequenced. In this way, the relatively strong skill of reading is used to assist the relatively weaker comprehension skills. This technique also shows what the child really does and does not understand, which is important for a teacher to know because the autistic or PDD child's reading often suggests more comprehension than is really there.

Reading Interests of Older and Higher Functioning Children with Autism and PDD. Older autistic children often prefer reading calendars, atlases, phone books, and even encyclopedias. Nonfiction is definitely preferred to fiction. Jed, a twelve-year-old young man with PDD, an IQ in the 120s, and an eidetic ("photographic") memory has started to read *The Encyclopaedia Britannica*, beginning with "aardvarks." He plans to read the whole thing. Another patient of mine, Ellison, reads the toll-free "800" Yellow Pages at the library. He makes lists and then calls for free booklets and advertisements from architectural firms. (This young man knows the names, number of stories, and other vital statistics of all the major buildings in the San Francisco financial district even though he lives in a small town ninety miles away.) Autistic children, like other children, read for pleasure, but what gives them pleasure is something different from other children their age. Autistic children virtually never read stories with elaborate plots and highly developed characters, but they do read fact-filled material. Parents and teachers need to capitalize on the narrow, intense interests of such children and try to expand their reading range beyond the material they will spontaneously read on their own. On his own, a child may be happy reading the same book about whales over and over. There should be limited access to a book a child is perseverating on (for example, only getting to look at it for ten minutes during free time in the afternoon at school). Teachers should make an effort to reinforce forays into new topics— like getting a whale fancier to take out a library book on tropical fish, and then building a lesson plan of reading out loud and writing about it.

Writing Skills

Autistic and PDD children who read well often seem better able to express themselves in writing than in spoken language. One reason for this may be that the expressive language problems associated with autism may be partly related to the speed with which processing of spoken language should occur. With many teenage and young adult autistic people I talk to, I often feel that our conversations are taking place underwater, or in slow motion, or in zero gravity because their sentence formulations are so drawn out. The second probable explanation for why many higher functioning autistic people write better than they speak is that speaking is a more social activity than writing. All the language pragmatics and social interactional aspects of a conversation— which present enormous difficulties in autism—impinge upon the thinking of an autistic person when he speaks. When he writes, he can be alone. Therefore writing can be a good modality for encouraging expression in older, higher functioning autistic and PDD students. Interestingly, *Nobody, Nowhere*, the autobiography of Donna Williams, who describes herself as a high-functioning autistic, seems to support these propositions. In a radio interview about her book, Ms. Williams would accept only questions that she had seen written down in advance.

Writing about Facts. It is easiest for an autistic child to answer discrete, factual questions about a story he has read, or to report facts he has amassed on a special topic. Mitchell, age eight, a student of mine years ago, was obsessed with calendars. On the first day of the month he would run to reach the classroom first so that he could pull the old month off the calendar and announce the new month. He would read the name of the month in a loud monotone with a slight French accent (which he had presumably picked up from his mother). For the first several days of each month, he would be motivated to write essays about the month: "November has Thanksgiving. We eat turkey and gravy. The leaves turn color in November." His reward was to be allowed to read his compositions (which in fact were rather similar day to day), out loud. In this way, we were able to capitalize on Mitchell's love of calendars to promote his reading, writing, spelling, and grammatical skills. Writing about factual material is generally good, but can become self-stimulatory and/or perseverative: Another patient of mine, described earlier, is also into calendars. Each afternoon after he has finished his homework he is allowed to work on his "Calendar Project." He began with January 1, 1900, and is writing out every date along with its weekday for the entire century. Although this is a recreational rather than educational activity for him, it could be pushed in the direction of being somewhat more educational and less perseverative—like learning to use a keyboard while writing out the dates.

Experiential/"First Person" Writing. Initial writing exercises for an autistic student might consist of copying sentences about a favorite topic. At the next stage, the student might be encouraged to circle an appropriate ending to a sentence (for example, Fire trucks are _____red/purple.). Later it might be possible for the student to "compose" an essay by answering several questions in a row with the answers written as consecutive sentences. (For example, Q: Where did we go on our class trip yesterday? A: We went to Marine World. Q: What was the most interesting thing you saw? A: I saw Shamu the killer whale. Q: What was interesting about it? A: He jumped and splashed me.) Finally, the student might be able to write a short essay with only one prompt, such as "Write about where we went on our field trip, what you liked best, and why." Autistic children, unlike other children when they first start writing, are not really motivated to share their experiences with others. This goes all the way back to the way autistic children as toddlers don't show joint referencing—the desire to have others watch and acknowledge their activities. Therefore, the experience of sharing a point of view through writing has to be taught.

Most older, higher functioning people with autism or PDD write in a way that very literally conveys the world as you see them experiencing it. They do not write much about perceptions, feelings and emotions in themselves or others, or anything that would make you believe they experience human relationships in a more empathetic way than they are able to express verbally. For example, Richard, a long-time patient of mine, wrote an essay about big dogs when he was in ninth grade. He began with: "The big vicious dogs had large white teeth. They chased me across the park." When I asked him about dogs after reading the essay, the conversation was much more one-sided and monosyllabic: Q: "Richard, do you like big dogs?" A: "No." Q: "Do you ever see dogs at the park?" A: "Yes." Q: "Do they frighten you?" A: "Yes."

Teachers often send me samples of a student's writing to demonstrate their frustration in not being able to get better verbal participation from a student who may write better than others in his class. Getting the student to write on a topic he particularly likes, and then having him read it aloud and answer questions from another student, can help facilitate social interaction through writing.

Math Abilities

Rote Math Skills. Autistic and PDD children are often interested in counting at a very early age. Many count before they say other words. The first real mathematical milestone, however, is the emergence of *one-to-one correspondence*. This is when a child can count out objects one at a time, knowing that one number corresponds to one quantity. This is a very physically based concept, and autistic children do best with physical math.

Autistic children tend to acquire math concepts that can be conveyed on a visual level fairly well. I will always remember Marc, a deaf, autistic seven-year-old boy whom I worked with during my special education teaching internship. He could sit for hours doing addition and subtraction problems, but because he couldn't speak, no one had ever tried to explain multiplication to him. One day I noticed he had drawn eight pictures of Big Bird in eight boxes on a large piece of paper. In each picture, Big Bird had rotated slightly, and by the last picture, he had rotated completely around. The order of the pictures was marked by little balls drawn in the lower right corner of each picture—one for the first picture, two for the second and so on. With this in mind, I wrote a simple multiplication problem—3 × 2. Next to the 3, I drew three balls; next to the 2, I drew two balls. I counted the three balls once and crossed off one of the two balls next to the number 2. I drew three balls at the bottom of the problem next to where the answer would go. I repeated this, scratching off the second ball next to the number 2 when I was finished. There were six balls at the bottom and I wrote the number 6 for the answer. I set up the next problem. Marc took away the pencil and drew the right number of balls and the answer for the second problem without help. I double-checked with my supervising teacher whether Marc knew how to multiply. She said no. After that, Marc certainly did know how to multiply, and did so whenever I gave him problems. One problem that I couldn't solve in those days was how to fade his dependency on the prompt—the little balls—which he continued to draw and scratch off. Using physical manipulatives (like blocks) that could simply be taken away after a while probably would have worked with him.

Functional Math. The stage of math at which many autistic children stall is word problems. Even autistic children who can easily plow through piles of rote multiplication and division have difficulty when even simple math is embedded in a more human context. For example, a student who can tell you in a flash that nine divided by three is three is very likely to have a great deal more difficulty responding to "If Tom, Jack, and Jim equally divide nine dollars that they earned raking leaves, how much should each boy get?" Setting math into a more instrumental, self-related context can help an autistic child deal with word math. For example, "You have nine Nintendo cassettes and put them in three piles; how many in each pile?"

Going back to physical manipulatives for teaching word math can help autistic children a great deal. It is also important in math, just as in reading, that the child actually understand what he is doing before moving on to the next level. It is definitely possible to teach an autistic child to multiply before he can do word math addition problems, but what's the point? Some parents and teachers push a child to do rote math "at grade level." If the child cannot use the math functionally, little is being accomplished but a demonstration of the child's ability to memorize. As with reading, it is important to keep comprehension commensurate with performance.

Making the Transition to A Functional Academic Orientation

A small proportion of children diagnosed with autism or PDD really do function within a year or two of grade level. Among children with autism, by the fifth grade probably twenty-five percent are academically within two years of grade functioning in more than one subject; this figure drops to 10% by the end of high school. The reason for the drop-off rate is that command of all subjects requires more complex language and abstract reasoning skills. These higher level cognitive functions—formal operational thinking—normally emerge around ages twelve to fourteen. At this point, the gap between most children with autism or PDD and their agemates tends to widen. For autistic and PDD children in the top twenty-five percent cognitively, maintaining the regular elementary school curriculum makes sense. For the other seventy-five percent, curriculum focus needs to becomes more oriented to language, reading, and math operations needed in everyday functioning. By the end of middle school age (eighth grade), those in the top twenty-five percent who have begun to fall farther behind, should also be considered for a more functional curriculum. There are many jobs that require basic literacy skills, but do not require that the child has ever read *Lord of the Flies* or learned algebra or geometry.

By high school, many cognitively higher functioning students with autism or PDD need a curriculum that specifically ensures that their cognitive skills can be applied in practical ways. Even students with "savant" skills, who like being able to tell you whether February 19, 2002, comes on a Tuesday, might not realize that if he's worked three hours for six dollars an hour, he's being cheated if he gets paid with a five-dollar and a ten-dollar bill. Small challenges like waiting for a bus may be frustrating for an autistic young person if someone else is sitting where he last sat in the bus shelter, the bus comes off schedule, or he finds he doesn't have exact change. While these are small challenges that two thirteen-year-old girls off to the shopping mall together could easily handle, an adult autistic person of normal intelligence might ruminate and complain for days after such a disruption in his routine.

For the autistic young adult, using intellectual capacity to apply skills in context and in a practical way is a whole additional area of learning. Generally, instruction programs that take advantage of the substantial rote memories of cognitively higher functioning autistic people by role-playing steps in common daily transactions can be helpful.

IQ and Adaptive Functioning. IQ is not as well related to the young person's level of *adaptive* functioning in autistic teenagers and young adults as it is in nonhandicapped people, or even in mentally retarded people without autism or PDD. Adaptive functioning, which was initially discussed in Chapter 5, is measured by how well an individual is able to use the intelligence he or she has to function in daily life. Like IQ, adaptive functioning can be measured with specific tests, but unlike IQ, adaptive functioning can be taught. Adaptive tasks that quite intelligent autistic people may need help with include self-care—like being forced to shower each day (whether they see a reason to or not), doing laundry, and keeping their bedrooms clean (when Mom has gotten old enough to retire from her job as the maid), and preparing simple, varied meals (instead of following an impulse to eat exactly the same thing every day at exactly the same time). It seems reasonable to expect that someone who can tell you everything you ever wanted to know about aardvarks (and more) should be able to do these simple tasks by the time he's eighteen, but with autistic young people, this is often not the case. Daily living skills outside the home often require special teaching too. Being able to read elevations, temperatures, sea depths, population densities, and distances in miles and kilometers off a topographical map of India does not ensure that you can use the map of the London Underground even if you've taken it five days a week since you were five-years-old. By the early teen years, it can be very helpful to make an adaptive behavior assessment of a cognitively higher functioning teen with autism or PDD, and develop specific plans for teaching specific adaptive behaviors.

Vocational Choices for Higher Functioning Young People with Autism and PDD

For children with autism and PDD in the top twenty-five percent, the beginning of high school (ninth grade) is a good time to begin to develop special talents into some sort of job skill. This is not to say that 100% of the curriculum needs to be focused this way, but there should be a particular effort to help the student do well in an area in which he feels he excels. This is good for self-esteem as well as being functional and adaptive to challenges the student will confront later. For example, a student who draws with an excellent sense of detail and proportion might begin to learn drafting and computer-assisted design. A student who is interested in plants might learn horticultural skills. A young man who is fascinated with electricity might learn skills related to electronic assembly or repair.

Because autism constitutes an additional barrier to functioning, autistic people seldom hold jobs at the level that could simply be predicted by their level of intelligence. Unfortunately, even the brightest autistic people tend to be overwhelmed by the social and decision-making aspects of most forms of employment. Many are happier working at jobs below their cognitive ability, but that allow them time to pursue their special interests. Careful vocational testing as well as discussions with the young person should be the basis of deciding on a specific area of vocational training. Higher functioning autistic people also need to be encouraged to examine realistically what kind of job they might be able to get. Even routine jobs in crowded places (like wiping tables at McDonald's or retrieving shopping carts a Safeway) tend to go awry. One of the therapists in our clinic interviewed a young man with Asperger's syndrome who had lost his job bagging purchases at K-Mart in his first week on the job because he held his ears and ran out of the store every time the bell announcing in-store specials went off.

Calibrating Expectations

One of my main concerns is that, often, too much is expected of higher functioning autistic and PDD adolescents as they approach high school age. High expectations, expectations to "get normal," tend to exacerbate the preexisting strain of social interaction rather than resolve it. Even among those in the highest functioning subgroup of individuals with autistic spectrum disorders—those diagnosed with Asperger's syndrome (see Chapter 5)—in the late teen or early adult years almost one-third develop psychiatric disorders that are believed to be the result of a poor ability to cope with the strains of daily living. Parents who work hard for years to teach their children sometimes find it hard to be less demanding as the teenage years are reached.

The vast majority of parents of such young people *can* see how the child's happiness will be compromised if they push harder. The watershed for parents of this subgroup of children is when they realize that their children need an opportunity to function closer to their social mental age than to their cognitive mental age. This is because in day-to-day life, the ability to function independently and on-the-job social skills are at least as important as the actual technical skills that are needed. For example, if an autistic person is adding information to a computer database, that person also needs to know when to ask questions about irregularities he may encounter, when to ask for new work, how to manage his time if he is asked to suddently shift from one task to another, and who in the company hierarchy to go to with different kinds of concerns, and so on. Many higher functioning autistic people who could operate the necessary data base software would have a great deal more difficulty fulfilling these other, more social tasks. So, as they get to be adults, many prefer jobs that are less intellectually challenging, but also less socially complex.

Most higher functioning people with autism and PDD virtually always need to live and work in environments where some level of special dispensation is made for their handicap. This is important for parents of higher functioning autistic people to know, so they can plan realistically when it comes to choosing how academically oriented a school program will be, and what type of job-oriented training the academic program can lead toward.

A related problem is that many cognitively higher functioning autistic people are not motivated to work at all. At best, they come to accept going to work and doing their job as part of an expected routine; but, if asked, they won't say that they "like" their work. Left on their own, a number of autistic young adults I've seen will loll around at home, watching TV, eating, and doing little else. They do not become bored from lack of social stimulation. Usually the parents of such young people become frustrated after a couple of years spent watching their children lolling around, with only part-time and transitory jobs, or very occasionally community college courses. At that juncture, a vocational assessment followed by some decision-making on behalf of the young person with regard to a place to live and work or obtain further job training is called for.

By the time an autistic person is in his early twenties, I encourage parents to find an out-of-home living situation for him. Autistic young adults still need to be instrumentally motivated, and as long as they can count on their family members to cook, clean, and care for them, they are likely to remain fairly inactive.

Skills Training for More Cognitively Disabled Autistic Persons

"High," "Low," and "Medium" Functioning Autistic Children

Sometimes severely retarded autistic children are referred to as "low functioning" autistic children. While these children are "lower," than "higher" functioning autistic children, it can be a hard label to accept, especially if you feel your child is being labeled as on the bottom of the pile. One mother I know wrote an article in *The Advocate,* the newsletter of the Autism Society of America, expressing how bad she felt as the parent of a "low functioning" autistic boy in a support group of parents who all described their autistic children as "high functioning." I told her that I knew several of the other families in her support group and that, actually, most had "medium functioning" autistic children. Autism is on a spectrum, and the middle is a lot larger than either extreme. Many "medium functioning" autistic children face the same challenges as "lower functioning" autistic children, but need somewhat less intensive training to reach goals. If your child is described as a "low functioning autistic," just remember that there are many children in the middle, and the truly "high functioning" autistics who are talked about so much are actually fairly rare.

The hardest thing about diagnosing mental retardation along with autism is that it narrows a parent's vision of the child's future. After I explain that a child is significantly mentally retarded *and* autistic, I answer questions and watch as the parents realize first that the child will never marry, never go to a regular high school, never go to *any* "regular" school, will never learn to really read, and in fact may never use spoken language. I can't imagine anything that could engender deeper feelings of hopelessness. Sometimes as parents realize all the things their child will never be able to do, they begin to feel that the child will never be able to do *anything*. That type of feeling is clearly related to the seeming hopelessness of the situation, but is just a feeling and *not* the reality. All children learn as they grow. They learn at different rates, and they learn different things. All children with moderate to severe mental retardation learn more slowly, and autism does provide them with an additional handicap.

For the autistic child with moderate to severe mental retardation, language learning, usually through the use of communication boards or sign, is a major focus of early schooling. The second major focus of early schooling for children who are significantly developmentally disabled is work on adaptive functioning. Adaptive functioning goals need to be addressed both at school and at home. In the following sections we will talk about how these skills can be encouraged to develop in both settings and the need for consistency between these two settings.

School-Based Daily Living Skills Curricula

Adaptive functioning is taught in school under several headings: Daily Living Skills, Real Life Skills, Critical Skills, Adaptive Behavior, and so on. The content of an adaptive skills program is on helping the child be as independent as possible. In the early years, this focuses on self-help skills such as self-feeding, toileting or toilet-schedule training, and learning how to undress and dress. Another important aspect of adaptive skills training for young autistic children is learning how to participate in a routine and follow the rules of a group. (This is true for all preschool-aged children.)

When these initial skills have been mastered, adaptive skills curricula that are usually introduced around age ten to twelve focus on everyday living skills like preparing food, making beds, doing laundry, and helping with household cleaning and gardening tasks. By middle school or high school age, adaptive functioning curricula focus on vocational skills such as sorting, assembling, and packaging. In Chapter 5, we discussed a test called *The Vineland Adaptive Behavior Scales*, which is frequently used to assess how well an autistic person is doing in applying his intellectual capacities to everyday functioning. For lower functioning autistic adolescents, it is important to focus on how to develop the types of skills the Vineland test measures, and on the particular difficulties that autistic people encounter in the development of these skills.

Focusing on adaptive living skills for developmentally disabled children has a long history—in fact, a longer history than the trend in the 1920s through 1970s of institutionalizing the mentally retarded and caring for them custodially instead of teaching them to care for themselves. Before this century, when rates of literacy and schooling were much lower, nobody thought of using relatively scarce educational resources on the mentally retarded; back then, many normal children without mental retardation did not go to school but received training at home and on the job that enabled them to grow up to be useful citizens. At that time, it was not stigmatizing for a developmentally disabled child to lack formal education. Often, only the brightest children were sent to school anyway; or only the youngest children went to school—if there were enough older children who could work to support the family economically.

Even in the 1940s, some of Dr. Leo Kanner's original descriptions of autism included individuals who were treated with "rustification"—being sent to live in the country with friends or family. There, the autistic person could be trained to do a job he could do well, feel good about what he was doing, and have to deal relatively little with the stresses of a more complex society.

The modern history of formal adaptive education for the developmentally disabled really started with the work of Maria Montessori in Italy. Although Montessori's work is now well known as a preschool curriculum, she originally started with the idea of what is now thought of as a functional skills curriculum for developmentally disabled children. Features of the Montessori curriculum that are in evidence in preschools today, like a "housekeeping corner" in each room, originally were intended to give mentally retarded children an opportunity to practice skills they would need every day like sweeping, wiping up, and bathing small children.

The thing that is most helpful in keeping lower functioning autistic people out of highly restrictive institutional placements today is their level of self-care and overall adaptive functioning. Through various policy changes, the biggest state institutions for the severely mentally retarded are being closed, allowing former residents to be cared for in smaller, more home-like settings closer to their families. To be a good community member of such a group home, however, the autistic child needs to have been prepared with skills to function partly independently.

Home-Based Daily Living Skills for More Severely Affected Children

Early self-care skills include self-feeding and toilet training; both can present some particular problems for parents of autistic children. Even a severely mentally retarded autistic child can learn most basic self-care skills by the time he is five or six years old (although when he is two, parents can be quite skeptical). There are a couple of basic principles for teaching these skills: First, a high degree of consistency is needed in the demands put on the child. Second, each achievement will be made in small, gradual steps. Third, don't try to teach everything at once. Fourth, expect from your child only that which is appropriate for his mental age. In the following sections, we'll discuss some basic strategies for accomplishing self-help skills. An excellent resource on this topic is *The Me Book: Teaching Developmentally Disabled Children* by Dr. Ivar Lovaas, a behaviorally oriented guide to accomplishing early milestones in the education of autistic and other developmentally disabled children.

Feeding Difficulties

Self-Feeding Skills. There are certain cultural differences as to how early children are expected to feed themselves, but by eighteen months old, most children in most cultures are primarily feeding themselves non-messy finger foods. Because autistic children tend to prefer to do things for themselves if they can, finger-feeding is usually not delayed. If the child has specific problems in fine motor development, the feeding may be messy, but the autistic child will generally want to do it for himself. By the time a child has a mental age of around eighteen to twenty-four months, it is reasonable to begin working on self-feeding of messy foods (for example, applesauce, cereal with milk, yogurt, ice cream). It can be helpful to start with one favorite food in one setting. The child can be helped, hand-over-hand to, say, spoon ice cream into his mouth. If he refuses to hold the spoon, the ice cream shoud be placed out of sight (for five to ten seconds) and the trial repeated. If the holding of the spoon is refused several times, the ice cream should simply be put away. The worst thing to do at this point would be to feed the child the ice cream or let him feed it to himself without using the spoon. It would also be a good idea to wait at least a few minutes before offering the child something else he likes to eat or drink instead (like his bottle). For most autistic children, refusal to use a spoon or fork is not a matter of not having the coordination to hold a spoon or fork. (A child who can neatly pluck an M&M should have no trouble with a spoon.) Even a child who still holds a crayon with a full fist can use a baby spoon. Autistic chldren resist using spoons because they don't see why they should learn *your* way of eating when they already have *their* way of eating. Unlike a mentally retarded child who is not autistic, the autistic child is more interested in pleasing himself than in pleasing you, especially if your "pleasures" are at odds with his. The battle of the wills that can take place around self-feeding are not really that different from other children's "terrible two's" battles. All children, autistic or not, need to learn that parents are in a better position to make rules than they are, and that life does indeed have rules that need to be accepted. Sometimes it seems hard to impose rules on a mentally retarded or autistic child because you feel sorry for him. But not doing so doesn't help him, and it doesn't help you.

Food Fads. Part of the self-feeding battle is that some autistic children appear to develop very narrow food preferences. I say "appear" because food preferences are learned behaviors, and the child *can* learn to like something new. Narrow food preferences are most common in firstborns—parents of latter-borns have less time to fuss with food refusals, and tasty rejected foods get eaten by other siblings, leaving the food refuser with nothing to eat, or having to wait until others are done eating. So, for example, many autistic children eat things in school that they won't eat at home. That's because if it's snack time and you're hungry, and everyone gets grape juice and graham crackers, you'll drink grape juice and eat a graham cracker instead of just sitting at the snack table doing nothing. The same philosophy can be applied at home.

Often parents are concerned because their autistic child won't eat anything except milk and white bread, or anything but Hi-C, McDonald's french fries, and cheese pizza. There is usually no reason why an autistic child shouldn't be trained to eat a more well-rounded variety of foods. A very small number of autistic children do have oral-motor problems, usually evidenced by drooling or gagging, even when eating favorite foods. Such children may refuse foods that have to be chewed. Such children should be treated by an occupational therapist or speech and language pathologist who specializes in feeding problems.

The first step in expanding food choices is offering the child a reasonable, nutritious substitute for an exclusive food. For example, a child who will drink only Hi-C might be offered some watered-down orange juice or some apple juice. Offer it in whatever kind of container the child is used to (a training cup, a regular cup, bottle, etc.). Don't use the same exact container as the currently accepted food, or the child may begin to reject the food he does accept in that container. At first, if the child rejects if after one taste, put it away and offer it again several seconds later. After several rejections, put it away, and wait at least a half hour (and until any tantrum disappears) before offering the food the child does like. The next time the child wants Hi-C, juice should be offered again instead—a little more persistently. Wait longer until giving the food the child does like. The same rules go with solid foods. A tiny bit of the new food should be tried before the preferred food is given. Give the old food in limited quantity. Try the new food again. Gradually, the mix between new and old foods can be shifted. Don't worry that the child will starve. There are children who hold out and eat very little for two or even three days, but eventually they do eat some of what is offered. The tantrum that will inevitably result should be ignored. Walk away from it. When it diminishes a little in intensity, offer the new food again. Don't try this at family mealtime. Feed everyone else before or after.

Family Mealtimes. The next issue is how to get the autistic child to be a part of family mealtime. This is really a very individual family matter. If there are other siblings who would like to use dinner time to talk about school, friends, and activities, I usually vote for letting the autistic child do something else if he will disrupt the meal. The other children need routine and a planned, available time to communicate with parents, too. Jiff, seven-year-old brother of Joe, a very talkative ten-year-old with Asperger's syndrome, recently had a weekend with his mother while Joe visited his grandmother alone. Mrs. Carried, Jiff and Joe's mother, told me that one night at dinner Jiff said "This is s-o-o nice, Mom, I mean it's so quiet without Joe." A look of embarrassment and upset then crossed Jiff's face and he added, "I don't mean I don't love Joe. . . . That wouldn't be good." It can be hard for families to know what they're missing if they are always accommodating the special needs of their autistic child. Dinner time can sometimes be a good routine time of day for other family members to be together, especially if it can be done in a way so that the autistic child is happy too—like getting to eat first and watch a video while the rest of the family eats.

Many families who *would* like their autistic children to eat with the rest of the family describe how their autistic children "graze" from the table and never sit through a meal. Like other behavioral issues, this problem needs to be addressed in gradual steps. Begin by trying to have the child stay at the table for only a couple of minutes while he eats. Bring small toys to the table that he can play with right in front of him or at his high chair tray. If eating stops, and disruptive behavior seems imminent, put the child down before he misbehaves. Do not reward bad behavior with the desired removal from the table. Either let the child down before he fusses to leave the table, or quiet the child somewhat before releasing him. Prohibit grazing. Restrict eating during mealtimes to eating at the table. Again, the mental age rule applies. A child with an eighteen-month mental age usually *doesn't* stay at the table throughout a prolonged dinner.

In restaurants, be prepared to take shifts as you would for a younger child, restrict yourself to a fast-food outlet or a family restaurant, or don't bring a child who cannot stay contained for the normal duration of a mealtime. Do unto others as you would have them do unto you—if you were having dinner out without children. It's kind of cute if a three-year-old grabs a french fry from someone else's table. It is usually not appreciated if the child who does it is a ten-year-old.

Toilet Training

Nobody likes to change diapers, and doing it for four or five years for the same child gets onerous, especially if there are one or two younger sibling's in diapers, too. Many parents come to my clinic with the specific request for help on how to toilet train their autistic child. Toilet training autistic children is different from toilet training other children in a few ways. First, autistic children do not learn well from imitation, and so the usual strategies of taking Billy into the potty with Daddy, and taking Sarah into the potty with Mommy, make little impression. Second, autistic children usually have little interest in using the potty in order to be deemed a "Big girl!" or "Big boy!" What autistic children do have going for themselves when it comes to toilet training is that many will comply to get a prized food reward (like some chocolate), and a number will decide for themselves that they don't like being wet or dirty and decide to train themselves after very few "lessons." Also, many autistic children love to adhere to a routine, and so once using the toilet becomes a routine, they have relatively few accidents.

In American culture, most children are toilet trained at around age two to two-and-a-half, a little later for boys than for girls. Bladder training usually precedes bowel training, and day dryness precedes nighttime dryness. The same progression is usually true of autistic children. Readiness for toilet training is fairly strongly correlated with the mental age of the child, since both physical and cognitive systems must cooperate in the activity. Children with mental ages below two- to two-and-a-half years (in terms of performance IQ) are usually not fully ready for toilet training, irrespective of their chronological age.

Schedule Training. For autistic children who are at least three years old, we usually begin with what is referred to as *schedule training* or *timed toileting*. This means that the child is toileted on a schedule with the idea of catching the child in the act of doing the right thing, and reinforcing it. For schedule training to be really effective, it needs to be undertaken as a joint effort by home and school. Readiness for schedule training can best be determined by parents who begin to realize that the child goes with a dry diaper for periods of an hour or more. It also helps if the parents have an idea of when the diapers are usually wet or soiled. Some children give off pretty clear signals about their need to wet or soil their diaper, and these are important pieces of information for setting up a toileting schedule. Usually, when schedule training is begun, the child is taken to the toilet as soon as he wakes up in the morning, and again ten to fifteen minutes after having some juice or milk. In school, children are usually taken to the toilet when they arrive, before or after recess, after snacks, and any other time they look like they might have to "go." During each visit to the toilet, the child is helped to pull down his pants (the new pull-up diapers are a real boon to this stage), and sit (with supervision) for three to five minutes. Tricks like running the tap and pouring warm water over little boys' penises can help too. Any success should be met with intense verbal praise and an immediate (while still on the toilet) food reward. Some children catch on to schedule training right away and, before anyone realizes it, begin to take themselves to the toilet. One mother told me how, a few days into toilet training, she heard the toilet flush, and then realized that the only family member who wasn't in the room was her three-year-old autistic son. She went in the bathroom and there he was, pulling up his pants. For some autistic children, watching the toilet flush is a big reinforcer, and they come to see flushing as integral to the toileting routine.

Some parents and teachers report a considerable sense of frustration with other children who seem to withhold until their diapers are back on and *then* have a bowel movement. Two suggestions for these children are (1) watch them carefully and try to get them right back on the toilet again when they get ready to go, or (2) put a wet diaper back on for a few moments so it is slightly aversive, and then take the child to the potty, and change the diaper only after he has successfully sat on the potty for a few moments.

It is sometimes easier to accomplish schedule training at school than at home, because the school day is more routine, the bathrooms have multiple toilets, and the accompanying teachers or aides don't have to worry about what else is going on while they are involved in toilet training the way a parent at home does. But, if a child can learn to be dry in one setting, then he can learn to be dry in both. It is important that parents and teachers work closely on toilet training so that the behavior generalizes from school to home. To accomplish this, the verbal and situational cues for going and staying on the potty and using it appropriately need to be as consistent as possible. This means that the same type of potty seat and the same words and foods should be used in both settings until the child is equally reliable in both settings.

For most autistic children, consistent schedule training results in satisfactory toilet training within six months. Some children still take another year or more to be dry at night, or to be trained for both bladder and bowels. For lower functioning autistic children, complete toilet training may be difficult to accomplish until age eight, nine, or even ten. Usually, these children remain dependent upon a toilet schedule—they will go if taken, but seldom indicate a need to go, and if not asked or taken, continue to have accidents. A highly structured routine seems to be the best way to help such children be toilet trained as successfully as possible.

Bedtime Difficulties

Another major area of difficulty for many parents of young autistic children is getting them to go to bed at night and stay there. One part of this problem is that the disorder of autism is not uncommonly related to disturbances of sleep. Many autistic children seem to need much less sleep, routinely fall asleep quite late, refuse naps, and stay awake for long periods during the night. Some research has suggested this may be due to the function of certain brain neurotransmitters, but that's a "six of one, half a dozen of another" explanation for a parent whose child is still routinely awake at 11:30 P.M. There are behavioral strategies that improve sleep organization, if those fail, some medications that will be discussed in the next chapter.

Sleep difficulties can be managed using many of the same general behavioral strategies discussed in Chapter 11, as well as application of some of the same principles that have just been described for dealing with feeding and toilet problems. As with feeding and toilet problems, expectations for the child should be geared to the child's developmental level, and the battles may be fought the same way. For example, many non-autistic eighteen- to twenty-four-month-old "terrible two-year-olds" decide it's more fun to sleep in their parents' bed with them. Autistic children will do this too, but it can be a little harder for parents to reject, because the autistic child is often less resistant to contact and cuddlier when he's sleepy—giving parents a kind of closeness that's not always available when the child's fully awake. While there are cultural differences as to who in the family sleeps with whom, and at which ages, it's worth saying that a four-year-old autistic child who becomes accustomed to sleeping with parents may be quite hard to move out if he's still doing it at age eight—at which time he will take up more of the bed and may thrash about while he sleeps. If one parent is more amenable to having the child in bed with them than the other, then having the child in the parental bed many not be a good idea for the marital relationship.

A highly structured bedtime routine that includes taking the child to his own bed and staying with him for a while and reading, listening to music, or doing some other well-liked activity should be instituted. A young child may need to have a parent stay with him until he falls asleep. After a while, the parent may want to stay close to the bed rather than in the bed as the child falls asleep. There should, however, be a limit to how long the parent stays, and after that time, the child should be left in his room. Some autistic children are perfectly happy alone in their rooms, and will get up and play at all hours of the night, even in the complete dark. If your child does this, it's okay. He may just not be sleepy. There should, however, be a way to prevent the child from leaving the room—either one or two tiers of baby gates, a child-proof door-knob cover, or a hook-and-eye latch on the outside of the door. The method should depend on the age of the child and how determined she is to escape.

If the child will need to be left in her room to "cry it out," any potentially dangerous objects should be removed. (If there is a sibling in the room, he should be removed too—at least until the learning to sleep through the night lessons are completed.) Most children will give up on crying after less than an hour, and most don't persist in a protest pattern for more than five days. Typically, the protests grow less severe and less convincing each night. Some autistic children, however, can get really worked up, and cry for as long as five hours, or cry to the point of vomiting. If your child is one of these, a medication to promote falling asleep, or even a little pediatric cough syrup can help take the edge off.

It is not a good idea to let an autistic child have the run of the house at night. Eventually, the child will probably find something dangerous to get into—like a knife drawer that hasn't been closed far enough to engage the childproof latch, the stove, or the refrigerator. There is always a first time for the child to discover a new hazard.

Daily Living Skills for the More Cognitively Disabled Teenager and Young Adult

The next area of skills training is the area of everyday living skills or what in educational terms is sometimes referred to as critical skills. This includes those things that a person needs to do to provide for his or her own self-care—taking transportation, shopping, cleaning, cooking, doing laundry, maintaining one's house, and so on. On *The Vineland Adaptive Behavior Scales,* these skills are called daily living skills, and there are age norms associated with part or complete mastery of various skills. For children without developmental disabilities, daily living skills are learned incidentally and are never formally taught in school (except, thank goodness, driver's education).

For the developmentally disabled person, and the autistic person in particular, daily living skills have to be taught specifically and made part of a routine. Some of these skills are actually more easily taught to autistic people than are others—if you can capitalize on the desire for routine or sameness, or on having an instrumental need met. In this section we'll discuss the particular difficulties in teaching everyday living skills to autistic people and describe two model programs—one that helps lower functioning students achieve these goals, and another that helps higher functioning students do the same.

Most often, autistic young people do better with demands that they encounter in highly routinized situations than they do with demands that come up in situations that are in more flux. Daily living skills that can be carried out at home or in school (more familiar settings) are usually easier to achieve than those that need to be carried out in public places. Autistic people are often at least a little wary and uncomfortable in public places, and tend to find the unpredictable behavior of other people annoying and overstimulating rather than novel and interesting. Autistic people are more likely to excel at tasks where other people don't have to be around, or where they are doing something to satisfy themselves. Therefore household tasks like cooking tend to go over better than doing the laundry, and solo tasks like gardening are favored over cooperative tasks like moving furniture. Routine, repetitive tasks tend to be more likable than ones that present many decision points.

Exemplary Adult Programs

A Model Daily Living Skills Program for Teenagers and Young Adults with Autism and Severe Cognitive Disability

To give an example of what school should be like for severely handicapped adolescents, I'll describe a program that has excelled at teaching adaptive skills in context. This program was set up through one parent's efforts, and was the result of her determined effort to obtain an appropriate education for her own fifteen-year-old severely handicapped autistic daughter. Through persistent litigation against a school district that had sixteen-year-old severely handicapped (SH) students sitting all day and labeling the same ten flash cards, sorting colored rings, and tracing the alphabet, a program was created that allowed these students to learn how to behave like real teenagers and young adults. As a consultant to the litigation and the program development process, I was able to watch a truly wonderful transformation for these severely handicapped students.

The remodeled "classroom" looked more like a very large L-shaped studio apartment than a classroom. There was a kitchen area at the top of the L, a living room at the bottom of the L, and a bedroom/grooming room on the short side of the L, to which a bathroom was attached. All ten students, who were fifteen to twenty years old, were severely mentally retarded; two or three of them, including Celia, whose mother had pushed so hard to create the program, were also autistic. The class was staffed by a teacher and two or three aides. Peer tutors from a nearby high school also came in to help individual students. Under supervision, students could go into the kitchen to set the table for lunch or snacks, prepare sandwiches, pour drinks, and wash and put away dishes afterwards. Some students had begun to be able to cook in the microwave, first selecting appropriate ingredients from the refrigerator with the guidance of a teacher and a pictorial cookbook. In the livingroom area, other students were assigned activities like sorting and folding laundry they had washed by operating the laundry machines themselves. Other students could spend time in the living room when they had completed work assignments, and were allowed to choose activities like selecting and listening to music with headphones, looking at magazines, or working with a peer tutor on a computer program. In the grooming room, there were beds to make, and a closet and dresser to organize. Girls were helped to comb and arrange their hair, and a couple showed interest in using make-up. In the bathroom, there was a separate grooming station for each student, and an opportunity to be supervised at good dental hygiene. Outside the class, some students did gardening tasks around the grounds (two or three to one aide), and some did janitorial work in the cafeteria after the elementary students had lunch.

Most of the students in the program were still at the stage of emergent skills in most of these areas. But the difference in these same students from the year before was striking. There was no one spending long, long periods of time completely spaced out. There were many fewer behavioral outbursts in the classroom. There was more social interaction among the students around their activities. The teachers seemed less tense. The students had different activities that they did well, and which were becoming their contribution to their "community." As an example, Celia, had a couple of things she did particularly well. Like many autistic people, Celia loved to watch water run. If Celia did dishes, she could have the water run while she washed. If she went off-task and only watched the water, the water got turned off. So, Celia washed dishes. The teachers also discovered how to get Celia to make beds. Celia had a routine in which she loved to bounce coins or marbles or other small objects off semi-hard surfaces, catch them, and then flap excitedly. If Celia would make a bed neatly, she could then have five minutes of bouncing objects off the bed. Celia made beds, and she made them smooth and tight so they would be good for bouncing. A year before, in the same class, Celia had sat through piles of flash cards giving one-word labels to pictures, occasionally interrupting herself to query "Go swing? Go swing?" or jumping up to raid the teacher's desk drawer where cookies were kept.

In other similar programs, autistic people tend to excel in food preparation since they enjoy being able to eat what they've made afterward. Others who like very routine, precise tasks find satisfaction with a specific task that is orderly, like stacking 144 small boxes into a larger box to make a gross of something. Others thrive on a task with a high sensory component of some sort, like operating a can-crusher for a recycling program or watering plants.

Severely handicapped students who can have the advantage of a good daily living skills program in their last few years of high school have a much better chance of making a successful transition to a group home living situation. From there, vocational options can be pursued using skills that have also been individually matched and developed as part of school preparation.

A Model Daily Living Skills Program for High-Functioning Teenagers and Young Adults with Autism, PDD, and Asperger's Syndrome

Earlier in this chapter, I described the top ten percent or so of young people with autism or PDD who continue to attend regular school classes for the most part and stay within a year or two of their grade levels in academic subjects. These students *do* graduate from high school meeting either full graduation requirements or the GED (Graduate Equivalent Degree) requirements that are used in some special education and adult education programs. In California, our two-year community colleges even have special classes for learning-disabled college students that the highest functioning people with autism, PDD, and Asperger's syndrome sometimes enroll in. Non-autistic students of the same age and academic level have few problems at this age with beginning to live and work independently. The high-functioning autistic young person, however, usually has difficulty using adaptive skills in an independent living setting, and is ill prepared to cope with the social and employment aspects of the "real world." Typically, these young people *do* know how to make their bed, do laundry, microwave a pizza, and brush their teeth adequately. Left on their own, however, many never make their bed, wear only disheveled clothes, eat mainly lots of junk food, and have chronic bad breath.

What the higher functioning young person with autism or PDD needs is *oversight* for their daily living functions, rather than the close supervision and prompting that the more severely handicapped autistic person needs to accomplish these daily goals. There are very few programs that provide this kind of model. Such programs are actually less numerous than programs for severely handicapped students. A very good one that I have visited serves multiply learning disabled, borderline IQ clients; in addition, a few people who have Asperger's syndrome or who are very high-functioning autistics have participated in the program. All clients in the program live in sets of garden apartments within a quarter-mile of the program's center, which is located on a residential boulevard in a suburban community. The sets of apartments are in complexes where the majority of tenants are not in the program, but are people who might be neighbors anywhere. The program's center is in a building that looks like a professional office building; it contains a livingroom-type recreation center, a physical activities center, a conference room–classroom, a computer training room, as well as administrative offices for the program. Clients have time to spend together in the recreation center and in one another's apartments. In the first year of the program, clients learn the skills they need for living independently in their apartments, like cooking, shopping, and cleaning. There are supervisors who can teach organizational skills like making a shopping list and following it, and a newer client can be an apartment-mate with a more experienced client who already has these skills. For newcomers, there is a daytime program for learning how to prepare a resume and how to go on a job interview. There are supported-employment counselors to identify and train clients for particular jobs. Some students take adult school or community college classes part-time and work part-time. Others who have been in the program the longest hold full-time jobs, and do their jobs with just a regular on-site supervisor. In fact, "graduates" of the program can choose to continue to live in the apartments even when fully and independently employed, and some do, saying that they prefer to come home to other people with disabilities because it is so tiring to try not to act "different" all day at work. For an autistic person, the likelihood of making friends is greater in the program than in a more mainstreamed setting, since odd behavior is more easily overlooked, and some of the clients are very socially gregarious (perhaps too much so by "normal" standards). One high-functioning autistic patient of mine who has attended this program, Van, was an excellent chess player and very good at math, and at nineteen was successfully taking high school geometry. Other students in the program began to be friends with Van when they realized that he could do their math homework for them. (He wasn't any good at explaining it; he would just do it and hand it back to them— which seemed quite okay with his new buddies.)

So far, programs like the one just described seem to be few and far between. One problem can be funding. Many of the clients are not able to be quite independent, but are also not considered impaired enough to be eligible for certain types of developmental disabilities funding. Possibly, as the cost-effectiveness of such programs can be demonstrated, special funding can be made available.

Programs for "Medium Functioning" Students In Between

We've described adaptive living programs for the lowest and the highest functioning students. Many autistic young people are somewhere in between; they are the "medium functioning" autistics that were described earlier in the chapter. Similarly, there are programs, both inside and outside of the school system, that are "in between." These programs provide many of the same learning opportunities as the SH program that was described, but are able to do so along with more of a focus on the acquisition of specific vocational skills.

Residential living for the more mildly retarded autistic young person usually involves some sort of group home, which often includes other mildly retarded people who are not autistic. Each young person, given his own strengths, can be helped to find a niche where he can function best as part of a group, and also in a way that allows him to have the opportunity to do some of the things that he finds pleasurable.

School and Post-School Vocational Skills Training

The final area that is addressed in the educational program of many children with autism and PDD is vocational training. As we have already discussed, deciding on the right time for the initiation of such a program is partly a function of how far a student has been able to go academically. Eventually, some form of vocational training is appropriate for almost all people diagnosed with autism or PDD.

Moderately Impaired People with Autism

More moderately impaired autistic people may need to have a vocational choice made for them. Often a workplace that provides significant amounts of isolation and routine, like a library, a stockroom, or a warehouse, works out well. Some moderately impaired people with autism do best in sheltered workshop settings designed for the developmentally disabled. Sheltered workshops can work particularly well for the individual who has some hard-to-extinguish stereotyped motor pattern or other oddity that might make him (and others) constantly aware of his handicapping condition in a non-sheltered work place. Some autistic adults do best in a sheltered workshop because they lack motivation: McGuire, a twenty-seven-year-old mute autistic man, was actually quite competent at assembling boxes. The problem was that when he finished assembling a pile of boxes, he'd just sit there indefinitely, not asking for more work, or trying to leave his work bench. If he was given more boxes, he'd assemble more. In beginning any kind of vocational placement, the initial number of hours per day and days per week should be kept very minimal at first and increased gradually as the individual learns about the work setting and the job requirements.

Initial resistance and lack of enthusiasm for a new job or any new setting is common in autistic people, and may mostly be a reflect of their dislike of things that are unfamiliar. A major problem in the vocational placement of people with autism is motivation. There is little drive to imitate others or aspire to the things that agemates work to earn money for—like cool running shoes, a CD player, cars, or money for dating. Most material goods often mean little to the autistic person because he doesn't care so much whether he fits in with others or is "different." (If he does care, he probably can't identify what about himself is perceived as "different.") Most autistic young adults are actually fairly happy to watch TV, have their mothers cook for them, and have time to pursue whatever special interest they might have. Aside from trying to entice the young person to earn money to support his special interest, it can be hard to come up with a reason he or she will want to perform well on a job. Making work a necessary part of the daily routine is usually the best solution. In my experience, parents who have the hardest time getting their autistic young people to cooperate in vocational training are those who have allowed them to stay home and watch game shows and videotapes for a couple of years after their schooling ended at age twenty-two. Such students often do best with a job training program after they have also been able to move away from the unstructured (more indulgent) home environment and into some sort of group living situation that makes more developmentally appropriate demands for self-care. The dynamic of resisting work can become a powerful aspect of the relationship with the parents and can be maintained by the aggravation that the young person is able to cause his parents with it.

School-Based Vocational Training Programs

School programs can and should provide a gradual transition to work by starting with in-class prevocational tasks (like sorting and assembling). Often, special education classes get "real" jobs like stuffing envelopes with report cards, collating pages of examinations for other classes, or doing maintenance work around the school. Absurdly, some of these programs have been closed or compromised by civil libertarians who feel that on-the-job training without pay for the developmentally disabled person constitutes forced labor (and not education), because the workers are not able to give their own informed consent to say they want to work. Since most of special education is too poorly funded to pay students, some programs just shut down. Sometimes instead, the students must do meaningless repetitive tasks that can't be accused of being "work," like stacking key blanks into a box that then gets dumped so the next student can do the same.

Sheltered workshops for disabled adults can run on a piecework or contract basis, paying the worker a percentage of the standard wage based on his or her efficiency. So, if a typical nondisabled worker can assemble fifty boxes an hour and would be paid eight dollars per hour for such a task, an autistic person in a sheltered workshop would be paid four dollars per hour if he works at fifty-percent efficiency, assembling twenty-five boxes per hour. Labor costs for the company that contracts with the sheltered workshop are the same as if it had contracted with an organization that used nondisabled laborers. However, sheltered workshops still need grants to cover the costs of the staff that provide supervision, as well as other costs such as transporting workers to and from the workshop.

As preparation for the "real" world, it's important that schools *do* give real tasks to students receiving vocational training, not just colored blocks, or items that get dumped and repackaged by one student as soon as another has finished his "turn." Autistic students often need to be taught a sense of accom-

plishment from the tasks they do, and the job should result in real consequences. Initially, pairing task completion with some other token or reward is
a way of teaching this. Some schools tally up token dollars and cents that result
in real payments that the students can use on a field trip to a restaurant, the
bowling alley, or the movies at the end of the week. These programs are
usually funded by parents or some sort of fund-raising effort by the agency.

It is also important that a student be taught vocational skills that can be
directly used in a "real" work setting: A good community coordinator is important to this type of program, so that meaningful piecework can be obtained for
the students; in turn, students may eventually be able to land jobs with the
same or similar employers who contract with the vocational training programs.

Chapter Summary

In this chapter as well as the previous four, we have discussed many aspects of
educating autistic children. The school environment is a significant support
and positive influence on the lives of autistic children as they grow and develop. In most cases, the school also is a source of significant support for
families with the special stresses they face in parenting a child with disabilities.
In the next two chapters, we'll focus on other approaches to treating autism—
through psychopharmacology and through various non-mainstream treatments that are used even though data on their efficacy are absent.

◆ ◆ ◆

CHAPTER 14

Psychoactive Medications

When Are Drugs Used to Treat Autism and PDD?

What role do psychoactive medications have in the treatment of children with autism or PDD? The short answer is that psychoactive medications treat *symptoms*. There are no medications that have been found effective in the treatment of autism as a whole. This is because autism is not just one thing, but a syndrome—or collection of symptoms, as we discussed in Chapter 1. Autism is a collection of overlapping groups of symptoms that vary from child to child. When medications are used to treat an autistic child, they are used to treat a particular symptom or group of related symptoms. Symptoms of autism and PDD that sometimes improve with the introduction of medications include hyperactivity, short attention span, stereotyped motor movements, self-injurious behaviors (SIBs), aggressiveness, social withdrawal, excessive anxiety, and poor sleep. Although all of these problems can occur in autistic children, none are symptoms unique to autism, nor are any of the medications used with children with autism or PDD used only for children with these two diagnoses. There are no separate medications that are used only for autism or only for PDD.

Most medications used to treat autism were developed primarily to treat some other disorder, and then tried on autistic children or adults because of overlap in certain symptoms. This means that there are few drugs that drug companies have tested specifically to determine how well they work to treat autism. However, once the U.S. Food and Drug Administration (FDA) approves a drug for use in one population for one particular set of symptoms, doctors are free to use their own judgment to decide how to prescribe it for other populations or other types of symptoms. In the medical research literature, and in the child psychopharmacology literature in particular, there are many reports of how various psychoactive drugs have worked in treating autistic children. This literature develops as researchers decide, for one reason or another, to try different existing or new drugs to treat autistic children.

When Are Medications Usually Started?

Getting a diagnosis of autism or PDD doesn't necessarily mean that medications should be started right away. In fact, even when the child has symptoms that could respond to drug treatment (such as those already mentioned, which all autistic children have to some extent), it is almost always preferable to try to treat specific symptoms with behavioral approaches first. Exceptions to this rule are children who are so grossly hyperactive that they pose a danger to themselves or younger siblings, and the very small number of mentally retarded autistic children with severe self-injurious behaviors (SIBs). Most often, behavioral methods make a bigger dent in lowering the rate of negative behavior than medications do.

Medications used to treat autism or PDD *do not* cure symptoms, that is, make them go away entirely and forever. Often, symptoms are masked by psychoactive medications, the same way symptoms are masked in some chronic diseases like diabetes or hypertension, making the disease almost invisible when the patient is under good control by the medication; however, the symptoms will reappear if the medication is discontinued. When psychoactive medications are combined with behavioral treatments and educational approaches, hopefully, more lasting effects are produced. Extended periods of good behavioral control plus increased accessibility to teaching may lead to new learned behaviors that are maintained as the child matures; he can then be given a trial period with the medication reduced or withdrawn.

There is no evidence from any study that any medication that has been tried for autistic children in any way alters the underlying neurological causes of the disorder. We still know little about what autism looks like on a molecular or neuronal level. There is no evidence that any medication can provide lasting improvements in brain function or structure.

Homeopathic Interventions

Every couple of years, some new "cure"/explanation for autism arises from the more homeopathically inclined. I am not saying that homeopathic treatments are synonymous with "quack" cures, but some are. (If you could cure autism just by eliminating milk products from the diet, we'd have many fewer autistic children!) For a few years, there was a run on Nystatin (an antifungal agent) fueled by the assumption that autism was caused by candidiasis, a common vaginal yeast infection. (If all the women with candida infections at conception had autistic children, there would be a lot *more* autistic children!) Then there was the book *Fighting for Tony*, about how one mom cured her son of autism by treating his "cerebral allergy" to milk (which presumably made his brain swell and made him act autistic). I've yet to find an allergist or neurologist who can make any sense out of the concept of a "cerebral allergy." Caveat emptor!

Parent Concerns about Putting Children on Psychoactive Medications. For many if not all parents, the decision to try a psychoactive medication can be very difficult at first. All medications have at least some serious risks, and parents worry about putting their autistic child at any additional risk. Knowledge about the particular side effects of a particular medication for a particular child may allay this worry on a rational level, but nevertheless many parents remain uncomfortable, because accepting the need for medication means reaching a new level of realization that the child's problems are severe. This realization may cut painfully into successful defensive denial of the child's problems. For other parents, facing the severity of a behavior means feeling like a failure because neither normal good parenting nor even special approaches the parents may have tried has made the problem behavior significantly better.

Sometimes, it is teachers, therapists, or other caregivers who first suggest that the parents look into the issue of medication. In these cases, parents may feel angry—it is as if the professionals are giving up on the child, or saying, in effect, that the treatments they are giving are not entirely helpful. Usually, this is *not* what is being said. What is being said is that the professional feels that a medication might help the child get past certain interfering problems and be more teachable. However, to parents who may not yet have had time to fully accept that the child's problems are real and permanent, suggestions to give medication can feel like an insult directed at the child, the parent, or both.

"Zombies." Probably the biggest fear that most parents have about medication is that it will make their child act "like a zombie" or "doped up." No parents want their child in a psychopharmacological straitjacket. Properly administered, the effects of a psychoactive drug *do not* create excessive sedation. The child shouldn't appear sleepy or "spaced out." Well-administered medications should dampen interfering behaviors like hyperactivity, poor attention span, repetitive behaviors, or aggressiveness. It can be helpful to think of these behaviors as driven by motors—psychoactive medications keep the motors from running at too many RPMs. A psychoactive medication isn't meant to be a punishment for bad behavior. A well-trained psychopharmacologist does not think like the evil nurse in *One Flew Over the Cuckoo's Nest.*

Obtaining Consultation about Psychoactive Medications

There are some pediatricians who will prescribe psychoactive medications for children with autism or PDD, and some who won't. Pediatricians who have not had any special training in developmental disabilities and who may not have any other autistic children in their practices often prescribe Ritalin or a related drug used to treat hyperactive children (who are far more common than children with autism or PDD). As we will see, Ritalin or another "stimulant" drug is usually not the first choice for autistic children, although very occasionally, it sometimes does help an autistic child's hyperactivity.

Most pediatricians prefer to refer medication issues involving autistic children to a child psychiatrist or other child psychopharmacology specialist (such as a child neurologist), or to work in consultation with such a person. There are a small number of pediatricians who have done additional training in developmental or behavioral pediatrics, and these pediatrician–developmental specialists are often well qualified to handle medication issues on their own—especially if they have received specialized training in working with children with developmental disabilities.

A physician who is a specialist in giving psychoactive medications to children will know the latest research on side effects, new medications, and baseline tests that need to be made to determine if the child has any unseen health problems that might make the use of a particular medication unadvisable. Some drugs require that blood be drawn periodically to determine just how much is kept in the child's system since there can be great individual differences in how fast a medication is used up or how efficiently it is stored. Some medications require periodic monitoring via electroencephalograms (EEGs) or electrocardiograms (EKGs) to determine whether any bad side effects are accruing. Giving a child a psychoactive medication may be very helpful to his functioning, but it *is* a serious medical intervention. It's not like giving a vitamin pill in the morning, although it may become that routine. It's important to keep up any necessary monitoring of the physical effects of any drug that the doctor suggests.

In our clinic, we have encountered a very small number of parents who have medicated their children on their own. Mostly these are parents who are on psychoactive medications themselves and become convinced that their child has what they have—only worse. Typically, such parents start giving their child some of what they themselves are taking, such as Prozac (fluoxetine) or Tofranil (imipramine). Needless to say, this is *not* a good idea at all! Children metabolize medications at different rates than adults and may have different side effects. Children can be slowed down with medications that make adults speed up. It is important to learn how a particular medication may affect a child differently from an adult.

A Child's Age and the Use of Medications. As already discussed, it usually isn't advisable to start using a medication until some behavior interventions have been tried first. Generally, very few autistic children under three years old are on psychoactive medications. There are different classes of medications, and some of these classes of drugs tend to be tried with younger children first, because they are less likely to have side effects. In the three- to five-year-old group, the most hyperactive, negative, or agitated children may be treated with an antidepressant or a stimulant. Neuroleptics (sometimes referred to as antipsychotics because they were first developed to treat psychosis) are usually not introduced until the child is five, and even then only quite occasionally, until age ten or so. Many autistic people who eventually *are* treated with neuroleptics receive them for the first time during or after puberty. There are no absolute rules for prescribing various types of medications at certain ages. That is why a really experienced child psychopharmacology specialist can be very helpful. Such a clinician can draw from extensive clinical experience to meet the needs of a particular child.

Designing a Medication Trial

Putting a child on a medication should always be considered an experiment. Like any good experiment, there should be a design in place before the experiment starts, and there should be objective ways of measuring possible success and possible failure of the experiment.

Deciding What to Treat. The first step in designing a medication trial is deciding what behaviors the medication is to be used to change. There are five main criteria for deciding whether a particular problem area of behavior should be treated with a psychoactive medication:

CRITERIA FOR USING A PSYCHOACTIVE MEDICATION

1. *Is there any behavior that is such a problem that the child is frequently injuring himself or others?* This could include intentional or non-intentional aggression to others.
2. *Have behavioral approaches been tried, with little or marginal success?* Behavioral methods should almost always be tried first to see how much of the severity of the behavior problem can be reduced without resorting to medications.
3. *Are the problem behaviors present in more than one setting?* If the problem behavior is a reaction to a particular setting (for example, day care versus home), then the setting may need to be changed rather than the child. However if the child is "good" at home because no limits are imposed, but "bad" at school because there are rules to be followed, medications *may* be indicated.
4. *Do the behaviors to be treated interfere with the child's ability to learn?* Physical hyperactivity and inability to pay attention are the two most common of these.
5. *Are the potential benefits of the drug likely to compare favorbly with possible short- or long-term side effects?*

If the answer to one or more of these questions is yes, then a medication trial may be appropriate. Answering these questions fully is something that needs to be done through a fairly in-depth discussion between parents and doctors, taking into account the child's history and current behavior. An experienced clinician can help parents, teachers, and others involved in caring for the child to decide how out-of-range a particular child's behavior is. In a child who has not yet received any or much intervention(s), the clinician should be able to tell about how much the problem behavior may be expected to improve with intervention, and how much of the behavior is *so* excessive that it would be worthwhile to consider a medication immediately. A good clinician makes such a judgment by carefully observing the child's activity, attention, and ability to organize himself, both at times when the child is doing something of his own choosing as well as when he is being asked to do something by someone else. The decision to treat a child with medications should be made with input from parents, teachers, and others working with the child, as well as the opinion of the doctor. Parents also need to understand that no one can give their child a psychoactive medication without their knowledge, and as long as the child is in their full custody, a medication cannot be given without parental consent.

Collecting Baseline Behavioral Data Before a Medication Trial. The first step in planning a medication trial, then, is getting various people involved in the care of the child to agree on the target behavior(s) that a medication might help. The second step is to obtain baseline data. At best, this means writing down how often and for how long the child exhibits the problem behavior. If, for example, the child repeatedly asks questions that he knows the answer to, it might be helpful to mark down each time he does that, at school and at home, for a week, before beginning a new medication designed to reduce obsessive behavior. If the child is very hyperactive, it would be helpful if his mother and his teacher could each rate, on a five-point scale, whether the child had a "very bad day," a "not great day," an "average day," a "pretty good day," or an "excellent day." This record should be accumulated for a week or more before beginning a new medication. Sometimes teachers send home these types of reports anyway (as discussed in Chapter 10), and these can be used to track overall changes. It is also helpful if both parents can make separate, independent ratings of the problem behavior, even though they might be with the child for different parts of the day. The idea is to have an objective record for measuring behavior change on and off the medication.

Blind Trials. Once the decision has been made to use a medication, everyone hopes it will be helpful. This sets us all up to experience a placebo effect. A *placebo effect* occurs when taking an inactive medication—without knowing it is inactive—causes perceived differences in the target behavior, or actually results in change to the target behavior, just because the individual feels he or she is being treated. With autistic and PDD children, at least, we don't have to worry about the latter kind of placebo effect. They won't act better if given a placebo just because they hope to change themselves. However, those around the child may very well fell they are perceiving subtle changes due to the medication because they hope for it to have at least some effect. It is important to think about a possible placebo effect because imagining an effect that is not really substantially there may prevent moving on to different doses or other medications that may in fact, be more helpful.

When new psychoactive drugs are first tested for the U.S. Food and Drug Administration, the most rigorous test of a medication is considered to be a "double-blind crossover" study. In a double-blind crossover study, neither the doctor nor the patient knows if what is being administered is placebo or real medication. At some point, after the drug has had enough time to make the expected changes, the patient is "crossed over" on to the opposite treatment—real medication if the patient has been on placebo, placebo if the patient has been on medication. Records of behavior and physical function are taken throughout the trial and examined for changes in the two halves of the study—preferably before the person analyzing the data knows which treatment is which. In real life, we usually can't be that rigorous, but it helps to try.

We usually recommend that at least one significant caregiver remain unaware that the child is to be given a trial of medication or when it is that the medication is actually being used. The "blind" caregiver could be the parent who doesn't give the medication, a teacher, or even a friend or relative who knows the child well and sees him frequently. Actual record keeping of target behavior is preferable but not always possible. For example, a good way to go about a new medication trial is to begin a new drug in March and, by the end of April, say to the teacher: "My son's been on a new medication recently. Can you tell any differences in his behavior if you compare January and February to March and April?" As a first go, it is helpful *not* to say in which of these two-month time periods the drug was given, or even what drug was used (as special education teachers usually have some ideas about what certain medications are supposed to do). Try to arrange a time to sit down with the teacher and review behavior records and classwork that might further indicate changes in activity, attention, or other target behaviors.

Effects of Drugs versus Education and Maturation. Although it can be difficult to estimate, it is also important to acknowledge that a child's functioning should improve as a result of good education and maturation. Not all improvements a child shows when on a medication are due to the medication. Some medications make a child more accessible to learning but do not promote the emergence of specific skills like understanding language more or speaking, or learning to read, or developing friendships. Because of these difficulties in separating the results of drug treatment from other treatments, it is usually a good idea to begin a new medication at a time when other aspects in the child's life are *not* changing. Starting a new school and a new medication at the same time is, for example, a bad idea. Similarly, starting a new medication just when school lets out for the summer, and the child's whole routine is changing is not a good idea either. Changing just one thing at a time enhances the likelihood of accurately assessing positive (or negative) effects due to the medication alone.

Medications Most Often Used for Children
with Autism or PDD

The battery of medications used to treat autistic children is expanding, but still not large. There are a few basic classes of drugs that may be generally appropriate ("indicated") or inappropriate ("contraindicated") depending on the child's age, risk for different side effects, and previous history with psychoactive medications. Although risks and side effects vary with different medications, it is important to understand that when medications are selected and monitored carefully, the overall level of risk is quite low. More children die from self-inflicted injuries than from psychoactive drugs. Most drug side effects are totally reversible as soon as the medication is stopped.

New drugs come into use with autistic and PDD children in various ways. Some have been approved for use in adults, are used mainly in adults, and then slowly gain a foothold in the treatment of children. Eventually, specific studies are made to determine whether the drug affects children in ways that could not have been predicted, given what was already known about the drug's pharmacology and history of use in adults. A doctor who prescribes medications should be able to inform you about what is and is not known about a particular medication.

Sometimes when a new medication is first introduced, everyone jumps on the bandwagon, and the drug is proclaimed the long-awaited panacea. The "panacea" stage usually doesn't last very long, however. Often, initial reports of a drug's efficacy and safety are based on a small series of cases; these may include children who also happened to be attending a very good school at the time, or who were residents on a very structured, well-organized inpatient unit since these are the types of settings where research is often carried out. In the early 1980s, Pondimin (fenfluramine) enjoyed a blaze of glory under just such circumstances. A large multicenter trial was initiated (our clinic participated in this study), but soon it became clear that the medication helped relatively few children; that it didn't help many very much; and that it offered no real advantages over anything in the existing pharmacopeia. We would all like to see new medications be developed that work better than the ones we have now. Unfortunately, *wanting* a drug to work has no effect on its true efficacy. Generally, trying a drug with a proven track record for improving the behaviors you are concerned about is a better approach than trying the newest medication to come down the pike.

Classes of Medications

There are several classes and subclasses of medications used to treat children with autism or PDD. Usually, at first, just one medication at a time is used. Over time, other medications may be used to accrue some additional gain, to treat an additional set of symptoms, or to counteract certain side effects of other drugs. As medications are used in combination, the pharmacology grows more complex, and it becomes especially important to consult with someone whose expertise includes psychoactive medications, such as a child psychiatrist or child neurologist.

Drug Treatment of Autism versus PDD

By and large there is not a separate psychopharmacology of autism and of PDD. In general, hyperactivity and poor attention span are difficulties experienced by both children with autism and children with PDD. Autistic children display behavioral outbursts, agitation, and withdrawal more often than children with PDD and are somewhat more likely to receive medications that address those symptoms. Children with PDD, compared with autistic children, are more likely to show features of anxiety and compulsiveness and, when older, depression; and they are more likely to receive medications that address those symptoms.

Correct medication depends on the particular child's difficulties. Different medications work in different ways. In this book, we won't go into what makes different medications work when they are effective. Interested parents or teachers can ask their child's doctor for explanations or references.

Antidepressant Medications

There are a variety of antidepressants that work on a range of autistic symptoms; some are listed in Table 6. Although, as the name implies, antidepressants are medications originally developed to counter the effects of depression, they work differently in developmentally disabled children. By and large, tricyclic antidepressants are the kind of antidepressant most frequently used in treating children with autism or PDD; these children may benefit from reduction in gross motor hyperactivity, improved attention span, and a reduction in

Table 6 Antidepressant Medications Used to Treat Autism and PDD

Medication (Trade Name/ Generic)	Most Likely Benefits	Possible Benefits	Side Effects/ Problems
Tofranil (imipramine)	Increased attention, less hyperactivity	Decreased anxiety; inhibits enuresis	Very rare cardiac complications
Norpramin, Pertofrane (desipramine)	Increased attention, less hyperactivity	Decreased anxiety	Very rare cardiac complications
Prozac (fluoxetine)	Decreased compulsive, repetitive behaviors	Decreased anxiety, depression	Very rare cardiac complications
Anafranil (clomipramine)	Decreased compulsive, repetitive behaviors	Decreased anxiety, panic, depression	May lower seizure threshold
Desyrel (trazodone)	Helps child sleep through night	Increased daytime calmness	Occasional nausea

anxiety, if it is present. Tricyclic antidepressants may also normalize sleep patterns. Relatively few side effects are associated with antidepressants; however, an initial EKG should be obtained before a child is treated with Tofranil (imipramine) or Norpramin (desipramine); blood levels of the drug will need to be monitored periodically. Tofranil is the single most frequently used antidepressant for children with autism or PDD and the most widely studied. It takes a couple of weeks to show results (as blood levels of the medication rise), and it may take a while to work out an optimal dose. Norpramin works in a way that is very similar to Tofranil. A side benefit of Tofranil is that it may help a child with certain kinds of enuresis (bed-wetting). Tofranil is not helpful in initial toilet training but may help a child who has been dry during the day for a long period of time but still wets the bed at night, or a child who once had a period of complete toilet training, but has regressed.

A second type of antidepressant is one that more often helps children with PDD (and some children with autism) by reducing the frequency and intensity of compulsive repetitive behaviors, obsessionality, anxiety, and possibly depression. Medications such as Prozac (fluoxetine) and Anafranil (clomipramine) seem to sometimes help these behaviors. Prozac has been widely used to treat depression in adults and has had tremendous press coverage—some of it bad, mainly because of cases where people took more than the amount prescribed, or took Prozac in combination with other medications. Monitored and used as prescribed, it is quite a safe medication. It is not known whether the repetitive motor and sensory behaviors that younger and more retarded autistic children show have the same neurological basis as the repetitive routines and rituals exhibited by individuals with obsessive-compulsive disorders, but fluoxetine and clomipramine are sometimes also used to treat these.

Drugs that Promote Sleepiness. Another antidepressant medication that is occasionally used with autistic children, especially young autistic children, is Desyrel (trazodone). Autistic children have an increased incidence of sleep disturbance that can include long periods of night-waking, very prolonged onset of sleep, and early rising. This is not a winning combination for any parent's sanity (as we discussed in the last chapter). Desyrel, given before bed, helps the child get sleepy and remain asleep. Other medications given at night—such as the neuroleptics (and tricyclic antidepressants, as already mentioned)—also can promote sleepiness in the first hours after they are given, but Desyrel provides an alternative for better sleep when a neuroleptic is not otherwise needed, or where the neuroleptic works in some ways, but does not promote sleepiness.

Stimulant Medications

Stimulant medications have an opposite (paradoxical) effect in most children than they do in adults. Therefore stimulants slow hyperactive children down. Stimulant medications have been studied widely in hyperactive children—

Table 7 Stimulant Medications Used to Treat Autism and PDD

Medication (Trade Name/ Generic)	Most Likely Benefits	Possible Benefits	Side Effects/ Problems
Ritalin (methylphenidate)	Less hyperactivity, increased attention	Well studied in children	May lower seizure threshold; decreased appetite
Dexidrene (dextroamphetamine)	—	Less hyperactivity	Not as frequently used with children
Cylert (pemoline)	Best in postpubertal teens; longer acting	Less hyperactivity; increased attention	Modest or uneven results in prepubertal children

children with attention deficit hyperactivity disorder (ADHD). Ritalin (methylphenidate) is the most effective stimulant for slowing down children with ADHD; Dexedrine (dextroamphetamine) often works, too. Occasionally, Ritalin or Dexedrine has the same beneficial effects for autistic children, but most doctors who frequently treat autistic children with medications put it way down on their list of choices. In autistic children, use of stimulants can also be associated with an increase in stereotyped motor movements and the development of tics. (Tics, however, almost always disappear if the stimulant medication is stopped.) A very small proportion of autistic children respond to Ritalin with such increased activity that they are never given a second dose. Some have a terrific "rebound" from Ritalin, slowing down and paying better attention when it is in their systems, but becoming twice as active when it wears off (typically in the late afternoon). Another reason why a stimulant may not be the best choice for a particular autistic child is that stimulants tend to increase the child's ability to attend to one thing. Some autistic children already have stimulus overselectivity, meaning that they will pay attention to one thing, or one aspect of one thing, for far too long, even when not on medication. A medication like Ritalin may make this tendency even more pronounced.

For those autistic and PDD children who do respond well to stimulant medication, Ritalin has the advantage of being short-acting—it works within twenty to thirty minutes, and a dose is usually no longer clinically apparent after about four hours. Some parents with more mildly affected children like the effects of Ritalin because they can give it on school days after breakfast and lunch and it lasts just long enough to improve classroom attention. Ritalin tends to decrease appetite, so it is often given *after* a meal. Ritalin can also slow down physical growth slightly if given daily for a long period of time, so children on Ritalin need (if possible) to be given periodic medication-free holidays so they can catch up to their growth curves. A child on Ritalin should have his height and weight curves monitored regularly.

There is also a longer acting stimulant, Cylert (pemoline). Many doctors and parents prefer a stimulant that's longer than Ritalin because it evens out the roller-coaster effect of going on and off medication that a child may experience at different times in the day if he takes Ritalin, once, twice, or three times per day. However, in prepubertal children, most of a dose of Cylert is metabolized in the early part of the day, leaving the child virtually unmedicated by afternoon. For some children, it is preferable to give a dose of Ritalin later in the day—or just change to Ritalin altogether (if Ritalin is at all effective). In postpubertal children, Cylert is usually more effectively long-acting. Ritalin and Dexedrine both have long-acting forms, but there is relatively little evidence they are effective. The benefits and drawbacks of using these stimulant medications for treating autism or PDD are summarized in Table 7.

Neuroleptic Medications

Neuroleptic medications, also sometimes referred to as antipsychotic medications, have been fairly well studied in the treatment of autistic children. Neuroleptics are usually tried after other medications have provided less than satisfactory results, or when the child shows severely agitated, aggressive, or self-injurious behavior. In a subset of individuals, neuroleptics are the most likely to produce side effects, although at low doses, and in young children, side effects are less common than with higher doses and with older people. The advantage of neuroleptic medications is that they are the most effective at subduing negative behavioral outbursts that have no clear causes in the environment around the child. Children with outburst behavior often tend to be hyperactive, and neuroleptics are also effective in treating hyperactivity.

Dyskinesias. The major side effect concern with neuroleptics is the development of unusual involuntary body movements. One type of movement disorder is dyskinesia, which most often includes characteristic movements of the mouth, tongue, or fingers. One form of dyskinesia is called tardive (later-occurring) dyskinesia; it tends to develop after at least three months of neuroleptic treatment and may take the form of choreoathetoid movements (characteristic slithering movements of the neck, body, or extremities) or involuntary tics and grunts (which are a form of respiratory tic). Some of the movements children may develop as a result of neuroleptic treatment may look quite similar to the motor stereotypies that a large percentage of autistic children already have. Preexisting motor stereotypies should be carefully noted by the doctor giving neuroleptic medication before starting a new drug so that any later dyskinetic *side effects* can be distinguished from *preexisting* stereotyped motor movements. Another, more rare motor side effect of neuroleptics in children include dystonias, which are involuntary slow muscle contractions.

Although the development of dyskinetic syndromes are very disturbing to many parents, it should be remembered that about seventy-five to eighty percent of autistic and PDD children never develop any dyskinetic side effects, and there are adjunctive (simultaneous, preventive) treatments for those who do. Younger children (who are less often treated with neuroleptics) seem less at risk for dyskinesias. If a doctor is particularly concerned about the development of a dyskinesia, an additional medication such as Cogentin (benztropine) or even Benadryl (an antihistamine) may be given as well to prevent the emergence of motor side effects. If dyskinetic motor movements do develop as a result of treatment with a neurolepic, they almost always disappear if the drug is withdrawn in a gradual fashion.

Frequently Used Neuroleptics. Two neuroleptics in particular—Haldol and Mellaril—are used with autistic children (Table 8). Although they have similar major effects, their side effects differ. They also differ in potency—which means that one must be given in higher doses than the other to achieve the same result. Because the risk of side effects increases with dosage, if more neuroleptic medication is needed to achieve the desired behavioral change, at a certain point, a lower dose of a higher potency neuroleptic may be preferable to a higher dose of a lower potency neuroleptic. The two neuroleptics most often used with autistic children will be discussed here, but it is not uncommon for doctors to try other neuroleptics to get more "in-between" potency.

Mellaril. The first neuroleptic that is commonly used with autistic and PDD children is Mellaril (thioridazine), which is considered a lower potency neuroleptic. It is sometimes used when a child or teenager has a mild amount of erratic behavior such as extreme uncontrollable silliness or sudden bouts of agitation that interfere with the child's ability to learn or function in a classroom or other setting.

Sometimes Mellaril is used with PDD children who have unusual ideas that preoccupy them to the point that parents and teachers feel uncertain if the child knows what is really real. For example, one young man went through a couple of years of being preoccupied with trucks to the degree that he would refer to his eyelids as windshield wipers, and his body as the trailer. While a little bit of this is normal in three- and four-year-old boys, doing it persistently for a couple of years and never stepping out of one's "role" suggests a more fragile sort of mental organization that might benefit from a medication with antipsychotic properties. Mellaril is also fairly sedating when it is first taken, so if the child takes his daily dose just before bedtime, and if his parents are lucky, the child will sleep better and longer.

Table 8 Neuroleptic Medications Most Often Used with Autistic Children

Medication (Trade Name/ Generic)	Most Likely Benefits	Possible Benefits	Side Effects/ Problems
Haldol (haloperidol)	Less withdrawal; fewer stereotypies, less hyperactivity and agitatation	Possibly increased teachability due to improved attention	Lower seizure threshold; weight gain; sedation
Mellaril (thioridazine)	Less hyperactivity and agitation.	Less withdrawal	Lower seizure threshold; weight gain; sedation

Haldol. A second neuroleptic frequently used with autistic children is Haldol (haloperidol). If behavior is a really big problem, some doctors prefer to give a little bit of a higher potency neuroleptic like Haldol than a lot of a lower potency neuroleptic like Mellaril. Most often, Haldol is tried only after trials of one or more medications like Tofranil, Ritalin, or Anafranil have failed to produce the needed results. When hyperactivity is not significantly diminished by the above drugs—or only results in greater increases in agitation and irritability—then Haldol may be considered. Usually Haldol is started at a very low dose once or twice a day because some children are very sensitive to Haldol and respond markedly to even a very tiny dose. The psychopharmacologist's rule for Haldol is "start low and build slow." Periodic drug holidays every four to six months (times when the child is tapered from his or her medication) helps slow down the buildup of tolerance, too. Haldol is used to treat unremitting frenetic activity, bizarre or highly disorganized, unfocused behavior, as well as severe aggressive outbursts directed at self or others. Although nobody wants to chemically straitjacket any child, Haldol is often used when the child's activity level, coupled with lack of judgment, frequently produces behaviors that may be self-endangering or a danger to others. Used properly, Haldol need not be oversedating, although young people on significant doses of Haldol may be slightly more slow moving and slow to react than similarly disabled young people on no medication at all. Possible good effects of Haldol for autistic children include greater social awareness and less active resistance to social initiations.

Other Medications Used to Treat Autism and PDD

A variety of other medications are also used to treat autism and PDD (Table 9). They come from several drug classes, and each is used for slightly different reasons. A little bit about each medication that has frequently been used with autistic or PDD children will be described, along with why and when it may be helpful.

Tegretol. Tegretol (carbamazepine) is an anticonvulsant medication developed to treat seizures. It can also be helpful in treating autistic children who are not hyperactive overall but *are* subject to episodic outbursts of aggression. Tegretol may also be an effective alternative to a neuroleptic like Mellaril or Haldol, especially if there is concern about development of dyskinetic motor movements. The effectiveness and likelihood of a positive response to Tegretol is not as high as for a neuroleptic, but if it *does* work for a particular child, all the better. However, Tegretol does require regular blood drawing to monitor drug levels, and one quite rare side effect is suppression of the body's ability to make certain blood cells.

Trexan. Trexan (naltrexone) is one of the newer drugs to be studied for use with autistic children. It is a good medication to use even with fairly young

Table 9 Other Medications Used to Treat Children with Autism and PDD

Medication (Trade Name/ Generic)	Most Likely Benefits	Possible Benefits	Side Effects/ Problems
Tegretol (carbamazepine) (anticonvulsant)	Less hyperactivity, fewer behavioral outbursts	Treats possible "behavioral" seizures	Occasional effects on liver function and, rarely, bone marrow
Trexan (naltrexone)	Less hyperactivity, less negative behavior	Fewer stereotypies; less withdrawal	Low response rate, but good if it works
Pondimin (fenfluramine)		Less hyperactivity, better attention	Low response rate, mild benefits
BuSpar (buspirone) (anti-anxiety)		Decreased anxiety	Rare
Lithane (lithium)	Fewer episodic anger outbursts	Less moodiness	Occasional gastric distress, weight gain; thirst, acne

children because it has few known side effects, but produces many of the same gains that children make from treatment with Haldol. The reports of its greatest success come from one center where children who are treated with naltrexone also receive other high-quality treatments; this may explain why elsewhere the response rate to naltrexone is fairly low—one in five to seven children. However, it may be well worth trying before settling for a neuroleptic.

Pondimin. Pondimin (fenfluramine), mentioned earlier, had its heyday in the 1980's, when it first appeared to be successful in a very small series of autistic children; subsequent results with a much larger sample were much less satisfactory. Basically, fenfluramine seems to work the way a mild stimulant does for some autistic children—producing less hyperactivity, fewer stereotyped motor movements, and increased attention span. The problem is that the response rate to fenfluramine is very low (similar to naltrexone), and some children who do respond seem to develop a tolerance to it fairly quickly. In addition, fenfluramine was originally developed as a diet aid, and therefore has marked appetite-suppressing effects—many children develop poor appetites and can fall off their growth curves a bit while on this medication (as with other stimulants).

BuSpar. BuSpar (buspirone) is an antianxiety medication that may be effective in children with PDD and in some autistic children for whom chronic anxiety is a major factor. Some PDD children in particular, especially as they approach and go through puberty, develop chronic, high levels of anxiety or phobic symptoms that may result in a lack of interest in exploring things around them. BuSpar may also be helpful in very withdrawn, seemingly fearful individuals. We have seen a whole group of teens with autism or Asperger's syndrome in our clinic who never talk above a whisper; it seems almost as if they wish they could disappear (which they sometimes seem to be trying to do by closing their eyes when they talk to you, or by falling asleep as soon as they are left alone). If extreme withdrawal symptoms seem to be made worse by anxiety, an antianxiety medication may be helpful. BuSpar alone is usually not highly effective with PDD children or adolescents, but it is sometimes useful in combination with another medication that addresses other aspects of the child's difficulties.

Lithium. Lithium is frequently used to treat affective disorders in adults and tends to creep into the drug treatment regimen of adult autistic people far more often than for children. Like Tegretol, it may be an alternative to a neuroleptic for a child who cannot tolerate a nueroleptic. Lithium is really most appropriate for autistic people who have episodic, sometimes manic outbursts of negative activity that cannot be contained by those around them. For example, one of our young adult higher functioning autistic patients responded fairly well to lithium after becoming increasingly paranoid and finally developing the delusion he was a Ninja warrior—which resulted in him karate-kicking through the safety glass window of the door to the locked inpatient unit where he was being treated. Occasionally, lithium is helpful for autistic children with persistent aggressive behaviors. As with Tegretol, lithium blood levels must be monitored regularly. Although safe when used appropriately, lithium is highly toxic in overdose, and might not be a good choice in a household where the medication cannot be securely stored away from the autistic child.

Finding the Right Drug for a Particular Child. A number of other medications are prescribed for autistic children. Most are related to one of those already highlighted. A particular physician may prefer one medication over another based on his or her own experience. The main thing to remember is that there is a great deal of hit-and-miss, trial-and-error work in finding the right medication or combination of medications for a particular child. (Physicians prefer to call this "empirical trials.")

Some parents get quite frightened by one adverse drug reaction and back off from the whole issue of medication for an extended period of time. One bad reaction to one medication *certainly* does *not* mean that all other medications will cause bad effects. What is important is to try to understand what a particular prescribed medication is supposed to be doing for your child, and to objectively track whether, in reality, the expected benefits accrue.

B Vitamins. An offshoot of some of the psychopharmacological treatments that have been tried for autism is the use of high dosages of B complex vitamins. It has been suggested that B vitamins in high doses have some of the same psychopharmacological effects on autistic children as a mild stimulant medication would—namely, they may well quell physical hyperactivity and lead to a better ability to concentrate. A small number of autistic children seem to have a positive response to B vitamins, most have no response, and another small group (who may not benefit when on B vitamins) seem to grow more irritable when they stop taking them. Although some supporting research on the effects of high doses of B vitamins on the behavior of autistic children has been published, controversy surrounds the way some of the research has been carried out.

Some parents who hesitate to put a young child on a psychoactive drug feel more comfortable with trying a high dose of a vitamin first. This is understandable. However, excessive doses of B vitamins can have negative side effects too and, just like psychoactive medications, should be monitored by a pediatrician or child psychiatrist. In my personal experience, high doses of B vitamins occasionally make a child somewhat calmer and reduce problem behaviors that are related to the child being excessively active or overexcited. If B vitamins work for your child, fine—but don't expect them to work in lieu of other special educational or behavioral treatments that need to be ongoing at the same time.

Monitoring a Child's Benefits from Medication

Drug Holidays

Drug holidays are periods of time when the child comes off his medication for a while. There are a variety of reasons why and when drug holidays may be needed. A main reason for drug holidays is to see if the child still needs to be on the medication. Some symptoms that a medication is treating may spontaneously remit with age (such as hyperactivity) or get better with increased cognitive skill (such as attention span). More adaptive behavior patterns that a child may have been able to learn while on a medication may be sustainable off the medication if the new, good behavior pattern is well established. The only way to see if this is true is to take the child (usually gradually) off the medication and see how things go. If the child's target behaviors clearly begin to deteriorate as the medication is withdrawn, you may want to give up the idea of a drug-free period and return to the full treatment level. A drug holiday is not a good idea if it means the return of old negative behavior patterns, as this can destroy a lot of hard-earned achievements the child has made in self-control. For the child him- or herself, it can be scary to suddenly feel out-of-control again after having become accustomed to feeling more in control.

When parents do opt for drug holidays, it is usually during school summer vacation or holiday breaks. If the child is under less pressure to follow limits, he may tolerate removal of the drug better. On the other hand, the break in the child's routine that is associated with the end of school, or a holiday, may be *more* stressful a time for an autistic or PDD child, and precisely the *wrong* time to attempt a drug holiday. For some children, tapering a drug during school time (without telling teachers) is an opportunity to gather convincing data as to whether the medication is really being effective in school performance. If the "Josh had a bad day" note and a frowning face sticker come home day after day, you can be fairly certain that withdrawal of the medication is not being helpful to the child.

Some parents try to use medications only as often as they think the drug is needed. For some medications such as Tofranil, this is not really sensible because the medication takes weeks to reach effective levels in the blood anyway. More often, with a stimulant such as Ritalin (or even with Haldol) parents will adjust the dosage, play around with it, giving it only if the child starts to have a bad day or if there is going to be an activity that is likely to be particularly stressful for the child. I personally do not like such an approach. It puts the child on an unpredictable cycle of ups and downs, and being "on meds" can start to feel a lot like being punished. A child needs an opportunity to adjust to the mental state of being medicated and learn how to function well in that mental state. The child may subjectively prefer his unmedicated state, but it may not be helpful to his ability to function: For example, some children who benefit by being less hyperactive and being able to pay much better attention on Ritalin may find being on medication a "boring feeling" compared to the giddy, almost drunk state of being unmedicated.

Changes in doses should always be done in consultation with the treating physician. I know of more than one occasion when a frantic parent, desperate for a medication straitjacket, has unintentionally given her child an overdose. The effects of medications are not always linear (meaning that twice as much medication may not have just twice the effect). Dosage depends on the child's age and weight, as well as response, and tinkering with a complicated set of factors that are considered to determine the dose of a psychoactive medication, without consulting a doctor, is asking for trouble.

Recognizing When to Change Medications

Even the most "day and night" medication may begin to fail some day. The onset of puberty is the main time when previously effective medications may start to wane. The stimulants often fail to maintain effectiveness through puberty, and the neuroleptics may need major dose adjustments. Some medications like Cylert may work better after puberty (have a more long-lasting effect) and should be worth trying again.

Autistic adolescents, like all adolescents, can get quite wild; however, autistic adolescents sometimes express this in physically destructive ways (compared to the verbally abusive style preferred by so many of their non-autistic adolescent siblings). Therefore, adolescence is often the time when medications are first needed in order to help stop the child from acting out aggressively against others or him- or herself.

Around late latency (at nine or ten years of age) and into early adolescence, many children with PDD or Asperger's syndrome can begin to develop seriously fixed obsessional behaviors—such as talking endlessly about skyscrapers, fireplace equipment, or keys and locks. If and when an obsessional cluster of symptoms appears, adding a drug like Prozac may help quell the urge to fill all available time with thoughts and discussions about the favored topic. As we have discussed before, it is important to help the autistic individual go beyond his one topic (not just because he can become a pest to others), but because he is inhibiting his own ability to learn other things.

Compliance: Getting Medications to Be Taken

Once you have identified a medication to try, the next issue is figuring out how you are going to get the child to take it. Only a few of the medications we have discussed come in liquid form (Haldol, Tegretol, Prozac, and lithium are exceptions), and only a few come in gelatin capsules (for example, Tofranil and Prozac), or as chewables (Tegretol). Most often parents are faced with getting the child to take a pill. A few children will do this willingly. A few more will simply chew it up if you hand it to them—one of the rare situations in which having a child who puts everything into his mouth comes in handy.

For a child who gags on pills, spits them out, or refuses to put them in his mouth, there are a few pointers. One is that you can crush the pill (you can buy pill crushers in any pharmacy) and put it in a favorite liquid like orange juice, or embed it in a spoonful of something the child finds yummy, like ice cream. The more finely it's crushed, and the stronger tasting the food, the less likely it will be detected. The prescribing physician can tell you if a particular medicine tastes bitter (like Pondimin), so you can be prepared to mix it with something with a stronger counteracting taste like peanut butter or cheese spread. When the child won't take a pill easily by just swallowing it, the main problem is knowing how much medication actually got in. Therefore it's important to mix the medication with just a small amount of food (for example, one teaspoon of ice cream—not the whole bowl) so you can supervise the consumption of that portion. Most children, however, will learn to swallow pills if you persist in giving the pill with fluids, and it may be worth the initial effort to work on this skill.

Higher functioning children may resist taking their medications as they get older. Someone who is hyperactive does not necessarily enjoy feeling less hyperactive, even if others around him or her do benefit from having that person act more calmly. As the child, teenager, or young adult reaches this stage, it is important that taking the medication be made part of a routine. It is important that someone be responsible for routinely observing that the medication was really taken and not thrown out, spit out, or "cheeked" until no one was looking. A child who takes a psychoactive medication needs to feel it is as much a part of his daily routine as brushing his teeth, and not just something that is intermittently monitored when he or she has been acting bad.

Long-Term Management of Medication

All children who receive psychoactive medications should have ongoing medical management. Depending on the medication, this will mean different types of tests at different intervals. It is very important that any doctor who prescribes medications have access to all other information on the child's health status, and that the child never receive medications from different doctors at the same time without each doctor knowing what the others are doing. This is true even if one of the doctors is administering homeopathic treatments like megavitamins. Medications can interact with one another in specific ways to produce side effects that might not be seen with either medication alone. The doctor who prescribes a psychoactive medication definitely needs to know if the child is taking medicines for other physical ailments, as not all medications mix safely with one another.

Chapter Summary

In this chapter, we have discussed the use of psychoactive medications for children with autism and PDD. In deciding to use medications, a careful evaluation of the child's behaviors both at home and in the classroom needs to be made, and behavioral methods of changing behavior should usually be tried first. In addition to special education and medication, some parents and teachers also reach out for new treatments and apparent cures for autism that emerge from outside the mainstream of special education or medical practice. In the next chapter, we talk about some of these and how to assess their efficacy.

CHAPTER 15

♦ ♦ ♦

Non-Mainstream Treatments for Autism

There are a number of treatments for autism that are fairly controversial because they became widespread even before—or in spite of—scientific data about their effectiveness. Some of these treatments wax and wane in popularity, and some are just a flash in the pan. At most times, there are one or two nontraditional forms of treatment for autism that are particularly popular, and a certain percentage of parents decide to try one or more of these just in case it does help their child. In this chapter we'll discuss a number of non-mainstream treatments including facilitated communication, auditory training, the "Options" method, holding therapy, allergy treatments, and special diets.

Evaluating Non-Mainstream Treatments

What usually makes a treatment for autism controversial is professionals on one side insisting the treatment makes no sense, and a dramatic testimonial or two on the other claiming that the treatment made all the difference in the world for one particular child. The truth of the matter is that there are wide individual differences among autistic children. There are children who are misdiagnosed autistic, who may instead have severe language disorders, severe emotional problems, or childhood schizophrenia. Among all these children, there *are* likely to be a *few* children who, because of their particular constellation of strengths and weaknesses and because of the cause of their particular variant of autism or PDD, *do* respond to a particular treatment that is quite likely to be unhelpful to the vast majority of autistic children. Whenever a new treatment for autism starts to come into use it is important to ask "Does this make sense?" and "Did the child who got better have any of the same problems as my child?" When it comes to "miracle" cures for autism, it's a seller's market and the buyer must beware.

When a particular child does respond to a new and inexplicably helpful treatment, it would be more useful to ask "Why did this work with this child?" and "How exactly was it helpful?" and "What else could explain the apparent success?" rather than declaring a field day for the new treatment. Unfortunately, many families are so eager to find new things that may be helpful, that it is easy to buy into the claims of a particular treatment without taking time to think it through, or talk about it with a professional they can trust.

If It Sounds Too Good To Be True, It Probably Is

The accumulation of knowledge occurs gradually and logically. Some knowledge (less) accrues through inspirations of genius. However, much of what we have come to understand about autism and PDD that is truly helpful is knowledge that has been acquired gradually, logically, and slowly. Unfortunately, there have been no big breakthroughs in the treatment of autistic children. Maybe the next treatment to come along will be a breakthrough, but more likely it will not be. Accomplishing behavior change is arduous, fairly hard work. *But,* every year there is at least one flash in the pan when it comes to the treatment of autistic children. Not surprisingly, parents of all developmentally disabled children are subject to wanting miracle cures. Parents of autistic children may be more prone to such beliefs because their children *look* so normal. Without doubt, almost every treatment that has come along for any developmental disability has been tried on autistic children.

Every year there is some new idea about treating autism that involves a technique that "works" for no real scientific reason. Sometimes, the new treatment is first written about as an individual case, or as a small series of cases. Sometimes, the methodology for the new technique is spread through photocopied articles that have never been published in any scientific journal (because, as the author inevitably explains, he or she is challenging all the ideas held by the Autism Establishment who wish to preserve faith and funding for their own weak treatments). In recent years, various new "discoveries" in treating and understanding autism have been first disseminated through sources like *Reader's Digest,* and television programs like *Prime Time Live* and *20/20.* These information sources are in business to make money, which means attracting readers and viewers with sexy headlines and promises of new frontiers and medical breakthroughs. For commercial television, making money is at least as important as being right (as long as you don't get sued—because that would *cost* money).

The general public, who do not live with, or even see real autistic children, lap up the television networks' views on autism, integrating it into their existing knowledge about autism, which is largely based on Dustin Hoffman's performance in the movie *Rain Man.* The success of *Rain Man* marked the beginning of media's awareness that autism was a topic that could attract viewers and boost ratings, and since then, media attention to unvalidated treatments for autism has markedly increased.

To me, propagating misinformation among parents of autistic children is like taking candy from babies—it's easy to do and it's nasty. Parents and teachers of children with autism and PDD want very much to see the children they care for get better. Nothing about my work gives me more pleasure than to have a re-visit with an autistic child who is doing amazingly better than when I saw him last. But it is very important to me that the gains be real ones.

Like faith healing, many non-mainstream treatments for autism have a powerful appeal to the unconscious. Because autistic children almost always look quite normal, it is easy to maintain the belief, on an irrational, unconscious level, that there is a normal little person inside the autistic exterior, struggling to emerge whole. I think of this as the "homunculus theory of autism." Treatments that appeal to the homunculus theory of autism exploit a very vulnerable group of people—caregivers of developmentally disabled children. To my mind, promoters of such treatments are up there with televangelists who oversell religious retirement communities and keep the change, and used car salesmen who set back odometers 50,000 miles.

Ferreting Out the Fluke Cures. How do you know if a new treatment for autism has any validity? How do you even know if those who *are* scientifically informed think a treatment is a reasonable approach? Why not try it anyway? What if it only helps one out of a hundred children and your child is the one?

There are many treatments for autism that have grown up out of weak theoretical justifications. But if such a treatment works, and we know it works because of scientifically valid experiments, it helps revise a theory about autism. So a treatment for autism without any real theoretical foundation is, in and of itself, not so bad. What is bad is a lack of case-controlled evidence that something works on someone other than the child who has been featured in a sensational book, magazine article, or television program.

As we discussed in Chapter 14 in reviewing the use of psychoactive medications for autism, there are drugs that may be helpful even though the reasons they may be helpful are not entirely clear from a medical point of view. Therefore, it definitely *is* important to keep an open mind to new treatments. But keeping an open mind to new treatments means that it is important to explore alternative hypotheses as to why a new treatment may *not* be working: Sometimes when children improve, there is a strong bias to attribute positive change to the nearest treatment that has been introduced, rather than considering that improvement may be due to the cumulative effect of some other ongoing treatment, like special education.

With these warnings in mind, let's get specific. What *are* these various treatments that in the long run seem to perform less well than advertised? They fit into some basic categories like diets, therapies purported to promote neurological changes, and social-interactional interventions. We'll discuss the treatments that have received the most attention and examine evidence (or lack thereof) that they are efficacious. Most of these treatments may work somewhat for a very small number of children under very specific circumstances. Sometimes, a treatment may help, but maybe not in the way intended (for example, a strict diet may help a mother finally get control of the range of foods she can insist that her child eat). With any particular treatment, it is important to understand how much a particular child is likely to be helped, and in which ways, before proceeding full steam ahead into any new treatment program that raises high hopes. Some treatments come to be seen as a panacea for every difficulty the autistic child has.

No treatment for autism or PDD has ever been shown to help all aspects of the disorder, because, as we have discussed in earlier chapters, autism and PDD constitute a syndrome. Not all children have all symptoms, and some children are affected by some symptoms more than other children are. It is quite likely that, as a group, autistic spectrum disorders have a variety of causes and, as such, really aren't likely to have one cure. Therefore, treatments are really symptom specific. It would be more reasonable for new, non-mainstream treatments, just like other established treatments, to improve one thing (like communication) but not another (like sociability). Although areas of development like communication and sociability are not entirely separate, most treatments that do have some efficacy will have greater effects in one area compared to others. Do be particularly leery of treatments that claim to treat autism as a whole, as well as treatments that do radically different things for some autistic children than others (like eradicate toe-walking in one child and improve eye contact in another).

"Think Twice" Treatments

Facilitated Communication

One of the most controversial treatments for autism to come along in many years is "facilitated communication," or F/C as it is often called. F/C involves holding a child's hand, index finger pointed out, and "steadying" it to enable the child to type on a computer keyboard or portable communication device, or pick letters from an alphabet on a sheet of paper. The method was originally devised to help children with severe neuromotor disorders like cerebral palsy (CP) to communicate. Some children with CP have significant hand tremors (palsy), and so the facilitator was introduced to help the child steady his own movements. In addition, some CP children can't speak or can only make a limited number of sounds because they have poor control over the movements of their mouth, jaw, and tongue. Originally, F/C was refined by a therapist in Australia working with CP children; at some point, she tried it on autistic children, too, and found that it seemed to produce similar results despite the fact the autistic children appeared to have good fine motor coordination (and would seem to have no need to have their hand steadied to hit specific keys on a keyboard). By the early 1990s, the technique was brought to the United States by a special educator who promoted it heavily as something that virtually all autistic and, in fact, virtually all mentally retarded children could learn as well.

The American promotor of F/C felt that the child's previous level of functioning could be either high or low; it didn't matter. Through F/C, many children regarded as severely retarded and/or autistic could allegedly reveal inner worlds that operated with normal, near-normal, or even above-normal intelligence. Most "demonstrated" that they could read and type as soon as they were facilitated at a keyboard. Unlike normal children, autistic children who were facilitated did not need a period of years to learn to read or write, and many cases of children reading and writing above their chronological ages were reported. In addition, it was claimed that F/C could not be scientifically tested, because doing an experiment (like showing a child and a facilitator different pictures and then having the child type what he alone had seen) would force the facilitator to violate the child's trust in him or her—and without trust, the facilitation could not occur. Proponents of F/C insisted that it was the child and not the facilitator who controlled the child's hand movements as they typed letters, and pointed to a couple of cases where children eventually learned to type independently or only with a gentle touch from the facilitator. Critics of F/C countered that it was the facilitator and not the child who was unconsciously composing the typed messages, and that through behavioral conditionings, even subtle shifts in gentle pressure could be telling certain children whether they were heading for a "right" key or a "wrong" key.

The American promotor of F/C was able to have his program and students featured in the *New York Times Magazine.* Several months later, some of the very same children appeared again, along with some others—this time on *Prime Time Live,* a national network television program. The *Prime Time Live* presentation tested the limits of reality, showing a severely retarded autistic young man who facilitated with one hand being held to a keyboard while seemingly disattending and flapping his other hand. Through his facilitator, he expressed that he did not need to look at the keyboard because he could picture where each letter was without looking (or orienting his hands on the keyboard as a touch-typist would). Following these testimonials, F/C reached its kindling point and spread across the United States. Following this publicity, F/C became increasingly widespread among parents, teachers, and speech and language pathologists. Many who "saw," "believed."

Nevertheless, the numbers of critics grew, and many of their criticisms were empirically tested in well-designed experiments. Experiments with F/C uniformly showed that if the facilitator and child were fed different visual or auditory information, and the child was then asked to provide a facilitated response about that information, the response provided would *never* be based on what the child had seen or heard, but would either be a wrong response or a response based on what the facilitator had seen or heard. The experiments on F/C seemed to indicate that some facilitators were more direct than others at moving between their own perceptions and communication attributed to the child. But the experiments uniformly suggested that the typed content would come from the facilitator's mind, and not the child's. This, then, would explain how children who were previously considered to have a mental age of two years, could read, write, and spell like an adult. One study showed that if you asked two facilitators to ask two children the same questions and compared their responses, transcripts of the accuracy of the typing, the child's percentage of relevant responses, and the sophistication of language were more similar according to who the facilitator was, not which child was responding to the questions.

In some cases, F/C began to be used in schools to replace methods of communication the child could already do well—like use a communication board, sign, or in some cases, even talk. Through F/C, inordinate numbers of allegations of child abuse by parents and caregivers (though never against facilitators) began to emerge. Ironically, F/C began to produce results that turned against the very people who had brought it to life.

At this point, the data on F/C are fairly clear: While there are probably a tiny number of children who communicate better after F/C, the vast majority of children are not helped. Children who are likely to actually benefit from F/C probably are ones who do need to have their hands held to steady tremors, and who otherwise are cognitively normal or perhaps only mildly impaired. There are a few cognitively higher functioning mute autistic and PDD children who can learn to read, and therefore to type, and therefore to express themselves without oral means. Such children should need little or no "hand-holding" to begin typing. By and large, facilitated communication is a hoax that unfortunately has managed to deceive many parents and teachers because it appeals to a longing for a normal child to be "inside."

Auditory Training

Another unusual treatment for autism that has appeared in the last few years is called auditory training. The purpose of auditory training is to teach an autistic person to hear more fully and more accurately. The rationale is that because some autistic people are hypersensitive to some sounds while sometimes seeming not to respond to other sounds, they need training in how to listen. While there is some general sense in this, the approach to accomplishing this is strange. Proponents of auditory training promote the idea that someone can be taught to hear better by listening to specially recorded music through headphones. First, the patient is given an audiogram (a hearing test), to determine whether there are frequencies at which perception of sound is either hypo- or hyperacute. Next, music recorded on CDs (compact disks), which are already digitalized, are redigitalized to eliminate frequencies associated with hyperacuity, or to emphasize frequencies associated with hypoacuity. Over a period of sessions, the listening experience is systematically altered through further redigitalizing, and is supposed to result in a more normal audiogram at the completion of treatment. The treatments can be given up to several times a week, and sometimes treatment is "completed" in a few weeks. The treatment usually costs hundreds of dollars. There are many photocopied and re-photocopied lists of parent testimonials around, but no case-controlled scientific studies that show if and how auditory training really works. In consulting with colleagues who are audiology specialists, I have been able to obtain no explanation whatsoever why this method should work. Instead, each audiologist I've questioned about auditory training has asked me if there is something about autism that might explain why it should work, because there is no explanation he or she can proffer based on existing knowledge in the field of audiology.

The successful "results" of auditory training on a possibly autistic girl were first published in *Reader's Digest*. Five or so years later, there are still no scientific reports to support the efficacy of this treatment; although a couple of experimental studies have been undertaken, there have been only equivocal results.

Dietary Regimens

Many claims have been made about the relationship between diet and behavior. On an everday level, we are all aware that imbibing foods with psychoactive substances in them—like coffee with caffeine, or beer and wine with alcohol—can change the way we feel and behave. Initially, hyperactivity in children was linked to excessive sugar consumption, and this made some sense because sugar is metabolically available as energy more readily than carbohydrates, fats, or proteins. However, very careful, large-scale research has shown that sugar and hyperactivity are not linked. Although, on a case by case basis, a small number of people may be very sensitive to sugar and do feel an intense burst of energy after having a candy bar or a can of soda this is not true for most hypersensitive children.

The only significant relationship between diet and developmental disorders that has ever been scientifically demonstrated is the effect of dietary phenylalanine on the development of phenylketonuria (PKU), a mental retardation syndrome caused by a genetic defect that renders an individual unable to metabolize the amino acid phenylalanine, which can build to toxic levels in the brain.

Many diet-based claims about behavior and developmentally disabled children have gone way beyond the logical connections that can be drawn between certain foods like coffee, sugar, and alcoholic beverages, and subsequent mood or arousal states. Proponents of various dietary treatments often claim that developmental disorders may be caused by specific food allergies, or lack of the right substances in the diet at the right times.

In fact, parents of children with autism or PDD have not been so much affected by diet treatments as have parents of hyperactive children. The best known "behavior diet" is the Feingold diet, which, after years of being around, still lacks one well-done scientifically controlled study that shows that it makes a significant difference. (And, as mentioned earlier, a recent excellent large study has disproved Feingold's contentions.) Some diets are based on the idea that the autistic child has undetected allergies that cause an allergic reaction— and that the allergic reaction is the child's autistic behavior, rather than sneezing, a rash, or a cough, as is common with almost all allergies. This is a big leap of faith. It makes *some* sense to believe that a child who is allergic to something may act irritably when, for example, he has an undetected milk allergy, drinks some milk, and then develops some gastric distress. However, various testimonials have put forth the idea that a change in diet can affect the essential nature of the child's autistic symptoms, or how well he can learn. An example of this, mentioned in the last chapter, was one mother (a nurse, no less) who wrote a book claiming that her son's autism was due to a "cerebral milk allergy," and that when milk was removed from his diet, he became normal.

Among the diets I've seen wax and wane in popularity with parents of autistic children are sugar-free diets, wheat-free diets, preservative-free diets, red dye–free diets, and rotation diets (in which a small number of foods are eaten in concentration for a week or more, and then the diet is "rotated" to another set of foods). Undoubtedly, some children *are* allergic to some of the things that get removed from their meals in the course of these various forms of dietary treatment. They probably do feel somewhat better as a result. However, there is no evidence that diets can cause or alleviate symptoms of autism.

My position on these diets is that (1) there are individual differences in how children can respond to any dietary change, (2) most dietary changes don't do much, and (3) most diets can't hurt, but (4) if you are going to undertake a dietary change, be clear ahead of time about what changes you expect in the child. Diet changes, like the medication changes discussed in Chapter 14, should be entered into with an open mind and, if possible, with an informed observer who knows the child but is blind to the diet change. Be careful to consider whether concomitant learning through schooling, or other changes in the child's life, might not explain any improvements instead. Always change one thing at a time: Don't start a new diet the same week as a new school or a new medication.

Most diets are—more or less—a bother. It is already hard enough raising an autistic child. There is no point in making your life even more constrained if you don't have to. Diets can have a certain appeal because they can give you a distinct intervention to do with the child on a daily basis. However, the more such interventions you add, especially without proof of efficacy, the more complex (and tiring) your life is likely to become. Make sure you can see some benefit if you go with a dietary change. Keep your mind open.

Autism and Yeast Infections: Candidiasis and Nystatin

Candidiasis (candida yeast infection) is a ubiquitous form of vaginal yeast infection that many women contract during their childbearing years. Candidiasis may be so mild that the woman is unaware that she is infected, and she may not seek treatment. Several years ago, it was noted anecdotally that many mothers of autistic children reported having been treated for candidiasis. Looking back on what might have gone wrong to cause their child's autism, some mothers asked whether undetected candida yeast infections in pregnancy might have been the culprit. To date, it is clear that many mothers of autistic children did have candida infections during pregnancy, but there is no clear evidence that they have had such infections at a rate that is higher than the general population. This means that many more women who also had candida infections went on to have normal children. Nevertheless, in the early and mid-1980s the idea caught on that autistic children might benefit from being treated with Nystatin, the medication used to treat candida infections in women with this type of vaginal yeast infection. Nystatin was often recommended for the child whether or not a mother could document having candidiasis in her pregnancy and also whether or not the child showed signs of candidiasis. I was never able to ascertain the logic of this treatment (although the appeal of a straightforward "cure" was certainly clear). In fact, when this treatment was at its peak of popularity I received one telephone call from a rather dubious allergist asking the blood serotonin level of a child we were following. (Blood serotonin levels have no clinical significance as far as any treatment for autism goes, but at the time we were studying the effect of a particular medication on serotonin.) Out of curiosity, I asked this allergist how he planned to use the information I would give him about the serotonin level in his Nystatin treatment plan. He said he felt it was important to consider the "full picture." I thought he was a charlatan and told the patient's mother so. The mother gave the treatment with Nystatin a go anyway, but gave up after a couple of months because it apparently made no difference. This case illustrated for me the way in which such snake oil salesmen try to legitimize their endeavors by insinuating their warp into the context of acceptable standards of care.

The downside of useless interventions such as Nystatin treatments is that children not only fail to get better, but as with other non-mainstream cures, parental hopes are falsely raised and then deflated. Some parents will tell me that they prefer to have their hopes falsely raised than to never have experienced that period of increased hopefulness. That's fair enough. But it's also important to go into questionable long-shot treatments with one's eyes open. In pursuing a treatment like the Nystatin/candida connection, parents also can risk investing sometimes scarce financial resources for medicine that will not work.

Holding Therapy

Shades of Bruno Bettleheim! A New York psychiatrist, working primarily with an outmoded psychogenic (that is, parent-caused) view of autism, decided that if parents held their autistic children (very tightly), the children would emerge from their autistic worlds because they would finally know they were loved. The ideas behind holding therapy were lent credence through the work of Niko Tinbergen, a Nobel laureate and one of the founding fathers of the field of animal ethology, who in his declining years advocated holding therapy in an otherwise rather interesting book—an ethological analysis of the behavior of autistic children, which he co-authored with his wife, who had taught autistic children for many years.

Like other unconventional treatments for autism, there was an alluring grain of truth to holding therapy—that perhaps contact-sensitive autistic children could be desensitized by high levels of physical contact. Holding therapy consisted of sessions where a parent would hold his or her (fairly small) autistic child face to face in a loving but rather immobilizing embrace until the child ceased to struggle and engaged in a period of calmness and at least brief eye contact. Some holding therapy approaches also involved having the parents shout to the child that the parents *did* love the child, but that the parent was angry that the child withheld his or her love, and that the child *must* give up his autistic aloneness and come out. Holding therapy sessions typically last from twenty to forty-five minutes. (The sessions tend to get shorter once the child gets the gist of what is going on—that is, he'll keep getting held until he stops struggling.) Since most autistic children who do like physical contact tend to strongly prefer it when *they* can be the ones to initiate and terminate the contact, holding therapy sessions tended to be rather violent.

When holding therapy first became popularized in the late 1980s we attempted to study it empirically in collaboration with a child psychotherapist who was offering it as a clinical treatment. The problem was that when it didn't work, the therapist would simply tell the parents that it was either because they weren't doing it often enough (four or five times a week was the standard in this study), or that their hearts weren't really in it when they did do it. One family we followed, the Wongs, wanted so much to have the procedure help their son that Mr. Wong quit his job as a manager in a computer firm for a year to stay home with four-year-old Brett and hold him three or four times a day. After a year, the benefits of holding therapy had not materialized, and Mr. Wong was having severe enough stress-related physical symptoms of his own that his internist recommended that he do something less stressful—namely, return to his full-time job—which (with my hearty endorsement) he did. Although children do grow calm after being held, and may even make brief eye contact, the effects do not seem to extend to the children becoming more social at other times.

Options Therapy

"Options" therapy came out of a book, *Son Rise,* that described the efforts of two parents, particularly the mother, to find their own way to treat their son whom they describe as autistic. (Over the years, I've run across a couple of the professionals who were among those alleged to have diagnosed the boy as autistic, and both remain uncertain that the boy actually was autistic before treatment.) Basically, in *Son Rise,* the mother shows her son that she accepts the boy's "world" as a bridge to the boy joining "her" world. The mother spends vast amounts of time confined with the boy in a small room, imitating whatever he does so that he'll realize she's there and that there are similarities between them. Demands are never placed on the child. After one particular breakthrough session in the room, the child begins to "emerge."

This therapy makes little sense developmentally. The way children learn *is* partly by having their actions mirrored back, but *also* by having those actions elaborated and connected to new things that the child has not discovered on his own. That's exactly what a mother does when a baby coos, and the mother repeats the baby's cooing noise, making it sound more like "ba-ba," and then says "bottle," and then showing the baby her bottle. If the mother never added any new information, and only mirrored the baby's own actions with different modulations, it would be like a hall of mirrors—and there would be little opportunity to learn about things that were not self-generated.

After the *Son Rise* book became popular, the couple who wrote the book set up an institute and began charging thousands of dollars for a brief workshop on how to use their method. "Options" is now promoted by parents and therapists who have been through the training. Like other non-mainstream treatments, there has never been any research showing the benefits of this approach on a controlled group of children who did or did not receive the therapy.

Sensory Integration Therapy

Sensory integration therapy has come into the treatment of autistic children from the field of physical therapy. Most autistic children do not have specific fine or gross motor physical deficits, so physical or occupational therapy is often not a recommended special education service. Even if the child has slight physical development delays, these problems usually receive less attention, because the communicative and social difficulties are so much greater. Nevertheless, sensory integration therapy is sometimes suggested because many autistic children do have sensory processing abnormalities like being overreactive to touch; are seemingly insensate to many painful stimuli; display hypersensitive hearing; or look at, smell, or tap things incessantly.

Sensory integration, as the name suggests, is supposed to provide ways in which the child will develop better modulated sensory responses, and as a result, (and here's the leap of faith) should become more social and communicative. There certainly is evidence that a sensory integration approach can help with the child's overresponsiveness to certain sensory stimuli. For example, a child who is hypersensitive to touch can benefit by being gently stroked with a very soft brush, and slowly introduced to stiffer brushes so that he can tolerate contact on various parts of his body. As the child grows to like the brushing, talking to the child or making eye contact can be added, so that, hopefully, making eye contact becomes more tolerable, too.

In behavioral terms, the positive effects of sensory integration can be described as "systematic desensitization." To this extent, a sensory integration approach may be helpful. However, there is no evidence that there *are* any corresponding neurological changes, as is sometimes implied by proponents of this approach. There is no evidence that there is subsequently better transfer of information across sensory modalities. In Chapter 11, we discussed "crossmodal transfer of information"—putting information in via a stronger sense channel to help it be comprehended by a weaker one. While sensory integration therapy may not perform as some advertise, in my clinical experience, its curriculum can be an appealing social interaction modality for autistic children who are attracted to the movement and tactile stimulation involved. Any applications of sensory integration therapy that make a particular autistic child more open to interaction are worth pursuing for that reason alone.

Chapter Summary

We've covered some of the main controversial therapies for autistic and PDD children. Looking back on this chapter, you may feel I've conveyed a sense of negativism about many alternative treatments. If this seems so, it's because I've seen too many parents invest time, money, and hope in treatments that they eventually give up on in cynical dismay. I also worry that time spent pursuing unproven treatments is time that is lost. This is especially a concern in the early years, when intervention is so critical.

Always examine new therapies carefully. Get a variety of opinions. Consider both the pros and cons. If you go for a new, unproven treatment, set your goals and constantly look for evidence of whether the goals are being met. Always consider alternative hypotheses; that is, other possible explanations for positive changes. Also remember that all autistic and PDD children improve somewhat with maturation. Get periodic, outside professional evaluations as benchmarks. Children with autism and PDD need both good intentions *and* good treatments to get better.

Afterword

My purpose in writing this book has been to help parents, caregivers, and teachers of children with autistic spectrum disorders to cope better with the disabilities they confront. The single greatest difficulty in writing this book has been in making "autism" and "PDD" real for each reader. The child or children each reader will have in mind will be different. Not all children with autism have the same constellation of symptoms. In addition, each autistic child, just like each child who is not autistic, has a unique personality that is his or her own. I hope you will think about what you have read here and realize that some information will not pertain now, and may never pertain to your child. Try to make sense of the parts that do ring true, and don't worry about the rest.

For most parents, "autism" is a word they've rarely even heard before someone starts suggesting their child may be autistic. Faced with a great unknown, reading helps make autism real. Once something becomes real through words, we feel we can begin to take effective action. Reading about autism, therefore, is a form of coping. The more coping you can do, the better. Read, meet doctors, ask questions, meet teachers, observe classrooms, watch therapists work with your child. Get ideas from wherever you can. Use those around you as resources. Don't hesitate to get others to help you understand how your own observations and theories about your child fit into what they say. In certain ways, a parent or a teacher who is with an autistic child daily is more of an expert on that particular child than any "autism expert."

If you read this, and you *do* feel your child may be autistic, and you haven't sought professional help yet, please do it. The earlier we can intervene, the more hope there is. If a child is autistic, even mildly autistic or your child is suspected of having a mild developmental disorder, it won't go away on its own. It can't hurt to get help.

The emotional stress of parenting a child with a disability can be nearly devastating for some parents—especially at first. Take care of yourself, too. Don't make the rigors of your child's treatment into some kind of punishment for yourself. Having an autistic child is a genetic or environmental event that in the vast majority of cases was beyond your control. Don't fall into a pattern of punishing yourself for it.

As a parent, above all, your child is your child. Even if your child is autistic, and you must undertake to become his or her teacher and advocate, you are still the only mother or father your child has. In his or her own way, each autistic child needs love and understanding as well as treatment. Each child, autistic or not, marches to the beat of his own drummer. Parenting an autistic child requires being able to hear that beat, and then teaching your child how to dance to it.

Index

AAMD Adaptive Behavior Scales, 105
Ability, islets of, 67–69
  performance intelligence and, 100–101
  quantification and, 69
Ability-grouped classes, 211–212
Abstract language, 272
Activities. See also Stereotyped motor behavior
  lack of engagement with, 60–61
  play. See Play
  unusual, intense interest in, 67–69
Adaptive functioning
  in Asperger's syndrome, 113, 118
  intelligence and, 283
  tests of, 104–105
  training in. See Daily living skills training
Adolescents. See also Classrooms; Special education
  book about, 189
  high-functioning, daily living skills training for, 296–297
  intelligence tests for, 103–104
  lower-functioning, daily living skills training for, 293–296
  medications for, 318–319
  medium-functioning, daily living skills training for, 297–298
  psychotherapy for, 146–147
Adults
  Asperger's syndrome in, 117–119
  book about, 189
  eligibility for developmental services, 170–171
  high-functioning, daily living skills training for, 296–297
  intelligence tests for, 104
  lower-functioning, daily living skills training for, 293–296
  medium-functioning, daily living skills training for, 297–298
  parents' concerns about, 133–134
  psychotherapy for, 146–147
  residential placement for, 160–161
Advocacy, 183–186
  advocates versus attorneys for, 183–184
  fair hearings and, 184–186
  when to go to, 185–186
  for IEP, 178, 183–184
    advocates versus attorneys for, 183–184
    mediation and, 184
The Advocate, 193
Affect. See Emotion(s); Emotional expression
Affection, physical, 31–32
African American families, coping with diagnosis by, 132–133
Age. See also specific age groups, i.e., School-aged children
  eligibility for developmental services and, 170–171
  expressive language, 90, 254
  medications and, 304–305
  mental, 97–98
  parental, parenting and, 140–141
  of parents, parenting and, 140–141
  receptive language, 90, 254
Allergies, as cause of autism, 302–303, 328
Aloofness, child abuse and, 31
Alpern-Boll Scales, 105
Alternative treatments. See Treatment interventions, nonmainstream

American sign language (ASL), 260
Americans with Disabilities Act, 176
Amniocentesis, detection of fragile X syndrome by, 120
Anafranil (clomipramine), 309, 310
Anger, as response to diagnosis, 130–131
Anticipatory reach, 45
Antidepressant medications, 309–310
Antipsychotic medications, 304–305, 311–314
    dyskinesias and, 312–313
Aphasia, 54
Appearance, of autistic children, 49
Arm-flapping (arm-waving), 75
Arousal, self-regulation of, repetitive movements as, 71–72
Asian American families, coping with diagnosis by, 132
Asperger's syndrome (AS), 110–119
    in adults, 117–119
    autism contrasted with, 113–116
        social impairments and, 113–115
        special interests and, 115–116
    book about, 189
    characteristics of, 21
    diagnosis of, 104, 112–113
    former terms used for, 112–113
    obsessive behaviors in, 319
    origins of diagnosis of, 111–112
    prevalence of, 12
    in younger children, 116–117
Assessment. *See also* Developmental evaluation; Diagnosis
    of attachment behavior, 34, 35–36
    of brain damage, 104
Association for Retarded Citizens, 194
Attachment behavior
    assessment of, 34, 35–36
    autistic development of, 33–36
    early, 26–27
    normal development of, 33
Attachment objects, 61–62
Attention
    getting and holding, 250–251
    physical exercise as method of focusing, 251–252
Attorneys. *See also* Advocacy
    IEP and, 178, 183–184
Audiologists, role in developmental evaluation, 90–91
Audiometry, sound field (play), 90
Auditory brain response (ABR), 90
Auditory evoked potential, 90
Auditory hypersensitivity, 77, 78
    auditory training and, 326–327

Auditory hyposensitivity, 77–78
Auditory processing, echolalia and, 55
Auditory training, 326–327
Aunts, roles for, 155–156
Authoritarian parenting, 141–142, 143
Autism
    Asperger's syndrome contrasted with, 113–116
        social impairments and, 113–115
        special interests and, 115–116
    association with fragile X syndrome, 13, 23
    association with mental retardation, 11–12, 97. *See also* Developmental evaluation, intelligence testing in; Mental retardation; Special education, mental retardation and
    behavioral versus physical markers of, 86–87
    causes of, 12–13, 302–303, 328–329
        blaming spouse for, 126–127, 138, 144
        understanding to promote coping with diagnosis, 126
    development over time, 106–107
    diagnosis of. *See* Coping with diagnosis; Developmental evaluation; Diagnosis
    diagnostic criteria for, 12–13
    eligibility for services and, 169–170
    inheritance of, 93, 126
    language deficits and, 255
    medications for, 309
    PDD,NOS distinguished from, 15–20
        communication and. *See* Communication; Language; Nonverbal communication; Verbal communication
        DSM-IV criteria and, 16–19
        ICD-10 criteria and, 19–20
        social development and. *See* Social development
    PDD,NOS distinguished from PDD,NOS, play and. *See* Play
    prevalence of, 12
    risk factors for, 12–13, 86, 92–93
        for autism and PDD,NOS, 12–13
    social relatedness and, 255
    sociopaths distinguished from, 29
    terminology for, 9–11
    treatment of. *See* Treatment interventions; *specific treatment approaches*
Autism (Schriebman), 188
Autism . . . Nature, Diagnosis and Treatment (Dawson), 191
Autism: A Guide for Parents and Professionals (Wing), 188

Autism: New Hope for a Cure (Tinbergen), 47

Autism: Understanding the Enigma (Frith), 188

Autism and Asperger's Syndrome (Frith), 112, 189

Autism Diagnostic Interview (ADI), 95–96

Autism Diagnostic Observation Schedule (ADOS), 94

Autism in Adolescence and Young Adults (Schopler and Mesibov), 189

Autism rating scales, 95–96

Autism Society of America (ASA), 85, 192–194

Autism Society of Canada, 194

Autistic classes, 210–211

Autistic disorder. *See* Autism

Autistic savants, 67–69
performance intelligence and, 100–101
quantification and, 69

Autistic spectrum disorders, 10

Aversives
mild, to reduce negative behavior, 237–238
physical, 240–241

Babies. *See* Infants and toddlers

Babysitters, 158–159

Bargaining, as response to diagnosis, 128

Baseline data, collecting before medication trial, 306

Bayley Scales of Infant Development (Bayley-II), 101–102

Beauty, of autistic children, 49

Bedtime difficulties, 292–293
medications promoting sleep for, 310

Behavioral assessment. *See under* Developmental evaluation

Behavioral testing, 86–87

Behavior control, teacher's aides for, 225

Behavior-focused observation, in classroom, 216–217

Behavior intervention services, 172–173

Behavior management, 231–242. *See also* Discipline
instrumental learning and, 232
reducing interfering negative behavior and, 236–242
accompanied time-outs for, 238–240
ignoring for, 236–237
mild aversives for, 237–238
physical aversives for, 240–241
restraint for, 241–242
spanking for, 241

reinforcement schedules for, 233–235
reward hierarchy for, 232–233
token economies for, 235–236

Behavior modification
application of. *See* Behavior management
myths about, 203

Beliefs, cultural, coping with diagnosis and, 131–133

Benadryl (diphenhydramine), 313

Benztropine (Cogentin), 312–313

Bereavement, as response to diagnosis, 122–123

Bilingual parents, early language development and, 264–265

Biting, of hands, 74

Blame, by spouse
parenting and, 138, 144
as response to diagnosis, 126–127

Blind medication trials, 306–307

Blood tests, for fragile X syndrome, 119

Body imitations, 38

Books
on Asperger's syndrome, 112
on autism, 47, 187–191
first-person accounts, 189–190
general information, 187–188
research-oriented, 190–191
special interest areas of, 189
treatment-oriented, 188, 189, 288
autobiographical, 279–280
on fragile X syndrome, 23

BOS, 94

Brain
autism and, 134–135
growth and development of, 198

Brain damage, assessment of, 104

Brain stem evoked response (BSER), 90

Bribes, avoiding using reinforcers as, 234

Brothers. *See* Siblings

Brothers and Sisters: A Special Part of Exceptional Families (Powell and Ogle), 189

Burnout, in children receiving intensive programs, 206–207

BuSpar (buspirone), 315–316

B vitamins, 316–317

Canada, autism society in, 194

Candidiasis, as cause of autism, 302, 328–329

Capacity, of autistic or PDD child, intensiveness of early intervention and, 205–206

Carbamazepine (Tegretol), 314, 315, 319

Caregivers. *See also* Parent(s)
  allegations of abuse by, facilitated commu-
    nication and, 326
  attachment to. *See* Attachment behavior
Case management, 171–172
Cattell Scales, 102
Change, resistance to, 65–67
Checklists, for behavioral assessment, 95–96
Child abuse, 144–145
  allegations of, facilitated communication
    and, 326
  aloofness and, 31
Childhood Autism Rating Scale (CARS), 96
Childhood disintegrative disorder (CDD),
    characteristics of, 22–23
Child neurologists
  medications prescribed by, 304
  role in developmental assessment, 91
Child pharmacology specialists, medications
    prescribed by, 304
Child psychiatrists
  medications prescribed by, 304
  role in developmental evaluation, 88, 89
Child psychologists, role in developmental
    evaluation, 88, 89
Children With Autism (Powers), 188
Circle time, 207–208
Classrooms, 209–230
  ability-grouped, 211–212
  designated autistic classes and, 210–211
  grouped by educational diagnosis, 210
  mainstreaming and full inclusion in, 225–
    230
    autistic and PDD children with hearing-
      impaired children, 264
    day care and social mainstreaming and,
      230
    limitations to, 226–227
    peer tutoring and, 229–230
    prerequisites to, 227
    purpose of, 227
    reverse mainstreaming and, 228
    shadow aides in, 228–229
  for PDD children, 212
  social skills development and mixed-
    disability classes and, 212–213
  structure of, 219–225
    child's adjustment to, 220–221
    contained classes versus changing classes
      and, 221–222
    need for structure and, 220
    reducing distractions and, 221
    teacher's aides and, 222–225
  teachers and, 213–215

  establishing relationship with, 214–215
  interviewing potential teachers and, 214
  teaching to the middle and, 213
  visits to, 215–219
    behavior-focused observation during,
      216–217
    emotional experience to seeing other
      handicapped children and, 216
    etiquette for, 217–218
    learning about instructional alternatives
      during, 216
    observation of teacher's aides' activities
      during, 223
    parent-teacher relationship and, 218–219
Clinicians. *See* Developmental evaluation,
    professionals' roles in; Professionals;
    specific professionals
Clomipramine (Anafranil), 309, 310
Cogentin (benztropine), 312–313
Cognitive functioning. *See* Developmental
    evaluation, intelligence testing in; In-
    telligence; Mental retardation
Comfort-seeking, 32–37
  autistic development of attachment behav-
    ior and, 33–36
  normal development of attachment behav-
    ior and, 33
  when child is hurt or ill, 36–37
Commands, follow-through on, 249–250
Communication, 43–59
  communication boards for. *See* Communi-
    cation boards
  of diagnosis, 124
    ambiguity in, 130
  emotional expression in, 48–50
    tone of voice and, 49–50
  expressive, communication boards for, 256
  nonverbal. *See* Nonverbal communication
  between parents, 122, 143–144
  teacher's aides to increase exposure to
    speech and language therapy goals
    and, 224–226
  verbal. *See* Language; Verbal communica-
    tion
Communication boards, 255–260
  choices between two options and, 258
  electronic, 259–260
  for expressive communication, 256
  role in language development, 258–259
  three-dimensional, 256
  two-dimensional, 255–256
  when to use, 256–257
Communication Problems in Autism (Schop-
    ler and Mesibov), 191

Communicatively handicapped (CH) educational track, 276
Compensatory stimulation, 198
Computer-assisted instruction (CAI), 244–246
software for, 244
Computer games, 246
Consistency, joint custody and, 140
Conversational skill, 58–59
language pragmatics and, 58–59, 267–272
Coping, by siblings. *See* Siblings, coping patterns of
Coping with diagnosis, 121–135
concerns about prognosis and, 133–135
biological versus psychological theories of causes of autism and, 134–135
fantasies about child's death and, 135
fear that child will never grow up and, 134
cultural beliefs about disability and, 131–133
defenses and acceptance of diagnosis and, 128–131
ambiguous communication of diagnosis and, 130
anger and frustration with doctors and, 130–131
denial and, 128–130
seeking alternative treatments and, 131
initial reactions and, 123–133
bargaining as, 128
blame and guilt as, 126–127
dissociation, disbelief, numbness, and saturation as, 125
hopelessness as, 125–126, 127
observations contradictory to diagnosis and, 124–125
outcry as, 125–126
understanding causes of autism to promote coping and, 126
of mental retardation, 286
natural defenses and grief and, 121–123
bereavement and, 122–123
Costs, of special education, 176, 177–178
Counseling, genetic, 93
Counting, 281
special interests involving, 69
Couples therapy, 147–148
Cultural beliefs about disabilities
coping with diagnosis and, 131–133
in mainstream American culture, 159–160
Custody, joint, 140
Cylert (pemoline), 311, 312, 318

Daily living skills training
for high-functioning adolescents and adults, 296–297
for lower-functioning persons, 285–294
adolescents and adults, 293–296
bedtime difficulties and, 292–293
feeding difficulties and, 288–290
home-based, 287–293
school-based curricula for, 286–287
toilet training, 290–292
for medium-functioning students, 297–298
Dangerous behavior, residential placement and, 161
Day care, social mainstreaming and, 230
Day treatment, 175
Death, of child, fantasies about, 135
Deep pressure stimulation, craving for, 80
Denial, as response to diagnosis, 128–130
Department of Developmental Services (DSS), 169
Desipramine (Norpramin; Pertofrane), 309, 310
Desyrel (trazodone), 309, 310
Detail scrutiny, 78–79
of hands, 75
Developmental delay. *See also* Mental retardation
use of term, 97
Developmental disabilities services. *See* Treatment interventions
Developmental disorders, definition of, 11–12
Developmental evaluation, 85–105
adaptive functioning tests in, 104–105
agencies providing, 172
behavioral assessment in, 94–96
autism rating scales for, 95–96
informal observation for, 94
standardized play sessions for, 94–95
behavioral testing in, 86–87
developmental history in, 91–93
genetic, 92
genetic counseling and, 93
of pregnancy, 92–93
for first IEP, 180–181
intelligence testing in, 96–104
accuracy of, 98–99
islets of ability and, 100–101
mental age scores and, 97–98
performance intelligence and, 100–101
psychologists and, 89
tests used for, 101–104
verbal intelligence and, 99–100
medical insurance coverage for, 186–187

Developmental evaluation (*cont.*)
    medical testing in, 87
    professionals' roles in, 88–91
        of audiologist, 90–91
        of child neurologist, 91
        of child psychiatrist, 88, 89
        of developmental evaluation team members, 88–89
        of pediatric geneticist, 91
        of psychologist, 88, 89
        of speech and language pathologist, 90
Dexedrine (dextroamphetamine), 311, 312
Diagnosis, 82–120
    acceptance of. *See* Coping with diagnosis
    of Asperger's syndrome, 104, 112–113
    changes in, 24
    communication of, ambiguity in, 130
    developmental evaluation for. *See* Developmental evaluation
    diagnostic criteria for autism and, 12–13
    differential, 105, 110–120
        Asperger's syndrome and, 110–119
        fragile X syndrome and, 119–120
    early, 84, 105–109
        development of autism over time and, 106
        home videos of toddlers and, 106–107
        Pervasive Developmental Disorders Screening Test for, 107–109
    educational, classes grouped by, 210
    fear of, 97
    labeling and, 82–84
    need for, 82, 83, 169–171
    of PDD,NOS, 16–17
    purpose of, 82
    reactions to. *See* Coping with diagnosis
    resources for, 84–85
    timing of, 84
Diagnosis and Assessment in Autism (Schopler and Mesibov), 191
Diagnostic and Statistical Manual of Mental Disorders, Fourth Edition (DSM-IV)
    criteria for Asperger's syndrome, 112–113
    criteria for autism and PDD,NOS, 16–19
    nonverbal intelligence and, 16–17
Dietary regimens, 327–328
Differential diagnosis. *See* Diagnosis, differential
Diphenhydramine (Benadryl), 313
Disability, cultural beliefs about, coping with diagnosis and, 131–133
Disability and the Family (Turnbull, Turnbull, Summers, and Roeder-Gordon), 189

Disbelief, as response to diagnosis, 125
Discipline. *See also* Behavior management
    fear of using, 136–137
    inappropriate punishment and, 31
    standards of behavior for autistic child and siblings and, 149
    teacher's aides for, 225
Dissociation, as response to diagnosis, 125
Distractions, reducing in classrooms, 221
Divorce, among parents of autistic and PDD children, 137–138
    joint custody and, 140
Doctors. *See specific specialties, i.e.* Psychiatrists
Double-blind crossover studies, 307
Drug holidays, 317–318
Drugs. *See* Medications; *specific drug names*
Dyskinesias, 312–313
Dysphasia, 54

Early intervention, 196–208
    infant stimulation programs, 172
    initiating, 196
    intensiveness of, 201–208
        burnout in children and, 206–207
        child's capacity and, 205–206
        family functioning and, 205
        group activities and, 207–208
        initiating intervention and, 206
        intensive method and, 201–204
        intrusive versus insistent methods and, 204
    need for research on, 197
    neuropsychological support for, 197–201
        learning and, 201
        skill development and, 198–201
    pediatricians as gatekeepers to, 196–197
Easter Seal Society, 194
Eating. *See* Feeding
E-2 Checklist, 96
Echolalia, 55–57
    delayed, 56–57
        functional, 56
        nondelayed, 56–57
    immediate, 54–55
        auditory processing and, 55
        pronoun reversal in, 55
Echopraxia, 64
Education. *See also* Classrooms; Special education
    books about, 188
    drug effects versus, 307
    IEP and. *See* Individual educational program (IEP)

parents as consumer watchdogs of, 163–
164
Educational diagnosis, classes grouped by,
210
EEGs, 91
The Effects of Autism on the Family (Schopler and Mesibov), 191
Electric shock, to reduce negative behavior,
240–241
Electronic communication boards, 259–260
Emergence: Labeled Autistic (Grandin), 190
Emotion(s), of others, perception of, 30–31
Emotional expression, 48–50
tone of voice and, 49–50
Employment, 283–285
Asperger's syndrome and, 118–119
calibrating expectations regarding, 285–286
job coaching and, 174
sheltered workshops and, 174–175
supported, 174
vocational training and, 174, 298–300
for moderately impaired people with au-
tism, 298–299
school-based programs for, 299–300
England, autistic society in, 194
ETHOS, 94
Etiquette, for classroom observation, 217–
218
Evaluation. *See* Assessment; Developmental
evaluation; Diagnosis
Experiential writing, 280–281
Explaining autism or PDD, to siblings, 148–
149
Expressive communication, communication
boards for, 256
Expressive language, 100
Expressive language age, 90, 254
Expressive relating, 27–29
hand-leading and, 28
social referencing and, 28–29
Eye contact, 46–47
language development and, 268–269

Facial cues, 46–47
eye contact, 46–47, 268–269
smiling, 46
Facilitated communication (F/C), 324–326
Facts, writing about, 280
Fair hearings, IEP and, 184–186
when to go to, 185–186
Families. *See also* Parent(s); Siblings
books about, 189
extended, 154–156
aunts' and uncles' roles and, 155–156

grandparents' roles and, 154–155
functioning of, intensiveness of early intervention and, 205
outings without autistic or PDD child for,
158–159
psychotherapy for, 148. *See also* Psychotherapy
residential placement and, 161–162
support groups for. *See* Support groups
Family mealtimes, 289–290
Family Pictures (Miller), 190
Family planning, parenting of autistic and
PDD children and, 138–139
Family therapy, 148
Fantasies, about child's death, 135
Fathers. *See* Parent(s); Parenting
Feeding, 288–290
family mealtimes and, 289–290
food fads and, 289
self-feeding skills and, 288–289
Feelings. *See* Emotion(s); Emotional expres-
sion
Feingold diet, 327–328
Fenfluramine (Pondimin), 308, 315, 319
Fine-motor ability, 100
Finger-flapping, 75
Fixations
on touch, taste, and smell senses, 79
visual, 75, 78–79
Fluoxetine (Prozac), 304, 309, 310, 319
Follow-through, on commands, 249–250
Food fads, 289
Fragile X syndrome, 119–120
association with autism, 13, 23
characteristics of, 23–24
prevalence of, 12
The Fragile X Syndrome (Hodnap and Leck-
man), 23
Friendships
lack of
Asperger's syndrome and, 114–115
autism and, 41–42
parental, roles for friends and, 156–
157
Frustration, as response to diagnosis,
130–131
Full inclusion. *See* Classrooms, mainstreaming and full inclusion in
Functional academic orientation, transition
to, 282–283
Functional skills. *See* Adaptive functioning
Future, concerns about. *See* Coping with
diagnosis, concerns about prognosis
and

Gender
  autism and PDD,NOS and, 12
  prevalence of autism and PDD,NOS and,
    12
  Rett syndrome and, 21
Generalization, problems with, 98
Genetic counseling, 93
Genetic factors
  in autism, 93, 126
  in fragile X syndrome, 119–120
Genetic history, 92
Geneticists, role in developmental assess-
    ment, 91
Gessell Scales, 102
Gestalt processing
  language, 247–248
  visual, 247
Gestures. *See* Nonverbal communication,
    gestures and
Goals, for IEPs, 181–183
  progress toward, 182–183
  setting, 181–182
Grandparents, roles for, 154–155
Grief, as response to diagnosis, 122–123
Gross-motor ability, 100
Group activities, importance of, 207–208
Group home programs, 160
Guilt, as response to diagnosis, 126–
    127

Haldol (haloperidol), 313, 314, 319
Halstead-Reitan battery, 104
Hand-biting, 74
*The Handbook of Autism and Pervasive
    Developmental Disorders* (Cohen,
    Donellan, and Paul), 191
Hand-flapping, 75
Hand-leading, 28, 45–46
Hand regard, 75
Head
  banging of. *See* Self-injurious behaviors
    (SIBs)
  hitting side of, 74
Hearing. *See also* Auditory *entries*
  assessment of, 90–91
Hearing-impaired children
  autistic, 263
  mainstreaming autistic and PDD children
    with, 264
Higashi School, 204, 251–252
Hitting, of side of head, 74
Holding therapy, 329–330
Homeopathic interventions, 302–303, 328–
    329

Hopelessness, as response to diagnosis, 125–
    126, 127
*How to Teach Autistic and Severely Handi-
    capped Children* (Koegel and
    Schriebman), 188
Hyperlexia, 278–279
Hypersensitivity, auditory, 77, 78
  auditory training and, 326–327
Hyposensitivity, auditory, 77–78

IDEA (Individuals with Disabilities Educa-
    tion Act) [Public Law 101-476], 176
Ignoring, to reduce negative behavior, 236–
    237
Illness, comfort-seeking behavior and, 36–37
Imagination
  lacking in play. *See* Play, lack of imagina-
    tion in
  language and, 65
Imipramine (Tofranil), 304, 309, 310, 319
Imitation, 37–39
  developmental aspects of, 39
  levels of, 38
  task modeling and, 246–247, 249
Individual differences
  in attachment behavior, 35–36
  in response to task modeling, 249
Individual educational program (IEP), 163,
    231
  determining content of, 179
  fair hearings and, 184–186
    when to go to, 185–186
  first, 164, 180–181
  goals and objectives on, 181–183
    progress rate and, 182–183
    setting realistically, 181–182
  mediation and, 184
  outside assessment for planning, 180–181
  professional advocacy for negotiation of,
    178
  triennial review of, 181
Individual Program Plan (IPP), 171, 184
Individuals with Disabilities Education Act
    (IDEA) [Public Law 101-476], 176
Infants and toddlers
  development of autism in, 106–107
  early intervention with. *See* Early inter-
    vention
  head-banging in, 72–73
  intelligence tests for, 101–102
  psychotherapy for, 145–146
Infant stimulation programs, 172
Informal observation, for behavioral assess-
    ment, 94

Information processing, cross-modal and
  multi-modal, 242–244
  tactile to verbal transfer of information
    and, 243–244
  visual to auditory transfer of information
    and, 242–243
Inheritance
  of autism, 93, 126
  of fragile X syndrome, 119–120
Injuries. *See also* Self-injurious behaviors
    (SIBs)
  comfort-seeking behavior and, 36–37
Institutional care, 160
Instructional methods, 242–252
  computer-assisted instruction, 244–246
  computer games as, 246
  cross-modal and multi-modal information
    processing and, 242–244
    tactile to verbal transfer of information
      and, 243–244
    visual to auditory transfer of information
      and, 242–243
  gestalt processing and, 247–248
    language, 247–248
    visual, 247
  helping autistic children to get the most
    from, 249–250
    follow-through on commands and, 249–
      250
    getting and holding child's attention
      and, 250–251
    physical exercise as method of focusing
      attention and, 251–252
    positive redirection and, 250
  individual differences in response to mod-
    eling and, 249
  for language skills. *See* Language instruc-
    tion
  learning about, 216
  task approximations and record keeping
    and, 248
  task complexity and, 248
  task modeling and, 246–247, 249
Instrumental language, 53–54
Instrumental learning, 232
Instrumental relating, 27–29
  hand-leading and, 28
  social referencing and
    in adults, 29–30
    in children, 28–29
Intelligence. *See also* Mental retardation
  adaptive functioning and, 283
  in Asperger's syndrome, 113
  nonverbal, 16–17

performance, 100–101
  testing of. *See* Developmental evaluation,
    intelligence testing in
  verbal, 99–100
Interests
  in play. *See* Play
  special
    in Asperger's syndrome, 115–116
    reading and, 279
    splinter skills and, 67–69
      performance intelligence and, 100–101
      quantification and, 69
International autism societies, 194
*International Classification of Disease, Tenth
  Edition (ICD-10)*, criteria for autism
    and PDD,NOS, 19–20
Interpersonal space, 47–48
Interviewing, of potential teachers, 214
IQ. *See* Developmental evaluation, intel-
  ligence testing in; Intelligence; Mental
  retardation
Islets of ability, 67–69, 100–101
Isolation, social, 26–27
  early attachment behavior and, 26–27

Jargon, 57
Job coaching, 174
Jobs. *See* Employment
Joint custody, 140
Journals, parent-teacher, 219

Kaufman ABC (K-ABC), 103

Language. *See also* Verbal communication
  in Asperger's syndrome, 116
  assessment of, 90
  early, in autistic and PDD children, 264–
    267
    in bilingual homes, 264–265
    language loss and, 265–267
  echolalia and. *See* Echolalia
  expressive, 100
  idiosyncratic word use and jargon and, 57–
    58
  imagination and, 65
  instrumental, 53–54
  loss of, 52–53, 265–267
    encouraging early vocal production and,
      266
    increasing oral-motor awareness and,
      266
    videotape viewing and, 266–267
  mutism and, 51–52
  onset of, 50–51

Language (*cont.*)
    pragmatics of, 58–59, 267–272
    receptive, 99–100
    teaching. *See* Language instruction
    verbal intelligence and, 99–100
Language development, autistic versus typi-
        cal, 253–255
    natural gestures to enhance communication
        "signal" and, 254–255
    talking to children at their language age
        and, 253–254
Language Gestalt processing, 247–248
Language instruction, 253–273
    autistic versus typical language develop-
        ment and, 253–255
        natural gestures to enhance communica-
            tion "signal" and, 254–255
        talking to children at their language age
            and, 253–254
    early oral language in autistic and PDD
        children and, 264–267
        in bilingual homes, 264–265
        language loss and, 265–267
    language pragmatics interventions for,
        267–272
        eye contact and, 268–269
        topic maintenance and topic elaboration
            and, 270–272
        turn-taking and, 269–270
    multiword language development and
        reading skills and, 272–273
        abstract language and, 272
        minimizing rote responding and, 272–
            273
    to nonverbal children, 255–262
        communication boards for, 255–260
        sign language for, 260–262
    "oral only" approach for, 262–264
        mainstreaming autistic and PDD chil-
            dren with hearing-impaired children
            and, 264
        signing as sole mode of communication
            and, 262–263
        social stigma attached to nonverbal
            methods of communication and, 262
Latino families, coping with diagnosis by,
        132
Lawyers. *See also* Advocacy
    IEP and, 178, 183–184
Learning. *See also* Classrooms; Individual
        educational program (IEP); Special
        education
    instrumental, 232
    neuropsychological theory of, 201

Learning disabled (LD) classes, 276
Learning handicapped (LH) classes, 276
Least restrictive environment (LRE), 176
Legal advocacy. *See* Advocacy
Let Me Hear Your Voice (Maurice), 190
Listening, training in, 326–327
Lithane (lithium), 315, 316, 319
Lovaas method, 201–204, 205–206
Luria-Nebraska battery, 104

Mainstreaming. *See* Classrooms, main-
        streaming and full inclusion in
March of Dimes, 194
Mascot role, siblings in, 153
Math skills, 281–282
    functional, 282
    rote, 281–282
Mealtimes. *See* Feeding
*The Me Book: Teaching Developmentally
        Disabled Children* (Lovaas), 188, 288
Mediation, IEP and, 184
Medical insurance, eligibility for services
        through, 186–187
Medical testing, 87
Medications, 301–320
    age of child and, 304–305
    Anafranil (clomipramine), 309, 310
    antidepressant, 309–310
    for autism versus PDD, 309
    Benadryl (diphenhydramine), 313
    BuSpar (buspirone), 315–316
    B vitamins, 316–317
    choice of, 316
    classes of, 308–309
    Cogentin (benztropine), 312–313
    Cylert (pemoline), 311, 312, 318
    designing trial of, 305–307
        baseline behavioral data for, 306
        blind trials and, 306–307
        criteria for use of medication and, 305–
            306
        drug effects versus education and matu-
            ration and, 307
    Desyrel (trazodone), 309, 310
    Dexedrine (dextroamphetamine), 311, 312
    drug effects versus maturation, 307
    Haldol (haloperidol), 313, 314, 319
    homeopathic interventions and, 302–303
    Lithane (lithium), 315, 316, 319
    long-term management of, 320
    Mellaril (thioridazine), 313
    monitoring child's benefits from, 317–320
        compliance and, 319
        drug holidays and, 317–318

recognizing when to change medications and, 318–319
neuroleptic (antipsychotic), 304–305, 311–314
  dyskinesias and, 312–313
Norpramin (desipramine), 309, 310
Nystatin, 302, 328–329
obtaining consultations about, 303–305
parents' concerns about, 303
Pertofrane (desipramine), 309, 310
placebo effect and, 306–307
Pondimin (fenfluramine), 308, 315, 319
Prozac (fluoxetine), 304, 309, 310, 319
Ritalin (methylphenidate), 303–304, 311, 312
role of, 301–302
sedation caused by, 303
stimulant, 310–311
Tegretol (carbamazepine), 314, 315, 319
timing of use of, 302
Tofranil (imipramine), 304, 309, 310, 319
Trexan (naltrexone), 314–315
Mellaril (thioridazine), 313
Mental age, 97–98
Mental retardation
  association with autism, 11–12, 97
  association with PDD,NOS, 11, 97
  determining degree of. *See* Developmental evaluation, intelligence testing in
  fear of diagnosis of, 97
  prognosis and, 133
  responses to diagnosis of, 286
  special education and. *See* Special education, mental retardation and
Merrill-Palmer Scales of Mental Development, 102–103
Methylphenidate (Ritalin), 303–304, 311, 312
Milk allergy, as cause of autism, 302–303, 328
Mind, theory of, 28, 44–45
Misinformation, about treatments, 322–323
Mixed-disability classes, social skills development and, 212–213
Montessori curriculum, 287
Mother(s). *See* Parent(s); Parenting
Motherese, 253–254
Motor behavior
  overreactivity to movement and, 79–81
  performance intelligence and, 100
  stereotyped. *See* Stereotyped motor behavior
Motor object imitation, 38
Movement. *See* Motor behavior; Stereotyped motor behavior

MRIs, 91
Mullens Early Learning Scales, 102
Mutism, 51–52

Naltrexone (Trexan), 314–315
National Autistic Society (England), 194
National Society for Autistic Children (NASC). *See* Autism Society of America (ASA)
Neglect, 144–145
Negotiating the Special Education Maze (Anderson, Chitwood, and Hayden), 188
Negotiation, of IEP. *See* Individual educational program (IEP)
Neuroleptic medications, 304–305, 311–314
  dyskinesias and, 312–313
Neurologists
  medications prescribed by, 304
  role in developmental assessment, 91
Neuropsychological tests, 104
Neuropsychological theories, early intervention and, 197–201
  learning and, 201
  skill development and, 198–201
Newsletter, of Autism Society of America, 193
Nobody, Nowhere (Williams), 190, 279–280
Nonverbal communication, 43–48
  facial cues and, 46–47
    eye contact, 46–47, 268–269
    smiling, 46
  gestures and, 45–46
    anticipatory reach, 45
    to enhance communication "signal," 254–255
    hand-leading, 45–46
    mute children's use of, differentiation of autism from language problems and, 52
    pointing, 45, 46
  interpersonal space and, 47–48
  theory of mind and, 44–45
Nonverbal intelligence, 16–17
Norpramin (desipramine), 309, 310
Numbers, special interests involving, 69
Numbness, as response to diagnosis, 125
Nystatin, 302, 328–329

Object(s)
  intense interest in, 67–69
  lack of engagement with, 60–61
  play with. *See* Play
  staring at, 75, 78–79
Object imitation, motor, 38

Objectives, for IEPs, 181–183
  progress toward, 182–183
  setting, 181–182
Object use, spontaneous, 38
Observation, of classrooms. *See* Classrooms,
    visits to
Obsessive behaviors
  motor rituals resembling, 76–77
  in PDD and Asperger's syndrome, 319
One-to-one correspondence, 281
Options therapy, 330–331
"Oral only" language approach. *See* Lan-
    guage instruction, "oral only" ap-
    proach for
Otacoustic emission testing, 90–91
Outcry, as response to diagnosis, 125–126
Overachievement, by siblings, 152–153
Overextension, 56

Pain reactions, diminished, in autistic chil-
    dren, 144, 241
Papooses, 242
Paraprofessionals. *See* Teacher's aides
Parent(s), 136–145. *See also* Parenting
  abusive, 31, 144–145
    allegations of, facilitated communication
      and, 326
  affection toward, 31–32
  attachment to. *See* Attachment behavior
  as cause of autism, 134
  choice of residential care and, 160–162
  classrooms visits by. *See* Classrooms, visits
      to
  communication between, 122, 143–144
  concerns about medications, 303
  as consumer watchdogs of child's educa-
    tion, 163–164
  coping with diagnosis. *See* Coping with
    diagnosis
  discipline by. *See* Discipline
  fear of diagnosis of mental retardation,
    97
  finding diagnostic services and, 85
  first recognition of problems by, 121–122
  friends of, roles for, 156–157
  holding therapy for demonstrating love for
    child and, 329–330
  IEP and. *See* Individual educational pro-
    gram (IEP)
  medications given to children by, 304
  misinformation about treatments given to,
    322–323
  outings without autistic or PDD child for,
    158–159

professionals' communication of diagnosis
    to, 124
  psychotherapy for. *See* Psychotherapy, for
    parents
  refrigerator, 134
  respite care and, 158–159, 172
  risk of child abuse and, 31
  stigma attached to, 157–158
  support groups for. *See* Support groups
  as teacher's aides, 223–224
  teacher's aides provided by, 178, 224
  teachers and. *See* Parent-teacher relation-
    ship
Parentification of siblings, 139–140, 150–151
Parenting, 136–143, 137–143
  age of parents and, 140–141
  divorce and joint custody and, 140
  length and strength of parents' relationship
    and, 137–138
  permissive versus authoritarian, 141–143
  planned versus unplanned and desired
    versus unwanted children and, 138–
    139
  single parents and, 139–140
Parent pairing, 192
Parent-teacher relationship
  building and maintaining, 218–219
    classroom visitation policy and, 218–219
    parent-teacher journals and, 219
  establishing, 214–215
PDD,NOS. *See* Pervasive developmental dis-
    order, not otherwise specified
    (PDD,NOS)
Pediatric geneticists, role in developmental
    assessment, 91
Pediatricians
  medications prescribed by, 303–304
  referrals provided by, 84–85
Peers. *See also* Friendships
  tutoring by, 229–230
Pemoline (Cylert), 311, 312, 318
Perception. *See also* Auditory *entries;* Hear-
    ing; Sensory function; Visual *entries*
  of others' emotions and feelings, 30–31
Performance intelligence (PIQ), 100–101
  splinter skills and, 100–101
Permissive parenting, 141–143
Perseveration, of sensory play, 62–63
Pertofrane (desipramine), 309, 310
Pervasive developmental disorder (PDD)
  non-autistic, 9, 20–24. *See also* Asperger's
    syndrome; Childhood disintegrative
    disorder; Fragile X syndrome; Perva-
    sive developmental disorder, not oth-

erwise specified (PDD,NOS); Rett syndrome
terminology for, 9–11
Pervasive developmental disorder, not otherwise specified (PDD,NOS)
association with mental retardation, 11, 97
autism distinguished from, 15–20
communication and. *See* Communication
DSM-IV criteria and, 16–19
ICD-10 criteria and, 19–20
play and. *See* Play
social development and. *See* Social development
behavioral versus physical markers of, 86–87
classrooms for, 212
definition of, 9–10
diagnosis of, 16–17. *See also* Developmental evaluation; Diagnosis
eligibility for services and, 169–170
language deficits and, 255
medications for, 309
obsessive behaviors in, 319
prevalence of, 12
risk factors for, 12–13, 86, 92–93
social relatedness and, 255
Pervasive Developmental Disorders Screening Test (PDDST), 107–109
Phenylketonuria (PKU), 327
Physical abuse, 144–145
allegations of, facilitated communication and, 326
aloofness and, 31
Physical affection, 31–32
Physical aversives, 240–241
Physical restraint, 241–242
Physicians. *See specific specialties, i.e.,* Psychiatrists
Pica, 79
Pills. *See also* Medications
getting child to take, 319
Placebo effect, 306
Play, 39–41, 60–65
attachment objects, 61–62
lack of imagination in, 64–67
need for sameness and, 65–67
playlalia (echopraxia) and, 64
relationship between imagination and language and, 65
playlalia (echopraxia) and, 64
sensory, 62–64
perseveration and, 62–63
preoccupation with parts of objects and, 63–64

with siblings, 40–41
standardized, for behavioral assessment, 94–95
Play audiometry, 90
Play-DOS, 94
Playlalia, 64
Pointing, 45, 46
Pondimin (fenfluramine), 308, 315, 319
Positive redirection, 250
Power-pads, for computer-assisted instruction, 245
Pregnancy, planned versus unplanned, parenting of autistic and PDD children and, 138–139
Pregnancy history, 92–93
Preoccupation, with parts of objects, 63–64
Preschoolers
Asperger's syndrome in, 116–117
computer-assisted instruction for, 245
early intervention with. *See* Early intervention
intelligence tests for, 102–103
mainstreaming of, 228–229
Processing delays, in language development, 253–254
Professionals. *See also specific professionals, i.e.,* Psychiatrists
anger and frustration with, as response to diagnosis, 130–131
communication of diagnosis by, 124
developmental evaluation and. *See under* Developmental evaluation
intelligence testing and, 98
Prognosis, concerns about. *See* Coping with diagnosis, concerns about prognosis and
Projective tests, 89
Project TEACCH, 214
Pronoun reversal, in echolalia, 55
Prosody, 49–50
Prozac (fluoxetine), 304, 309, 310, 319
Psychiatric disorders, in Asperger's syndrome, 119
Psychiatrists
medications prescribed by, 304
role in developmental evaluation, 88, 89
Psychoactive medications. *See* Medications
Psychological defenses, as response to diagnosis. *See* Coping with diagnosis
Psychologists, role in developmental evaluation, 88, 89
Psychotherapy, 145–148
for children with PDD or autism, 145–146

Psychotherapy (*cont.*)
 for higher functioning adolescents and
  young adults with PDD or autism,
  146–147
 for parents, 147–148
  couples therapy, 147–148
  family, 148
  individual, 147
 for siblings, family, 148
Public
 attitudes toward developmental disabilities, 159–160
 reactions to autistic or PDD children, 157–
  158
Public Law 94-142, 176–177
Public Law 99-457, 176
Public Law 101-476 (Individuals with Disabilities Education Act [IDEA]), 176
Punishment. *See also* Aversives
 inappropriate, 31
 time-outs as, 238–240

Quantification, special interests involving, 69

Rating scales, for autism, 95–96
Reading, 277–279
 hyperlexia and, 278–279
 interests of older and higher functioning
  children with autism and PDD and,
  279
Reasoning ability, 100
Receptive language, 99–100
Receptive language age, 90, 254
Record keeping, task approximations and,
 248
Redirection, positive, 250
Redundancy, 199
Referrals, for diagnosis, 84–85
Refrigerator parents, 134
Regional centers, 169–170
Reinforcement
 avoiding using reinforcers as bribes and,
  234
 reward hierarchy for, 232–233
 schedules of, 233–235
 social rewards for, 233
 token economies and, 235–236
Relating. *See* Expressive relating; Instrumen-
 tal relating
Repetitive movements. *See* Stereotyped motor behavior
Research
 books about, 190–191
 on early intervention, need for, 197

Residential placement, 159–162, 175
 attitudes toward developmentally disabled
  children and, 159–160
 timing and reasons for, 160–162
 types of, 160
Respite care, 172
 babysitters for, 158–159
Restraint, 241–242
Retardation. *See* Mental retardation
Rett syndrome
 characteristics of, 21–22
 prevalence of, 12
Rewards, for behavior management. *See* Behavior management; Reinforcement
Risk factors, for autism and PDD,NOS, 12–
 13, 86, 92–93
Ritalin (methylphenidate), 303–304, 311,
 312
Rituals, motor. *See* Stereotyped motor
 behavior
Rocking, 72
Rote math skills, 281–282
Rote memory, splinter skills and, 100–101
Routines
 in classroom, 220–221
 need for, 65–67
Rules
 disregard for, 29
 rigid, for social behavior, 30

Sameness. *See* Change, resistance to; Rou-
 tines
Saturation, as response to diagnosis, 125
Schedule training, 291–292
School-aged children. *See also* Classrooms;
  Individual educational program (IEP);
  Language instruction; Special educa-
  tion
 Asperger's syndrome in, 113–115
 intelligence tests for, 103–104
 psychotherapy for, 145–146
 residential placement for, 161
Scratching, 74
Sedation
 medications causing, 303
 for neurological testing, 91
See signing. *See* Sign language
Self-feeding skills, 288–289
Self-injurious behaviors (SIBs), 72–74
 in babies and toddlers, 72–73
 in older children, 73–74
 physical aversives to reduce, 240–241
Sensory function, 77–81. *See also* Auditory
 entries; Hearing; Visual *entries*

auditory hypersensitivity and hyposensitivity and, 77–78
fixations on touch, taste and smell and, 79
overreactivity to movement and, 79–81
play and, 62–64
  perseveration and, 62–63
  preoccupation with parts of objects and,
    63–64
visual fixations and, 75, 78–79
visual regard and, 75, 78–79
Sensory integration therapy, 331–332
Sensory play, 62–64
  perseveration and, 62–63
  preoccupation with parts of objects and,
    63–64
Separation, among parents of autistic and
  PDD children, 137–138
Services. *See* Special education; Treatment
  interventions; *specific services*
Severely handicapped (SH) educational track,
  276–277
Sex. *See* Gender
Sheltered workshops, 174–175
Shock, electric, to reduce negative behavior,
  240–241
Siblings, 148–154
  books about, 189
  coping patterns of, 150–154
    acting as family mascot as, 153
    overachievement as, 152–153
    parentification as, 139–140, 150–151
    withdrawal as, 151–152, 153–154
  explaining autism or PDD to, 148–149
  family therapy for, 148
  play with, 40–41
  standards of behavior for autistic child and,
    149
The Siege (Park), 190
Sign language, 260–263
  as sole mode of communication, 262–263
  stigma and, 262
  when to introduce, 260–262
Single parents, 139–140
Sisters. *See* Siblings
Sleep. *See* Bedtime difficulties
Smell, fixation on sense of, 79
Smiling, 46
Social attitudes, toward developmental disabilities, 159–160
Social development, 25–42
  adult disabilities of, 29–30
  in Asperger's syndrome, 113–115
  comfort-seeking patterns and. *See*
    Comfort-seeking

early signs of social isolation and, 26–27
  attachment behavior and, 26–27
imitation and, 37–39
  developmental aspects of, 39
instrumental versus expressive relating
  and, 27–29
  hand-leading and, 28
  social referencing and, 28–29, 106–107
lack of friendships and, 41–42
perception of others' emotional states and
  feelings and, aloofness and child abuse
  and, 31
perception of others' emotions and feelings
  and, 30–31
physical affection and, 31–32
play and, 39–41
  with siblings, 40–41
relating and. *See* Expressive relating; Instrumental relating
social referencing and, 28–30, 106–107
Social mainstreaming, 227
  day care and, 230
  shadow aides for, 228–229
Social referencing, 28–30
  in adults, 29–30
  in children, 28–29, 106–107
Social relatedness, in autism and PDD, 255
Social rewards, 233
Social skill development, computers for, 245–
  246
Social skills development, mixed-disability
  classes and, 212–213
Sociopaths, autistic people distinguished
  from, 29
Software, for computer-assisted instruction,
  244
Son Rise (book), 330–331
Sound field audiometry, 90
Space, interpersonal, 47–48
Spanking, 241
Special education, 176–183
  appropriate programs for, 176–177
    "best" education versus, 179–183
    defining, 179
  books about, 188
  classroom selection for. *See* Classrooms
  costs of, 176, 177–178
  eligibility for
    federally guaranteed rights and, 176–177
    legal issues and rights related to, 177
  higher functioning children and, 277–285
    teaching math skills to, 281–282
    teaching reading skills to, 277–279
    teaching writing skills to, 279–281

Special education (*cont.*)
    transition to functional academic orienta-
        tion and, 282–283
    vocational choices for, 283–285
    IEP and. *See* Individual educational pro-
        gram (IEP)
    instructional methods for. *See* Instructional
        methods; Language instruction
    mental retardation and, 274–277
        communicatively handicapped educa-
            tional track and, 276
        level of, curriculum focus and, 274–276
        level of functioning and, 285–286
        severely handicapped educational track
            and, 276–277
    vocational training and, 299–300
Special interests
    in Asperger's syndrome, 115–116
    reading and, 279
Speech. *See* Communication; Language; Lan-
    guage development; Verbal communi-
    cation
Speech and language pathologists
    role in developmental evaluation, 90
    teacher's aides to increase exposure to
        goals established by, 224–226
Splinter skills
    performance intelligence and, 100–101
    quantification and, 69
Spontaneous object use, 38
Standardized assessments, for behavioral as-
    sessment, 94–95
Stanford-Binet-II (SB-II), 103, 104
Staring, 75, 78–79
State Department of Developmental Services
    (DSS), 169
Stereotyped motor behavior, 70–77
    dyskinesias differentiated from, 312
    earliest, 72–73
    functions served by, 70–75
    hand regard and flapping, 75
    later, 75–77
    self-injurious, 73–74
Stigma
    nonverbal communication methods and,
        262
    parents of autistic children and, 157–158
Stimulant medications, 310–311
Stimulation
    compensatory, 198
    deep pressure, craving for, 80
    infant stimulation programs and, 172
    limiting in classroom, 221
    self-imposed limits on, 220

Successive approximations, 248
Supported employment, 174
Support groups, 85, 191–195
    benefits of, 191–192
    parent pairing and, 192
Syndromes, 14

Tactile detail scrutiny, 79
Tactile to verbal transfer of information, 243–
    244
Tardive dyskinesia, 312–313
Task complexity, 248
Task modeling, 246–247
    individual differences in response to, 249
Taste, fixation on sense of, 79
Teachers. *See* Classrooms, teachers and;
    Parent-teacher relationship
Teacher's aides, 222–225
    for behavior control, 225
    to increase exposure to speech and lan-
        guage therapy goals, 224–225
    observing activities of, 223
    parents as, 223–224
    privately funded, 178, 224
    shadow, for mainstreaming, 228–229
Teaching. *See also* Instructional methods;
    Language instruction; Special educa-
    tion
    to the middle, 213
Tegretol (carbamazepine), 314, 315, 319
Testing. *See also* Developmental evaluation
    neuropsychological, 104
    projective, 89
Theory of mind, 28, 44–45
Thioridazine (Mellaril), 313
Timed toileting, 291–292
Time-outs, accompanied, 238–240
Toddlers. *See* Infants and toddlers
Toe-walking, 72
Tofranil (imipramine), 304, 309, 310, 319
Toilet training, 290–292
    schedule training, 291–292
Token economies, 235–236
Tone of voice, 49–50
Topic elaboration, 270–272
Topic maintenance, 59, 270–272
Touch, fixation on sense of, 79
Transferability of function, 199
Transfer of information
    tactile to verbal, 243–244
    visual to auditory, 242–243
Trazodone (Desyrel), 309, 310
Treatment interventions, 169–176. *See also*
    specific interventions

advocacy for obtaining. *See* Advocacy
behavior intervention, 172–173
books about, 188–189
case management, 171–172
day treatment, 175
developmental evaluation. *See* Developmental evaluation
early. *See* Early intervention
eligibility for, 169–176
  diagnosis and, 169–171
  through medical insurance, 186–187
homeopathic, 302–303
infant stimulation programs, 172
job coaching, 174
limitations of, 175–176
medications. *See* Medications
nonmainstream, 302–303, 321–332
  auditory training, 326–327
  cautions about, 322–324
  dietary, 327–328
  evaluating, 321–324
  facilitated communication, 324–326
  holding therapy, 329–330
  Nystatin, 302, 328–329
  Options therapy, 330–331
  seeking as response to diagnosis, 131
  sensory integration therapy, 331–332
psychotherapy, 145–147
  for adolescents and young adults, 147–148
  for children, 145–146
residential. *See* Residential placement
respite care, 173
scarcity of, 167, 169
sheltered workshops, 174–175
special education. *See* Individual educational program (IEP); Special education
supported employment, 174
vocational training, 174
Treatment resources, 167–195
Trexan (naltrexone), 314–315
Tricyclic antidepressants, 309–310
Turn-taking, language development and, 269–270
Tutoring, by peers, 229–230

Uncles, roles for, 155–156

Verbal communication. *See also* Language; Language development; Language instruction
  conversational skill and, 58–59
  language pragmatics and, 58–59, 267–272
  tone of voice in, 49–50
Verbal intelligence (VIQ), 99–100
Videotape viewing, language development and, 266–267
Vineland Adaptive Behavior Scales (VABS), 105, 286–287, 294
Virtual disability, 98
Visiting classrooms. *See* Classrooms, visits to
Visual fixations, 75, 78–79
Visual Gestalt processing, 247
Visual-motor ability, 100
Visual regard, 75, 78–79
Visual-spatial ability, 100
Visual to auditory transfer of information, 242–243
Vitamin B, 316–317
Vocational skills training, 174, 298–300
  job coaching, 174
  for moderately impaired people with autism, 298–299
  school-based programs for, 299–300
Voice, tone of, 49–50

Walking, on toes, 72
Wechsler Adult Intelligence Scale–Revised (WAIS-R), 104
Wechsler Intelligence Scale for Children–III (WISC-III), 103–104
Wechsler Preschool and Primary Scales of Intelligence–Revised (WPPSI-R), 103
What About Me? Siblings of Developmentally Disabled Children (Siegel and Silverstein), 189
Wing, Lorna, 111
Withdrawal, of siblings, 151–152, 153–154
Words. *See also* Language; Language development; Language instruction; Verbal communication
  idiosyncratic use of, 57–58
Work. *See* Employment
Writing, 279–281
  about facts, 280
  experiential, 280–281